T0227289

Optimizing the Treatment of Upper Extremity Injuries in Athletes

Editor

KEVIN C. CHUNG

HAND CLINICS

www.hand.theclinics.com

Consulting Editor
KEVIN C. CHUNG

February 2017 • Volume 33 • Number 1

ELSEVIER

1600 John F. Kennedy Boulevard • Suite 1800 • Philadelphia, Pennsylvania, 19103-2899

http://www.theclinics.com

HAND CLINICS Volume 33, Number 1
February 2017 ISSN 0749-0712, ISBN-13: 978-0-323-52792-7

Editor: Lauren Boyle
Developmental Editor: Kristen Helm

Hand Clinics (ISSN 0749-0712) is published quarterly by Elsevier Inc., 360 Park Avenue South, New York, NY 10010-1710. Months of publication are February, May, August, and November. Business and Editorial Offices: 1600 John F. Kennedy Blvd., Ste. 1800, Philadelphia, PA 19103-2899. Customer Service Office: 3251 Riverport Lane, Maryland Heights, MO 63043. Periodicals postage paid at New York, NY and at additional mailing offices. Subscription price is $398.00 per year (domestic individuals), $721.00 per year (domestic institutions), $100.00 per year (domestic students/residents), $454.00 per year (Canadian individuals), $839.00 per year (Canadian institutions), $541.00 per year (international individuals), $839.00 per year (international institutions), and $256.00 per year (international and Canadian students/residents). Foreign air speed delivery is included in all *Clinics* subscription prices. All prices are subject to change without notice. **POSTMASTER:** Send address changes to *Hand Clinics*, Elsevier Health Sciences Division, Subscription Customer Service, 3251 Riverport Lane, Maryland Heights, MO 63043. Customer Service (orders, claims, online, change of address): Elsevier Health Sciences Division, Subscription **Customer Service, 3251 Riverport Lane, Maryland Heights, MO 63043. Tel: 1-800-654-2452 (U.S. and Canada); 314-447-8871 (outside U.S. and Canada). Fax: 314-447-8029. E-mail: journalscustomerservice-usa@elsevier.com (for print support); journalsonlinesupport-usa@elsevier.com (for online support).**

Reprints. For copies of 100 or more of articles in this publication, please contact the Commercial Reprints Department, Elsevier Inc., 360 Park Avenue South, New York, New York 10010-1710. Tel.: 212-633-3874; Fax: 212-633-3820; E-mail: reprints@elsevier.com.

Hand Clinics is covered in *MEDLINE/PubMed (Index Medicus), Current Contents/Clinical Medicine, EMBASE/Excerpta Medica,* and *ISI/BIOMED.*

Contributors

CONSULTING EDITOR

KEVIN C. CHUNG, MD, MS
Chief of Hand Surgery, University of Michigan
Health System, Charles B.G. De Nancrede
Professor of Plastic Surgery and Orthopaedic
Surgery, Assistant Dean for Faculty Affairs,
Associate Director of Global REACH,
University of Michigan Medical School,
Ann Arbor, Michigan

EDITOR

KEVIN C. CHUNG, MD, MS
Chief of Hand Surgery, University of Michigan
Health System, Charles B.G. De Nancrede
Professor of Plastic Surgery and Orthopaedic
Surgery, Assistant Dean for Faculty Affairs,
Associate Director of Global REACH,
University of Michigan Medical School,
Ann Arbor, Michigan

AUTHORS

DANIEL AVERY, MD
Fellow, Department of Orthopaedic Surgery,
University of Connecticut Health Center,
Farmington, Connecticut

ASHEESH BEDI, MD
Harold and Helen W. Gehring Early Career
Professor, Department of Orthopaedic
Surgery, Shoulder and Sports Medicine,
University of Michigan, Ann Arbor, Michigan

JACOB W. BRUBACHER, MD
Department of Orthopaedic Surgery, Duke
University, Durham, North Carolina

MICHELLE G. CARLSON, MD
Associate Attending Orthopaedic Surgeon,
Hospital for Special Surgery; Associate
Professor of Clinical Orthopaedic Surgery, Weill
Cornell Medical College, New York, New York

PAUL S. CEDERNA, MD
Professor of Surgery, Section of Plastic
Surgery, Section Head, University of Michigan
Medical School, Ann Arbor, Michigan

HO-JUN CHEON, MD
Director, W Institute for Hand and
Reconstructive Microsurgery, W Hospital,
Daegu, Korea

KEVIN C. CHUNG, MD, MS
Chief of Hand Surgery, University of Michigan
Health System, Charles B.G. De Nancrede
Professor of Plastic Surgery and Orthopaedic
Surgery, Assistant Dean for Faculty Affairs,
Associate Director of Global REACH,
University of Michigan Medical School,
Ann Arbor, Michigan

WILLIAM H.J. CHUNG
Research Assistant, Comprehensive Hand
Center, University of Michigan, North Campus
Research Complex, Ann Arbor, Michigan

JEFF M. COPPAGE, MD
Hand Surgery Fellow, Hospital for Special
Surgery, New York, New York

CHARLES A. DALY, MD
Resident, Department of Orthopaedic Surgery,
Emory University School of Medicine, Atlanta,
Georgia

JIMMY H. DARUWALLA, MD
Resident, Department of Orthopaedic Surgery,
Emory University School of Medicine, Atlanta,
Georgia

BENJAMIN TODD DRURY, MD
Texas Orthopedic Specialists, Bedford, Texas

KATE E. ELZINGA, MD, FRCSC
Section of Plastic Surgery, Hand Surgery
Fellow, Division of Plastic Surgery, University of
Michigan Health System, University of
Michigan, Ann Arbor, Michigan

JOHN R. FOWLER, MD
Assistant Professor, Department of
Orthopaedics, University of Pittsburgh,
Pittsburgh, Pennsylvania

MICHAEL S. GART, MD
Division of Plastic and Reconstructive Surgery,
Northwestern University Feinberg School of
Medicine, Chicago, Illinois

STEVEN C. HAASE, MD, FACS
Associate Professor, Departments of Surgery
and Orthopaedic Surgery, University of
Michigan Health System, Ann Arbor, Michigan

TIFFANY R. KADOW, MD
Resident, Department of Orthopaedics,
University of Pittsburgh, Pittsburgh,
Pennsylvania

JONG-MIN KIM, MD
Director, W Institute for Hand and
Reconstructive Microsurgery, W Hospital,
Daegu, Korea

ELIZABETH A. KING, MD
Hand and Upper Extremity Surgery Fellow,
Department of Orthopaedic Surgery, TriHealth
Hospital System, University of Cincinnati,
Cincinnati, Ohio

MEGHAN E. LARK, BS
Research Associate, Section of Plastic
Surgery, Department of Surgery, University
of Michigan Health System, Ann Arbor,
Michigan

JEFFREY NATHAN LAWTON, MD
Service Chief, Hand and Upper Extremity;
Associate Professor, Department of
Orthopaedic Surgery, University of Michigan,
Ann Arbor, Michigan

SIMON LEE, MD
Resident, Department of Orthopaedic
Surgery, University of Michigan, Ann Arbor,
Michigan

YOUNG-KEUN LEE, MD, PhD
Clinical Professor, Department of Orthopaedic
Surgery, Chonbuk National University Hospital,
Jeonju, Jeollabuk-do, Korea

THOMAS P. LEHMAN, MD
Associate Professor of Orthopedic Surgery,
Director of Hand Surgery, University of
Oklahoma Health Sciences Center, Oklahoma
City, Oklahoma

FRASER J. LEVERSEDGE, MD
Associate Professor & Vice-Chair; Director,
Hand, Upper Extremity & Microvascular
Surgery Fellowship, Department of
Orthopaedic Surgery, Duke University,
Durham, North Carolina

JOHN R. LIEN, MD
Assistant Professor, Section of Plastic Surgery,
Department of Orthopaedic Surgery, University
of Michigan, Ann Arbor, Michigan

RYAN A. MLYNAREK, MD
Resident, Department of Orthopaedic
Surgery, University of Michigan, Ann Arbor,
Michigan

MARK S. MORRIS, MD
Resident, Department of Orthopaedic
Surgery, University of Michigan, Ann Arbor,
Michigan

DAVID T. NETSCHER, MD
Clinical Professor, Division of Plastic
Surgery, Department of Orthopedic Surgery,
Baylor College of Medicine; Adjunct
Professor, Weill Medical College, Cornell
University, Houston Methodist Hospital,
Houston, Texas

KAGAN OZER, MD
Clinical Associate Professor, Department of
Orthopaedic Surgery, University of Michigan,
Ann Arbor, Michigan

DANG T. PHAM, MD
Resident, Department of Surgery, Houston
Methodist Hospital, Weill Medical College,
Cornell University, Houston, Texas

GHAZI RAYAN, MD
Clinical Professor of Orthopedic Surgery,
University of Oklahoma Health Sciences
Center, Oklahoma City, Oklahoma

JOHN G. SEILER III, MD
Professor, Georgia Hand, Shoulder & Elbow,
Atlanta, Georgia

EON SHIN, MD
The Philadelphia Hand Center, Sidney Kimmel
Medical College, Thomas Jefferson University,
Philadelphia, Pennsylvania

KIMBERLY GOLDIE STAINES, ORT, CHT
Department of Physical Medicine and
Rehabilitation, Michael E. DeBakey Veterans
Affairs Medical Center, Houston, Texas

JARED R. THOMAS, MD
Sr. Resident Surgeon, Department of
Orthopaedic Surgery, University of Michigan,
Ann Arbor, Michigan

RICK TOSTI, MD
Department of Orthopaedic Surgery,
Massachusetts General Hospital, Harvard
Medical School, Boston, Massachusetts

THOMAS A. WIEDRICH, MD
Department of Orthopedic Surgery, Chicago
Center for Surgery of the Hand, Northwestern
University Feinberg School of Medicine,
Chicago, Illinois

JENNIFER MORIATIS WOLF, MD
Professor, Department of Orthopaedic Surgery
and Rehabilitation, University of Chicago
Hospitals, Chicago, Illinois

MEGAN R. WOLF, MD
Orthopaedic Surgery Resident, Department of
Orthopaedic Surgery, University of
Connecticut Health Center, Farmington,
Connecticut

SANG-HYUN WOO, MD, PhD
President, W Institute for Hand and
Reconstructive Microsurgery, W Hospital,
Daegu, Korea

Contents

Although football is one of the most popular sports in America, its high injury incidence places concern on the injury prevention and safety of its players. This article investigates the perspectives of two National Collegiate Athletic Association Division 1 football coaches on promoting injury management and player safety while maintaining a highly competitive team. Through obtaining their coaching philosophy team management topics, effective strategies that contribute to a team culture prioritizing player well-being were identified. Interactions of football coaches with physicians and medical specialists are explored to highlight strengths that can optimize the care and treatment of football athletes.

Return-to-play (RTP) decisions often represent a challenge to physicians caring for athletes. The multifaceted and unique nature of each RTP decision makes standardization of the decision-making process impossible and demands of the physician thoughtful consideration of all competing interests and variables. Such difficult medical decisions are further complicated by unique ethical and legal considerations. Although no concrete RTP recommendations are available, the consensus of experienced team physicians and knowledge of the rules and regulations that apply to RTP are helpful guides to treating the various upper extremity injuries that occur in elite athletes.

The overhead pitching motion is a coordinated sequence of movements that subjects the shoulder to extreme forces. The ultimate goal of this complex, dynamic activity is to generate high ball velocity and accuracy. In doing so, repetitive throwing can cause adaptive and pathologic changes in the thrower's shoulder. This article reviews the relevant shoulder anatomy, the kinetic chain, and throwing mechanics, as well as common shoulder injuries and surgical options for the treating orthopedic surgeon.

Although rare, biceps and triceps tendon ruptures constitute significant injuries that can lead to profound disability if left untreated, especially in the athletic population. Biceps rupture is more common than triceps rupture, with both resulting from a forceful eccentric load. Surgical repair is the treatment method of choice for tendinous ruptures in athletes. Nonoperative management is rarely indicated in this population and is typically reserved for individuals with partial ruptures that quickly regain strength and function. Surgical anatomy, evaluation, diagnosis, and surgical management of these injuries are covered in this article.

Medial elbow injuries in the throwing athlete are common and increasing in frequency. They occur due to repetitive supraphysiologic forces acting on the elbow during the overhead throw. Overuse and inadequate rest are salient risk factors for injury. Most athletes improve substantially with rest and nonoperative treatment, although some athletes may require surgical intervention to return to play. Because of advances in conservative and surgical treatments, outcomes after medial elbow injury have improved over time. Currently, most athletes are able to return to a high level of play after ulnar collateral ligament reconstruction and experience a low rate of complications.

Elbow dislocations are more common in athletes than in the general population. Simple elbow dislocations should be managed with early range of motion and early return to sport, even with high-level contact athletes. Patients with instability on examination or with complex elbow dislocations may require surgical intervention. Overall, the outcomes after simple elbow dislocations are excellent and athletes should be able to return to play without significant limitations.

Modern competitive diving—especially platform diving—applies dramatic stress to the upper extremity. Some stress occurs during handstand-style takeoffs, but more force is delivered to the hand, wrist, elbow, and shoulder during hands-first entry. Hand positions that minimize the amount of splash result in forceful wrist extension. This repetitive impact can lead to chronic upper extremity pain and acute injuries that require operative intervention. Many divers use taping and bracing to prevent or treat this type of injury, but these are only modestly effective. Although minor injuries can improve with conservative management, carpal fractures and ligamentous injuries often require operative intervention.

A thorough understanding of the swing phases and mechanisms of injury in golf allows accurate diagnosis, treatment, and future prevention of injuries. Recommended initial treatment starts with cessation of practice to rest the wrist, a splint or orthotic brace, and nonsteroidal antiinflammatory drug medication with corticosteroid injection and swing modification. Pisiform excision is the best treatment of the most severe chronic cases of pisiform ligament complex syndrome. Delayed diagnosis of hook of hamate fracture may lead to complications, including flexor tendon rupture. Prompt surgical resection is recommended to hasten return to sport and to prevent further complications.

Hand and wrist injuries in martial arts are typically a reflection of the combat nature of this discipline. In striking sports, the axial load mechanism of injury is common and causes fractures and dislocations; in grappling sports, sprain injuries and degenerative changes predominate. There is clear evidence to support that hand protection reduces the risk of hand injury. Traditional training in martial arts on proper technique and target selection in striking sports reduces the risk of hand injury, and is an important component of hand and wrist injury prevention.

Management of hand and wrist injuries for athletes often places emphasis on an expeditious return to sport. Arthroscopic techniques have the advantage of directly visualizing joint derangements and correcting them via a minimally invasive approach. This article discusses the evaluation and management of common wrist injuries treated with arthroscopy in athletes, including scapholunate and lunotriquetral injury, triangular fibrocartilage complex tears, hamatolunate impingement, and arthroscopic-assisted reduction of wrist fractures.

Finger injuries are common in athletes playing in professional ball sports. Understanding the intricate anatomy of the digit is necessary to properly diagnose and manage finger injuries. Unrecognized or poorly managed finger injuries can lead to chronic deformities that can affect an athlete's performance. Multiple factors and treatment options should be considered to provide the best functional outcome and rapid return to play for an athlete. This article discusses the mechanism of injury, diagnosis, treatment, and return-to-play recommendations for common finger injuries in ball sports.

Closed pulley ruptures are rare in the general population but occur more frequently in rock climbers due to biomechanical demands on the hand. Injuries present with pain and swelling over the affected pulley, and patients may feel or hear a pop at the time of injury. Sequential pulley ruptures are required for clinical bowstringing of the flexor tendons. Ultrasound confirms diagnosis of pulley rupture and evaluates degree of displacement of the flexor tendons. Isolated pulley ruptures frequently are treated conservatively with early functional rehabilitation. Sequential pulley ruptures require surgical reconstruction. Most climbers are able to return to their previous activity level.

Football and rugby athletes are at increased risk of finger injuries given the full-contact nature of these sports. Some players may return to play early with protective taping, splinting, and casting. Others require a longer rehabilitation period and prolonged time away from the field. The treating hand surgeon must weigh the benefits of early return to play for the current season and future playing career against the risks of reinjury and long-term morbidity, including post-traumatic arthritis and decreased range of motion and strength. Each player must be comprehensively assessed and managed with an individualized treatment plan.

Thumb injuries are common in athletes and present a challenging opportunity for upper extremity physicians. Common injuries include metacarpal base fractures (Bennett and Rolando types), ulnar and radial collateral ligament injuries, dislocation of the carpometacarpal and metacarpophalangeal joints, and phalanx fractures. This review, although not exhaustive, highlights some of the most common thumb injuries in athletes. The treating physician must balance pressure from athletes, parents, coaches, and executives to expedite return to play with the long-term well-being of the athlete. Operative treatment may expedite return to play; however, one must carefully weigh the added risks involved with surgical intervention.

Upper extremity tennis injuries are most commonly characterized as overuse injuries to the wrist, elbow, and shoulder. The complex anatomy of these structures and their interaction with biomechanical properties of tennis strokes contributes to the diagnostic challenges. A thorough understanding of tennis kinetics, in combination with the current literature surrounding diagnostic and treatment methods, will improve clinical decision-making.

Gymnastics is a unique sport, which loads the wrist and arms as weight-bearing extremities. Because of the load demands on the wrist in particular, stress fractures, physeal injury, and overuse syndromes may be observed. This spectrum of injury has been termed "gymnast's wrist," and incorporates such disorders as wrist capsulitis, ligamentous tears, triangular fibrocartilage complex tears, chondromalacia of the carpus, stress fractures, distal radius physeal arrest, and grip lock injury.

The form and function of the cyclist exposes the ulnar nerve to both traction and compressive forces at both the elbow and wrist. Prevention of ulnar neuropathy and treatment of early symptoms include bike fitting, avoidance of excessive or prolonged weight-bearing through the hands, and the use of padded gloves. For persisting or progressive symptoms, a thorough history and physical examination is essential to confirm the diagnosis and to rule out other sites of nerve compression. The majority of compression neuropathies in cyclists resolve after appropriate rest and conservative treatment; however, should symptoms persist, nerve decompression may be indicated.

Michael S. Gart and Thomas A. Wiedrich

The approach to rehabilitation of upper extremity injuries in athletes differs from traditional rehabilitation protocols. In general, athletes have higher functional demands and wish to return to competitive sport in a timely manner. Comprehensive rehabilitation must therefore be balanced with a timely and safe return to sport. Several rehabilitation programs and adjunctive therapies are available to hasten convalescence while minimizing the athlete's risks of reinjury. Here, we review techniques for soft tissue mobilization and strength training in athletic populations. We also discuss orthotics, taping, and alternative therapies used in rehabilitation and evaluate the evidence in support of these modalities.

HAND CLINICS

RELATED INTEREST

Orthopedic Clinics, October 2016 (Vol. 47, No. 4)
Sports-Related Injuries
James H. Calandruccio, Benjamin J. Grear, Benjamin M. Mauck, Jeffrey R. Sawyer, Patrick C. Toy, and John C. Weinlein, *Editors*
Available at: http://www.orthopedic.theclinics.com/

Clinics in Sports Medicine, January 2015 (Vol. 34, No. 1)
Sports Hand and Wrist Injuries
Jonathan Isaacs, *Editor*
Available at: http://www.sportsmed.theclinics.com/

THE CLINICS ARE AVAILABLE ONLINE!
Access your subscription at:
www.theclinics.com

Preface

Optimizing the Treatment of Upper Extremity Injuries in Athletes

 CrossMark

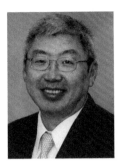

Kevin C. Chung, MD, MS
Editor

Sports are the essential fabric of the American life. As soon as a toddler is able to run, he or she is engaged in a number of sport activities ranging from T-ball, soccer, gymnastics, to a variety of racket sports. The intensity of our national sports programs and our affection for contact sports such as football make sports injury a common occurrence in athletes. Although many of these injuries are minor, a substantial number of these injuries are serious and can end the career of the athlete.

This issue on athletic injury is timely because it addresses many types of sports injuries and focuses not only on the treatments of these injuries but also on their prevention. The first article was written after an extensive interview with the coaches of one of the most recognized football programs in the country. My interviews with the head and assistant coaches at the University of Michigan, Jim Harbaugh and Jedd Fisch, provided thoughtful insight on preventing sports injuries in professional and college athletics. Both coaches have worked in the National Football League and in the college ranks and share their insight and philosophy regarding the prevention and treatment of injuries in high-performing athletes. In particular, Coach Harbaugh was the quarterback for the University of Michigan before continuing to play 14 years for several professional football teams. His perspective as a player is quite revealing, as he noted that playing hurt was part of his job, but he sought guidance from physicians about whether playing with certain injuries would jeopardize his football career.

I believe that the views presented by both coaches reflect concepts shared by all coaches ranging from professional to recreational sports. Coaches have a duty to protect their players and to present a culture of fair play, teamwork, and commitment to excellence without putting the players at risk. Even with these lofty goals, our society's collective interest should be to ensure that our athletes are able to perform at their full potential while simultaneously minimizing injuries through conditioning and preventive measures. The authors of articles in this issue are leading experts on treating injuries in athletes and have provided their lifelong experiences in managing these

Hand Clin 33 (2017) xiii–xiv
http://dx.doi.org/10.1016/j.hcl.2016.10.001
0749-0712/17/© 2016 Published by Elsevier Inc.

injuries effectively for safe return to competitive sports.

I am grateful that Coach Harbaugh and Coach Fisch took the effort to contribute to this issue. I am often struck by the infamous quote that "Winning isn't everything; it's the only thing," which is used to encourage players to strive for competition, but this quote does carry an unsavory connotation of winning at all costs. It is gratifying to me that our coaches at the University of Michigan do not subscribe to this overgeneralized opinion. Instead, they advocate that winning isn't everything; winning fairly without injuries to the players should be the most important goal.

I appreciate this opportunity to be editor of this outstanding issue, and I look forward to sharing this *Hand Clinics* issue with you.

Sincerely,

Kevin C. Chung, MD, MS
University of Michigan Health System
University of Michigan Medical School
2130 Taubman Center, SPC 5340
1500 East Medical Center Drive
Ann Arbor, MI 48109, USA

E-mail address:
kecchung@med.umich.edu

Treating the Football Athlete
Coaches' Perspective from the University of Michigan

Kevin C. Chung, MD, MS[a],*, Meghan E. Lark, BS[b],
Paul S. Cederna, MD[a]

KEYWORDS

- Football injuries • Concussion • Sports medicine • Coach philosophy • Athletes

KEY POINTS

- The management of player safety and injury prevention in collision sports is of public health concern.
- A football coach may have a large role in advocating for player safety and creating a team culture emphasizing healthy injury management.
- An athlete's well-being can be influenced by a coach's practice, game, and decision-making philosophy.
- Healthy football injury management can be maximized through optimal collaboration with medical professionals and use of resources.

INTRODUCTION

It is undisputed that football is one of the most popular sports in the United States, with approximately 3 million youth, 1 million high school, and 100,000 college participants annually.[1] The sport is known for its competitive emphasis on physicality and toughness, which contributes to the creation of the nation's most dynamic and specialized athletes. However, sports medicine research has demonstrated that football has one of the highest risks of overall injury of all American sports, and that this risk increases with the level of competition.[1–4] Epidemiologic studies evaluating injury rates at both collegiate and professional levels have shown that the majority of injuries are sustained as a result of high-energy player-to-player contact. The demonstrated high incidences of musculoskeletal and concussive injuries sustained by football players suggests that optimal injury management is of public health concern, especially in athletes at the highest levels of competition.[5]

From a medical standpoint, the football player is a unique patient. In addition to maintaining traditional patient–physician communication, a physician treating a highly competitive football player must balance communication within a wider

Disclosure: Research reported in this publication was supported by a Midcareer Investigator Award in Patient-Oriented Research (2K24 AR053120-06) to Dr K.C. Chung. The content is solely the responsibility of the authors and does not necessarily represent the official views of the National Institutes of Health. The authors do not have a conflict of interest to disclose.
a Section of Plastic Surgery, University of Michigan Medical School, Ann Arbor, MI 48109-5340, USA; b Section of Plastic Surgery, Department of Surgery, University of Michigan Health System, Ann Arbor, MI 48109-5340, USA
* Corresponding author. Section of Plastic Surgery, University of Michigan Health System, 2130 Taubman Center, SPC 5340, 1500 East Medical Center Drive, Ann Arbor, MI 48109-5340.
E-mail address: kecchung@umich.edu

Hand Clin 33 (2017) 1–8
http://dx.doi.org/10.1016/j.hcl.2016.08.001

network of stakeholders, which may include coaches, trainers, and other team-related staff. Research suggests that the roles of assistant and head coaches can extend beyond technical instruction and that, if an athlete perceives that their coach is supportive of responsible injury recognition and rehabilitation, they may be more likely to report an injury.[6] However, a coach's perspective on establishing a team culture valuing injury prevention is largely unexplored. This article aims to obtain the perspectives of Jim Harbaugh and Jedd Fisch (**Fig. 1**), head and assistant coaches of the University of Michigan football program, on the injury management of a highly competitive Division 1 football team within the National Collegiate Athletic Association (NCAA). We identify successful components of a competitive football team in relation to policy enforcement, coaching philosophy, and medical communication and investigate how these components can maximize the well-being of student-athletes (**Fig. 2**).

POLICY EVOLUTION

Policy administration is one of the most effective methods of protecting and advocating for the health and safety of football players. The majority of recent policy modifications and additions provide guidelines for the management of concussions and injuries to the head (**Fig. 3**), which consist of roughly 7% to 10% of all football injuries.[1,3,5] Concussions pose significant challenges to medical staff, in that they do not present with consistent symptoms. Although sideline tools such as the Sport Concussion Assessment Tool (SCAT) have been developed, an objective and universal

diagnostic tool does not exist.[7] Furthermore, concussion diagnosis strongly relies on the athlete's accurate reporting of symptoms, which can be hindered by factors such as inadequate understanding of concussion symptoms or concerns about losing playing time.[5,8] For these reasons, current trends in football research focus on the study of concussions in an effort to create management policies, playing rules, and practice guidelines that advocate for optimal player safety without sacrificing the physicality of the sport.

Football management associations at all levels have addressed the growing concern of concussion management through the development of a wide range of policies. In April 2010, the NCAA created the NCAA Concussion Policy and Legislation, which mandates implementation of a concussion management plan at each participating institution. This policy requires management plans to detail provisions of concussion education for all student-athletes, promptly removing athletes experiencing head trauma from competition, and prohibiting return to play for at least 24 hours.[9] Additionally, the policy mandates that all players diagnosed with a concussion be medically cleared by a physician before returning to athletic activities.[9] Jedd Fisch indicated that concussion awareness is a large component of the health policy evolution he has witnessed throughout his coaching experiences, and stated, "I could think of 2008, when we had some pretty significant concussions when I was at Denver, to now currently, and the concussion protocol has changed substantially. The return-to-play has also changed substantially, in regards to involving the independent neurologist, not the team doctor. If an athlete

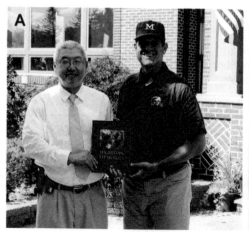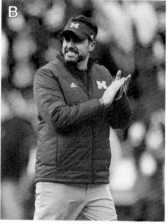

Fig. 1. (*A*) Jim Harbaugh, University of Michigan football head coach with Dr Kevin Chung. (*B*) Jedd Fisch, University of Michigan football passing game coordinator/quarterbacks/wide receivers coach. (*Courtesy of* [B] University of Michigan Football, Ann Arbor, MI; with permission.)

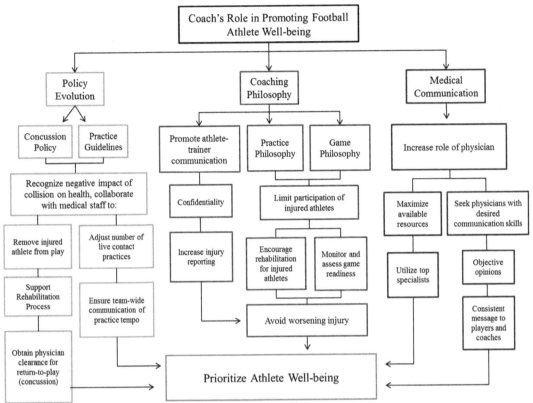

Fig. 2. Conceptual framework detailing multiple facets of the policy evolution, coaching philosophy, and medical communication involving a football team and how they contribute to prioritizing athlete well-being.

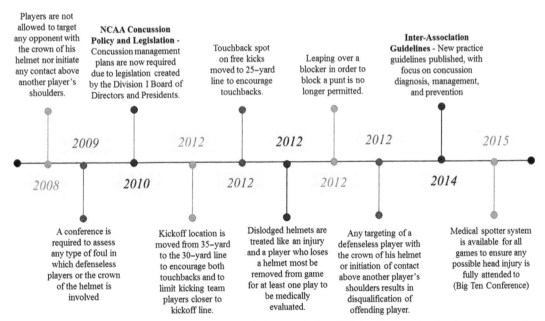

Fig. 3. Timeline of recent National Collegiate Athletic Association (NCAA) Division 1 rule changes promoting player safety. These events serve as a representation of some of the most significant changes that have been made regarding concussion and musculoskeletal injuries since 2008.

[after prior diagnosis of concussion] comes in with a headache, the return-to-play time is extended another few days or another week. It is important to trust the information that you're getting." Studies evaluating the effectiveness of the 2010 policy and similar policies enacted throughout all levels of play have indicated a consistent increase of concussion incidence, which is likely a result of improved concussion reporting and policy introduction increasing concussion diagnosis.[1,10,11] Research exploring institutional and trainer compliance with concussion education programs has demonstrated that players are being provided with concussion information; however, player internalization of the information requires further exploration.[12,13] Fisch's response indicates that, within the rapidly evolving concussion landscape, a coach's role requires trusting information provided by developing research and adjusting return to play in concordance with the advice of medical specialists.

In addition to shaping policy creation, sports medicine research and injury awareness have contributed to the modification and development of both football league- and conference-level playing rules. In the NCAA, the most recent rule modifications and additions involve prohibiting players from "targeting" or leading with the helmet when blocking or tackling and removing a player from the game for one play for medical evaluation if the player's helmet becomes dislodged during play.[14] Additionally, some conferences have implemented the use of a medical spotter positioned in the instant replay booth with direct communication to the field to alert the officials in the case of an unnoticed injured player.[15] Modifications of existing rules include expanding the definition of a "defenseless player," moving the kickoff line to encourage touchbacks, and increasing the penalty for targeting violations.[14] One study evaluated the effects of moving the kickoff line on injury rates and found that, after rule establishment, the incidence of injuries occurring during kickoff plays decreased significantly.[16] Results of this study suggest that the increasing development of rules and amendments for player protection can have a positive impact on injury reduction. When asked about the evolving rules of the game and increasing regulation, head coach Harbaugh responded, "Good officiating is critical to help protect the player. An official's first role is to protect the player, and their second role is to officiate the game." Harbaugh's responses suggest that, with the expansive landscape of football rules and interpretations reflected in game officiating, it can be important for coaches to recognize the emphasis on player safety that underlies rule creation.

Athletic medicine research related to concussion risk factors and epidemiology continues to fuel policymaking at all levels of football. In 2014, the NCAA released the "Inter-Association Guidelines" in which best practices for concussion diagnosis and management are detailed and expanded on through the incorporation of recent study results.[9] Although the high intensity and physicality of football heightens an athletes risk for a concussion, studies have found that more than one-half of concussions occur in practices, particularly those in which athletes are fully padded.[3,17–19] Although the NCAA does not regulate weekly frequencies of live contact practices, the association released "Practice Contact Guidelines" in 2014 that recommend limiting live contact practices to 2 per week.[20] When asked how these guidelines affect preparation for the physicality and live contact of a football game, Fisch insisted, "We do not need to hit as often to still have successful games and be a physical football team. I think that as long as everybody knows that a practice is live, and everybody is on the same page if a practice is not live, our risk of injury diminishes. When people are playing at different tempos or, for instance, playing at 100% speed and it's an 80% speed practice, that's when an injury can occur." Fisch's ideology not only stresses the importance of widespread communication in limited contact practices, but also demonstrates that quality practices can still be conducted in scenarios adjusted for injury prevention.

COACHES' PHILOSOPHY

At the most competitive level of play in a sport centered on tenacity and grit, it is often difficult for football players to remove themselves from competition when injured. An athlete's hesitation to report an injury has been linked to a variety of factors, such as fear of losing playing time, competitive pressure to win the game, reluctance to appear weak in front of coaches and teammates, or improper understanding of injuries.[21] Sociologic relationships that the player engages in are key factors in shaping perception of injury, and one of the most important is the athlete's relationship with their coaches.[22] Sports medicine research has indicated that an athlete's likelihood of reporting an injury, particularly serious injuries such as concussions, depends significantly on the coaching outlook and the value that the coaches place on injury prevention and rehabilitation.[6,22] Therefore, a coach's principles can play a large role in their athlete's well-being, and the creation of a team that values injury prevention; management may start at the level of the coach.

In managing his team, Harbaugh described his injury-reporting philosophy by saying, "we encourage our players to report any possible injury immediately so we can stop it from developing further. The athletes know that they have a duty to the team to report any injury because it affects the team." From being a former University of Michigan and National Football League (NFL) quarterback, Harbaugh understands the competitive drive that heavily influences a player's injury decisions, and explained that in his own injury occurrences, he "always wanted to know from doctors and trainers that, if I continued to play, would it just hurt, or would the injury get worse? If it just hurt, but I knew it wasn't going to get worse, then I wanted to find a way to still be able to play, which usually involved protecting the injury using taping or padding. Of course I always felt that with anything to do with the head, neck, spine, or heart; never keep playing through an injury in those particular areas. And others, for instance, particular soft tissue injuries such as pulled muscles, without a doubt if you keep playing you will injure it worse." These firsthand experiences are translated into Harbaugh's coaching philosophies emphasizing persistent athlete–trainer communication. Fisch added that a large part of integrating these ideals involves "discussion of the difference between being hurt and being injured. Our whole philosophy has always been that if you are injured, your job is to communicate that to the trainer to assess what type of injury it is and what type of medical treatment is needed." The role of athletic trainers can be impactful for injury management, as one study investigating the health education of athletes indicated that education about concussions and other injuries is most frequently provided by athletic trainers.[23] Fisch suggests that a main component of establishing a team culture of injury prevention starts with the coach's support of the trainer and the trust that the coach–trainer relationship entails. He added, "Our players feel that there's a confidentiality that occurs with the athletic trainers, and I hope that they can go to the trainers about everything so that they don't hide injuries. They do not have to go to the coach first; they can communicate player to trainer and trainer to player, which lets the trainer decide how substantial an injury is and whether the coaches need to be informed." This coaching outlook, in which coaches encourage frequent communication with athletic trainers and establish a route of direct trainer–coach communication for injuries, allows the football coach to place value on safe injury reporting practices and shape healthy team attitudes.

Coaches maintain an additional level of control in promoting health of their athletes through managing the participation of injured players during both practices and games. The high number of high-energy collisions in football practices and games places a mild or moderately injured athlete at risk of sustaining a more serious injury. With evidence suggesting a high prevalence of football injuries in practices, the process of the coaching staff in deciding whether previously injured athletes should contribute to practices falls under question.[3,17,24] When asked about the practice philosophy of head coach Harbaugh, Fisch stated, "One thing that I've noticed about Jim is that if an athlete feels as if they have an injury, they are out of [full contact] practice. He does not push the injured to become more injured, and instead encourages the injured to go get treatment. He would rather have a practice of 57 completely healthy athletes than a practice of 85 athletes in which 28 are hurt or injured." Harbaugh's insistence on practice participation of only healthy athletes protects those who are mildly injured from exacerbating their current injury. Further addressing the dangers of injured player participation, Fisch emphasized that "without a doubt, a player that cannot protect themselves is far more vulnerable than a player that at least has the ability to get out of harm's way." Harbaugh expanded on the roles of injured athletes during practices and explained, "We want to win every day, injured or not injured. Players who are rehabbing an injury or managing a limitation in practice want to win at what they're doing. Our players place a competitive mindset on coming back from an injury faster and better than anyone else, and an injury is looked at as an opportunity to come back better at techniques or fundamentals and stronger than one was before. The athlete is definitely not shut down when injured." The tenets of Harbaugh's philosophy aim to use his athletes' competitive drive as a positive gateway to injury rehabilitation rather than a barrier to injury reporting, which is exemplified by his daily practice values. Despite the pressures imposed on athletes by the competitive nature of football, these principles demonstrate that coaches can have a large role in steering the attitudes and responses of injured athletes in a direction that promotes healthy practices.

Although data suggest a higher incidence of practice-related injury in football, the intensity of football has been shown to produce a 6-fold increase in the risk of player injury.[3,24] This increased risk highlights the health benefits of coaches prioritizing game participation only to athletes who are healthy and able to remain healthy during live contact. In the University of Michigan football program, the protocol for assessing game readiness relies largely on the coaching staff's attentiveness to athletes' abilities and is achieved through Harbaugh's meritocracy principles, in which only athletes who perform the best in practices leading up to games are permitted to participate. Fisch stated, "The meritocracy philosophy comes into play in that we monitor everything. We monitor how many reps an athlete takes in practice and how many reps are taken in the weight room, and keep a running tally. Our athletes get rewarded for being able to participate and we do not put athletes on the field that give us the best chances to win, but did not participate all week. Athletes have to show that they're healthy, and that's another reason why our injury rates are so low." The outlook of Harbaugh and Fisch exemplifies the benefits of strict health evaluation of football players, which in turn can reduce injury rate and protect injured players that may be at higher risk of sustaining further injury.

A football coach's leadership is far-reaching and can affect not only the instruction of a team, but also the ideology of the players and their attitudes toward seeking medical care. The ideals of the University of Michigan football coaching staff, implemented in both practices and games, prioritize the health of the athlete through promoting injury reporting, restricting injured athlete participation, and conducting quantitative assessments of weekly capabilities. These actions contribute to the development of a team culture that values injury management and athlete–trainer communication in an effort to maximize player safety without sacrificing highly competitive gameplay.

MEDICAL COMMUNICATION

As the public awareness of football injuries such as concussions or anterior cruciate ligament (ACL) tears is increasing, the involvement of both team physicians and specialists in athletic medical care mirrors the same trend. In addition to incorporating team physician and specialist opinions into policy creation and return-to-play clearance,[9] football teams are expanding the role of medical professionals in the everyday treatment of athletic injuries. When asked about the greatest change witnessed in his own experiences of football, Fisch expressed, "Without a doubt, in the 20 years that I have been involved in collegiate and pro athletics, there has been a huge adjustment in terms of how much attention is being given to injuries. The communication between the training staff, medical staff, and coaches has been quadrupled, if not more." Fisch anecdotally described an example in which a quarterback suffered a significant laceration to the hand while scrambling in a game.

When the injury occurred, the team orthopedic surgeon and trainer performed initial wound management, and within 2 hours a hand surgeon was called in to examine the injury. The athlete's surgery took place one day later and in the 3 to 4 postoperative weeks, the hand surgeon made weekly visits to monitor the injury, and even traveled with the team until the stitches were removed. Increasing the physician's role in athletic treatment undoubtedly improves the quality of care administered to football players, although it may also add an additional level of communication in the multifactorial approach to athletic health care. For this reason, it is important to explore how physicians fit into the decision-making process, communication structure, and resource availability of football programs at the top levels of play.

At the collegiate and professional levels, a football player's health and injury status can often be a defining component of administration decisions concerning recruiting, eligibility, and career continuation. For these reasons, Fisch described the role of medical professionals in decision making as integral, and stated that in recruiting players with injuries, "we consult with an orthopedic surgeon and ask them questions regarding risk of injury, risk of repeating the same injury, risk of repeating an ACL injury if the player has already had 2 ACL injuries; it is a process similar to risk management." Harbaugh insists the same technique occurs for career- and season-ending injuries, and said that "those [decisions] are made with the doctors, families, and the player themselves. There's not much that I can bring to the table in terms of advice that can supersede a doctor. The decisions we make need to be beneficial for the individual, their career, or for the morale of the team. The health and welfare of our student-athletes is above the strong desire to win games." In both seeking out the opinion of medical experts and quantitative research, decision-making metrics can be provided to coaches, training staff, and athletes to make informed decisions that prioritize the athlete's well-being. Harbaugh's response suggests that although coaches do not have the expertise to make tough medical decisions, they can play a role in focusing decision making on player wellness instead of the competitive pressures of football.

Although a physician's involvement in athletics advances the level of care provided to football players, team physicians can frequently encounter challenges when navigating football injuries. Fisch described the ideal team physician as "someone who recognizes the importance of concierge medicine and understands that being a team physician is not a 9-to-5 job. Being a physician includes dealing with the paranoia of coaches, players, and parents, all constantly wanting to know when the athlete will be ready to play again. It is also important for team physicians to understand that player's livelihoods are based heavily on the decisions that are being made." The expectations of the many people involved in a player's medical treatment can impose immense pressures on team physicians, and in some cases have been shown to result in making unhealthy decisions for athletes.[25] To balance the high expectations and ensure the health of the athlete is always the first priority, Fisch stated that when choosing a team physician, "the number one most important quality is the delivery of a consistent message to player and to coach. Flaws and problems are sometimes a result of the player hearing one thing and the coach hearing another from the team physician, causing a player-coach disconnect. The best team physicians are the ones that can be objective and say 'Here is what I see, here is what I believe, let's make sure we're all on the same page.'" Harbaugh expressed similar views and stressed the importance of "open and direct communication. We operate a very open and direct culture here, good or bad news, I want to hear it." Harbaugh added, "As a coach, I didn't go to medical school, I don't have the expertise. So we try to surround our players with doctors that we trust, that are respected on boards and leaders in their field. We need to trust that our team is getting the best medical care possible." A physician's skill and expertise in their field are undoubtedly predictors of success in football team physicians; however, Fisch and Harbaugh's responses indicate that open and objective communicative strengths may be of similar importance.

Despite similarities in health policies and injury regulation between the NCAA and NFL, the resources available to athletes at the different levels of play are drastically different. Fisch suggests that the two greatest observed differences in injury management and prevention in the professional league are characterized by the involvement of agents in medical care and treatment guidance obtained from experienced teammates. He explained that, on a professional football team, an athlete sustaining an injury has "at least 1 or 2 teammates that have sustained the same injury as well, so the injured player can talk to them and they might make recommendations of which physicians provided the best care. Each athlete also has an agent that is extremely involved in the medical decision making for their client." At the professional level, it is easier for athletes to maximize the quality of the health care they receive, because of the extensive network of medical resources that exists within the players on a team.

In contrast, NCAA athletes rely on the trainers and medical staff provided for them at the university they attend. Instead of agents, collegiate athletes have parents who trust in the decisions of the collegiate-level medical care team. For collegiate student-athletes to maximize health care resources, Fisch insisted that they should "communicate and ask questions. Athletes should use all of the resources of the university they attend and need to understand that if they are at a program with a top medical school, then the program is likely to do a lot of research and they can ask the tough questions. The athlete should always be able to ask if there is a more experienced physician at their university that would be better in performing an operation or visiting for a second opinion." These opinions suggest that the medical environment of the university a football athlete attends can significantly affect the quality of care that the player receives. In commenting on the environment offered at his institution, Harbaugh emphasized, "We are very fortunate at the University of Michigan that we feel like we have the best in the country, it's hard to find better than what we have here."

SUMMARY

The highly publicized and competitive nature of football places a large importance on injury management for football players, particularly at collegiate and professional levels. Injuries are inevitable in contact sports, highlighting the necessity for a dynamic, integrative response prompted by coaches, trainers, and medical staff. Improvements in this response are reflected through evolving policies that are strongly rooted in sports medicine research and epidemiologic studies, with the most successful programs having flexible coaches that are able to adapt to policy evolution. Additionally, a coach's philosophy serves as a starting point for making significant advancements in the injury management of a competitive team, illustrated in how the coaches teach their players to report injury, seek rehabilitation, and manage a player's game readiness. Furthermore, this collaborative approach to medical treatment of football injuries flourishes at a university that can use top medical resources to support the health care needs of the nation's most competitive athletes.

ACKNOWLEDGMENTS

To the invaluable contribution of this article from Jim Harbaugh and Jedd Fisch, head and assistant football coaches, University of Michigan Football Program, Ann Arbor, Michigan.

REFERENCES

1. Lawrence DW, Hutchison MG, Comper P. Descriptive epidemiology of musculoskeletal injuries and concussions in the National football league, 2012-2014. Orthop J Sports Med 2015;3(5). 2325967115583653.
2. Dick R, Ferrara MS, Agel J, et al. Descriptive epidemiology of collegiate men's football injuries: National Collegiate Athletic Association injury surveillance system, 1988-1989 through 2003-2004. J Athl Train 2007;42(2):221–33.
3. Dompier TP, Kerr ZY, Marshall SW, et al. Incidence of concussion during practice and games in youth, high school, and collegiate American Football Players. JAMA Pediatr 2015;169(7):659–65.
4. Marar M, McIlvain NM, Fields SK, et al. Epidemiology of concussions among United States high school athletes in 20 sports. Am J Sports Med 2012;40(4):747–55.
5. Baugh CM, Kroshus E. Concussion management in US college football: progress and pitfalls. Concussion 2016;1(1):1–20.
6. Baugh CM, Kroshus E, Daneshvar DH, et al. Perceived coach support and concussion symptom-reporting: differences between freshmen and non-freshmen college football players. J Law Med Ethics 2014;42(3):314–22.
7. Chin EY, Nelson LD, Barr WB, et al. Reliability and validity of the sport concussion assessment Tool-3 (SCAT3) in high school and collegiate athletes. Am J Sports Med 2016;44(9):2276–85.
8. Torres DM, Galetta KM, Phillips HW, et al. Sports-related concussion: anonymous survey of a collegiate cohort. Neurol Clin Pract 2013;3(4):279–87.
9. National Collegiate Athletic Association. Guideline 2I: sports related concussion. 2014-2015. NCAA sports medicine handbook. Indianapolis (IN): National Collegiate Athletic Association; 2014.
10. Kilcoyne KG, Dickens JF, Svoboda SJ, et al. Reported concussion rates for three division I football programs: an evaluation of the new NCAA concussion policy. Sports Health 2014;6(5):402–5.
11. Lincoln AE, Caswell SV, Almquist JL, et al. Trends in concussion incidence in high school sports: a prospective 11-year study. Am J Sports Med 2011; 39(5):958–63.
12. Baugh CM, Kroshus E, Bourlas AP, et al. Requiring athletes to acknowledge receipt of concussion-related information and responsibility to report symptoms: a study of the prevalence, variation, and possible improvements. J Law Med Ethics 2014;42(3):297–313.
13. Kelly KC, Jordan EM, Joyner AB, et al. National Collegiate Athletic Association division I athletic trainers' concussion-management practice patterns. J Athl Train 2014;49(5):665–73.
14. National Collegiate Athletic Association. 2016 and 2017 NCAA Football Rules and Interpretations. Indianapolis (IN): National Collegiate Athletic Association; 2016–2017.
15. Big Ten Conference. 2015 Big ten football media days [press release]. Big Ten Conference, Chicago, 2015.
16. Ruestow PS, Duke TJ, Finley BL, et al. Effects of the NFL's amendments to the free kick rule on Injuries during the 2010 and 2011 Seasons. J Occup Environ Hyg 2015;12(12):875–82.
17. Zuckerman SL, Kerr ZY, Yengo-Kahn A, et al. Epidemiology of Sports-related concussion in NCAA athletes from 2009-2010 to 2013-2014: incidence, recurrence, and mechanisms. Am J Sports Med 2015;43(11):2654–62.
18. Houck Z, Asken B, Bauer R, et al. Epidemiology of sport-related concussion in an NCAA division I football bowl subdivision sample. Am J Sports Med 2016;44(9):2269–75.
19. Kerr ZY, Hayden R, Dompier TP, et al. Association of equipment worn and concussion injury rates in National Collegiate Athletic Association football practices: 2004-2005 to 2008-2009 academic years. Am J Sports Med 2015;43(5):1134–41.
20. National Collegiate Athletic Association. Appendix D: year-round football practice contact guidelines. 2014-2015 NCAA sports medicine handbook 25 edition. Indianapolis (IN): National Collegiate Athletic Association; 2014.
21. Kerr ZY, Register-Mihalik JK, Marshall SW, et al. Disclosure and non-disclosure of concussion and concussion symptoms in athletes: review and application of the socio-ecological framework. Brain Inj 2014;28(8):1009–21.
22. Kroshus E, Baugh CM, Hawrilenko MJ, et al. Determinants of coach communication about concussion safety in US collegiate sport. Ann Behav Med 2015; 49(4):532–41.
23. Kroshus E, Baugh CM. Concussion education in U.S. collegiate sport: what is happening and what do athletes want? Health Educ Behav 2016;43(2): 182–90.
24. Steiner ME, Berkstresser BD, Richardson L, et al. Full-contact practice and injuries in college football. Sports Health 2016;8(3):217–23.
25. Kroshus E, Baugh CM, Daneshvar DH, et al. Pressure on sports medicine clinicians to prematurely return collegiate athletes to play after concussion. J Athl Train 2015;50(9):944–51.

Expediting Professional Athletes' Return to Competition

Jeff M. Coppage, MD, Michelle G. Carlson, MD*

KEYWORDS

- Return to play • Protected return to play • Athlete • Professional athlete • Sports medicine • Hand
- Wrist

KEY POINTS

- Upper extremity injuries are common in elite athletes and are responsible for significant amounts of time away from sport.
- Return-to-play decisions can be difficult and demand careful consideration of many factors. Despite attempts to standardize the decision-making process, return to play considerations must be individualized to a given athlete and his or her injury.
- Return to play decisions for elite athletes have ethical and legal implications for the treating physician that must be carefully considered.
- There is variability in return-to-play protocols for given injuries based on the sport, position, and the nature of the injury.
- Return to play with protective equipment is highly variable, and league-specific regulations are outlined in this text and should be familiar to practitioners treating elite athletes.

INTRODUCTION

Injuries to the upper extremity are a common occurrence among professional athletes. Fifteen percent of injuries in the National Basketball Association (NBA)[1] and 50% of injuries in Major League Baseball[2] involve the upper extremity. Upper extremity injuries account for 18% of all injuries in the National Football League (NFL) and occur in 50% of NFL games.[3] Decisions regarding return to play (RTP) after upper extremity injuries represent an important and often challenging aspect of caring for elite athletes. Athletes with a prior injury are 4 times more likely to sustain another injury,[4] and premature RTP may result in complications and potentially permanent sequelae that would otherwise be preventable. The surgeon's recommendations regarding RTP must consider and balance many factors including the individual injury, athlete safety, timing and duration of time away from sport, short and long-term career considerations and ethical, legal, and financial issues.

The purpose of this article is to bring to light the multifaceted nature of RTP decisions. In addition to discussing individual injuries and treatment strategies to expedite RTP, the authors hope to provide the reader with an appreciation and understanding of other considerations that affect RTP decisions.

THE ROLE OF THE TEAM PHYSICIAN

Decisions regarding RTP are an integral part of the team physician's practice but may be less familiar to a consultant upper extremity surgeon. These decisions can be challenging because of many competing interests and parties including the athlete, coaches, trainers, agents, and

Disclosure Statement: None of the authors of this article have pertinent financial interests to disclose.
Hospital for Special Surgery, Hand and Upper Extremity, 523 East 72nd Street, 4th Floor, New York, NY 10021, USA
* Corresponding author.
E-mail address: carlsonm@hss.edu

Hand Clin 33 (2017) 9–18
http://dx.doi.org/10.1016/j.hcl.2016.08.002

organizations. The process of making recommendations regarding RTP has become more difficult in recent years because of the increasingly competitive culture of professional sports, rapidly changing medical technology and treatments, increased media involvement, and ever-increasing financial pressures to minimize missed participation in their sports activities. Furthermore, despite efforts to institute some degree of standardization to RTP decisions,[5–7] the process remains largely individualized to a specific injury in an athlete with a unique set of personal and professional circumstances that must be considered.

ETHICAL CONSIDERATIONS

A discussion of expediting athlete RTP would not be complete without mention of the ethical issues that are inherent in the current culture of elite athletics. Care of the elite athlete is complicated by attributes that are inherent to this patient population. The competitiveness of high-level athletics selects for highly motivated and committed individuals. These traits, although essential to elite performance, may serve as an obstacle to the delivery of ethical care. Athletes commonly pressure the physician into early RTP for a variety of reasons such as an inherent love for the sport, financial motivation, external pressure from peers and the organization, and perceived expectations to "play through it."

The relationship between an athlete's physician and his or her patient is unique because in modern-day professional athletics, the traditional doctor–patient dyad is probably more appropriately viewed as a doctor–patient–team triad[8] given the additional influences of the team on the athlete. Ethical standards such as informed consent, autonomy, and confidentiality become more difficult to apply to professional athletes. Informed consent is designed to protect patient autonomy by allowing an individual patient to make decisions based on his or her personal values. As more parties become involved in the medical decision-making process, the introduction of conflicting values and interests may sway the athlete to make decisions that are not aligned with his or her values and thus not allow for a truly autonomous decision. This is compounded by influences on the team physician. The position of team physician is considered one of considerable prestige and offers significant market advantages. This position establishes a relationship that has potential to introduce some degree of inherent conflict of interest for the physician. The team physician has incentives to maintain his or her affiliation with the team and take the team values and interests into consideration. This affiliation is further compounded by intense media attention to the injured athlete. The physician's decisions regarding RTP may be scrutinized by the media and the public and influence public opinion regarding the competence of the physician. The American Medical Association Code of Medical Ethics States that "The professional responsibility of the physician who serves in a medical capacity at an athletic contest or sporting event is to protect the health and safety of the contestants. The desire of spectators, promoters of the event, or even the injured athlete that he or she should not be removed from the contest should not be controlling. The physician's judgment should be governed only by medical considerations."[9] Although this is an agreed-upon tenet of athletic medicine, one can appreciate how the aforementioned pressures create challenges to dutiful execution of these principles.

Patient confidentiality is another area in which special considerations exist for the athlete. The physician has an obligation to keep all patient information confidential except in specific cases outlined by law.[10,11] Differences in the handling of the athlete's confidential medical information have been described depending on the relationship between the private physician and the physician who is employed by the athletic organization.[12] In the former relationship, the physician has no obligation to share the athlete's medical information with the athletic organization unless the information represents a potential harm to other players. In the latter relationship, the physician is an agent of the team and may be required to share information with the team even if the athlete requests that the information be kept confidential.[13] The impact of the Health Insurance Portability and Accountability Act (HIPAA) on this particular issue was analyzed by Magee and colleagues in 2003[14] who found that team physicians who care for professional athletes may disclose an athlete's medical information to the coaches and owners because the information is considered part of the athlete's employment record. Conversely, a physician who evaluates a professional athlete in his or her private office is bound by HIPAA confidentiality regulations. The issue of patient confidentiality for elite athletes has ramifications in the legal realm as well, which are outlined below.

LEGAL CONSIDERATIONS

In addition to the unique ethical environment of professional sports medicine, a special set of legal considerations exists. Although it is beyond the scope of this article to detail the many legal dilemmas that are germane to professional sports medicine, some legal principles and issues deserve mention. It is common for professional sports organizations to hire a physician or group of physicians to provide medical care to their athletes, and this care can be compensated or provided gratis.[15] Team physicians, by definition, have some degree of responsibility to the athletic organization; however, his or her primary responsibility is to provide for the physical well-being of the athletes. In providing such care, the team physician has a legal obligation to conform to the standard of care for their specialty training. However, there are often circumstances to be considered when treating elite athletes, which frequently lead to treatment decisions that may be different than those that would be made for a nonathlete or, as a 2013 *Washington Post* article stated, "there is medicine, and then there is National Football League medicine, and the practice of the two isn't always the same."[16] This statement raises the question of whether the standard of care for elite athletes should be distinct from those of nonathletes. One way in which the standard of care has been determined for elite athletes is the "customary medical practice standard" that uses expert testimony to provide proof of previously accepted medical practices. An alternative to the customary medical practice standard is the "acceptable practice standard" in which "acceptable or reasonable medical practices establish a physician's legal duty of care in treating athletes. In other words, what should have been done under the circumstances, not what is commonly done, determines the applicable standard."[15] Mitten[15] outlined potential advantages to the acceptable practice standard: "...it focuses on the current state of the medical art rather than on the historical conduct of sports medicine physicians, it enables the physician to deviate from an undesirable custom that is inconsistent with his best judgment, and thereby facilitates the development of sound sports medicine practices. Similarly, it permits physicians to adopt innovative treatments and rehabilitation procedures for athletes." Although some degree of ambiguity regarding the definition of standard of care in elite sports medicine will likely persist, other questions are also raised. Should there be differences in the standard of care for elite athletes versus nonathletes? Should the position of team physician be abolished such that athletes receive individual private medical care similar to that of the general population (with the same standards of care)? These questions remain largely unanswered.

Another legal issue at the forefront of elite athletics is medical confidentiality. The team physician has an obligation to inform the athlete that he or she is acting on behalf of the athletic organization and is providing medical care to the athlete, because it represents a conflict of interest.[15] HIPAA serves to shield an individual's protected health information (PHI) from third parties; the physicians generally require the patient's permission to disclose health information. Elite athletes and team physicians are subject to these regulations as well; however, there are special considerations. Disclosure of PHI in collegiate athletics is regulated by the Family Education Rights and Privacy Act (FERPA). HIPAA exempts FERPA-regulated activities as long as they are considered "traditional university operations," meaning that they fall within the realm of treatment.[17] Disclosure of collegiate athlete PHI to the coaches is considered a "traditional university operation," whereas disclosure of PHI to the media is considered a "nontraditional operation" and thus is subject to HIPAA regulations.[17] A different situation exists for professional athletics because FERPA regulations do not apply. With the introduction of HIPAA regulations, many professional organizations incorporated provisions allowing sharing of athletes PHI into the collective bargaining agreements (CBAs). Collective bargaining agreements are negotiated between the league and the players association and once agreed on, cannot be contested by individual players. The NBA CBA, for example, authorizes a team physician to "disclose all relevant medical information concerning a player to (i) the General Manager, coaches, and trainers of the team..." and the CBA also permits trainers, team officials, and athletic organizations to make PHI public.[17] Each professional sports organization has its own versions of CBAs and other contractual clauses that protect sharing of an athlete's PHI that would otherwise be prohibited by HIPAA regulations.

Many more legal issues beyond the scope of this article are relevant to the practice of sports medicine, and the professional team physician should be abreast of such legal considerations.

STANDARDIZING RETURN-TO-PLAY DECISIONS

The number of variables that play in to an RTP decision makes standardization of the RTP decision impossible. However, efforts have been made to standardize the process of making RTP decisions. Creighton and colleagues[6] presented a decision-based model that is designed to "clarify the processes that clinicians use consciously and subconsciously when making RTP decisions." Their model consists of 3 steps to making an RTP decision with various modifying factors that should be considered in each step. The first step is the Evaluation of Health Status, which assesses a variety of medical factors surrounding the athlete and the injury. The second step is the Evaluation of Participation Risk, which addresses portions of the decision-making process that pertain to the specific sport and activities required therein. The final step is Decision Modification to incorporate factors that are not related to the injury or specific sport such as external influences from family or team, legal issues, and financial considerations. Although this model helps the team physician by providing a structured process by which to conceptually organize RTP decisions, it also serves to emphasize the inescapable reliance on individualized decision making and physician expertise when making RTP decisions.

SPECIFIC INJURIES
Fractures and Fracture–Dislocations of the Phalanges

Phalangeal fractures take a variety of forms and each has different implications for treatment. Treatment depends largely on the characteristics and severity of the fracture, whether the digit can be protected during play, and the short-term, midterm, and long-term consequences of returning the athlete to play with a given injury.[18] Unless clear surgical indications such as an open injury, unstable fracture pattern, or articular involvement with displacement are present, consideration should be given in favor of nonoperative rather than operative management. The surgeon should consider whether surgical management will confer benefits to the athlete that nonoperative management cannot and whether these benefits will help the athlete achieve his or her goals with respect to RTP and long-term outcome. Graham[18] outlined a trend in his practice away from pinning and external fixators and toward open reduction internal fixation (ORIF) in athletes because the former do not provide an acceptable risk/benefit ratio to the elite athlete. The preference to avoid wire fixation in elite athlete was echoed by Gaston and Chadderdon.[19]

Variability is present among recommendations regarding RTP after phalangeal fractures and fracture–dislocations. For stable dislocations and fracture patterns, many team physicians advocate protected RTP between 0 to 4 weeks depending on the demands of the athlete and his or her sport.[20–23] A survey of 36 professional team physicians indicated that 94% recommended immediate protected RTP for stable proximal interphalangeal joint dislocations,[24] 30% recommended unprotected RTP at 4 weeks, 38%

recommended 4 to 8 weeks, and 8% recommended greater than 3 months. For operatively treated fractures, the surgeon must take the nature of the fracture, the strength of fixation, and the demands that will be placed on the individual athlete into consideration, but protected RTP can range from 1 to 4 weeks after surgery and unprotected RTP is typically 6 to 8 weeks.[20–22] Recommendations regarding proximal interphalangeal joint fracture–dislocations are highly variable based on individual injury pattern. Patients with operatively treated fracture dislocations typically return to protected play at around 4 to 8 weeks[25,26] (**Fig. 1**).

Metacarpal fractures

Metacarpal fractures are a common athletic injury, particularly in contact sports.[27,28] The anatomic location of the fracture (metacarpal head, neck shaft, or base) can have implications on treatment as can the degree of displacement (rotation, angulation, and shortening). Fortunately, most metacarpal fractures are minimally displaced.[29] Rettig and colleagues[30] reported that the mean time lost from athletic participation was 14 days. Athletes with nondisplaced or minimally displaced metacarpal fractures can generally return to protected play immediately or within days as long as they can perform adequately with the protective splint in place.[27] Athletes with displaced fractures treated with stable ORIF can return to protected play as early as 2 weeks postoperatively. For minimally displaced metacarpal fractures, 38% of team surgeons allow immediate return to protected play, 57% allow return to protected play at 3 to 4 weeks, and 73% allowed return to unprotected play between 4 and 8 weeks.[24]

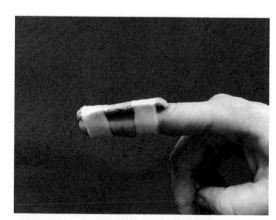

Fig. 1. Finger splint for finger fractures/dislocations. Foam is removed from an aluminum foam splint, and the metal is wrapped in moleskin. The splint can then be taped to the finger on the volar or dorsal surface.

Thumb metacarpophalangeal joint ulnar collateral ligament injuries

Injuries to the ulnar collateral ligament (UCL) of the thumb metacarpophalangeal joint are increasingly common in elite athletes and may cause significant limitations given the high level of function required.[31] Nonoperative management of acute UCL injuries is generally reserved for partial ligament injuries, whereas complete ruptures indicate operative repair.[32] For collegiate football players with complete UCL injuries, Werner and colleagues[33] recommended immediate repair for skill position players and delayed surgical repair at the end of the season for nonskill position players.

The nuances of the athlete's sport, position, risk for reinjury, and league rules must be considered when allowing an athlete to return to protected play after UCL injury. Time to RTP for athletes with partially ruptured ulnar collateral ligaments treated without surgery generally depends on the demands of the sport and whether the athlete can play with cast immobilization.[34] If able to play with cast immobilization, the athlete can often return within days of the injury once the acute swelling and pain has subsided. Typically a hand-based thumb spica splint (**Fig. 2**) or cast is prescribed for use at all times for 4 weeks. Protected range of motion exercises are started at 4 weeks followed by strengthening at 8 weeks.[32] Return to unprotected play often requires 8 or more weeks.[34]

Complete UCL ruptures in the elite athlete are an indication for surgical repair.[32–34] The timing of repair depends on several factors including time of injury from the end of the season, position, sport, and surgeon preference.[24,32,34] Werner and colleagues[33] recommended immediate repair for collegiate football players in a skill position and delayed repair after the end of the season for nonskill players. Approximately 38% of professional team physicians recommend immediate repair,

32% recommend repair at the end of the season if within 6 weeks, 8% recommend repair at the end of the season if within 3 months, and 19% recommend repair at the end of the season even if beyond 6 months from injury.[24] RTP after surgical repair of UCL injuries is variable and should be individualized to the player and the requirements for his or her sport. Some surgeons feel that athletes can return to protected play as early as 1 week after surgery provided that pain is controlled and the athlete can perform adequately with protective cast.[34] Werner and colleagues[33] described a protocol for complete UCL injuries in collegiate football players. They divided the players into 2 groups: skill players (quarterback, running back, wide receiver, and tight end) and nonskill players (offensive lineman, defensive lineman, linebackers). Skill players underwent immediate operative repair whereas nonskill players were returned to protected play and underwent repair at the end of the season. Postoperatively, nonskill players were allowed to return to protected play once pain controlled but skill player–protected RTP was delayed until after the initial 4-week period of immobilization because of demands of their positions. Most professional team physicians (64%) recommend waiting 3 months before return to unprotected play.[24]

Scaphoid fractures

The scaphoid is the most commonly fractured carpal bone and can result in significant short- and long-term limitations if not promptly treated.[35] Operative treatment of scaphoid fractures is preferred for high-level athletes because it allows for early range of motion and RTP with a union rate that approaches 100%.[36–40] Nonoperative management is usually reserved for fractures of the scaphoid tubercle.[41–43]

The nature of the fracture and the sport and individual demands of the athlete influence the time

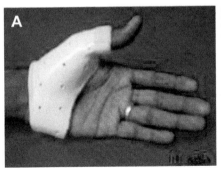 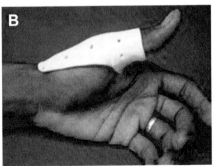

Fig. 2. Splints for return to protected play after thumb UCL injury. (*A*) Hand-based thumb spica for protected return to play. (*B*) Reduced cone splint can be taped on for play when decreased protection is allowed. (*From* Carlson MG. Commentary on RCL/UCL injury in basketball. Hand Clin 2012;28(3):374; with permission.)

Table 1
Protective play guidelines for collegiate and professional sports

Sport		Rules Governing Special Protective Equipment
Baseball	NCAA	No player may wear a nonstandard elbow protection pad, or any pad designed to protect the upper or lower arm, unless the player has an existing elbow or other arm injury and the team carries with it the following documentation: • A letter identifying the player and describing the nature of the injury and describing the proposed elbow protection pad • A physician's report diagnosing the injury • A physician's determination of length of time the protective pad will be necessary Any hard cast must be padded and covered.
	MLB	No player is permitted to wear an elbow protection pad that exceeds 10 inches in length, as measured when the pad is lying flat. A nylon pad shall surround the shell of any elbow protection equipment. A manufacturer's logo on the protection pad may appear in one location and shall not exceed one square inch. No player may wear a nonstandard elbow protection pad, or any pad designed to protect the upper or lower arm, unless the player has an existing elbow or other arm injury and the Club had obtained the prior approval of the Commissioner's Office to wear that particular nonstandard equipment. To obtain such prior approval, the Club will be requested to provide the following: • A letter identifying the player and describing the nature of the injury and describing the proposed elbow protection pad • A physician's report diagnosing the injury • A physician's estimate of length of time the protective pad will be necessary
Men's Basketball	NCAA	Elbow, hand, finger, wrist or forearm guards casts or braces made of fiberglass, plaster, metal or any other nonpliable substance are prohibited. Pliable (flexible or easily bent) material covered on all exterior sides and edges with no less than $1/2$-inch thickness of a slow-rebounding foam shall be used to immobilize and/or protect an injury. Equipment that could cut or cause an injury to another player is prohibited, without respect to whether the equipment is hard. Equipment that, in the referee's judgment, is dangerous to other players, may not be worn.
	NBA	The officials shall not permit any player to wear equipment which, in their judgment, is dangerous to other players. Any equipment that is of hard substance (casts, splints, guards, and braces) must be padded or foam covered and has no exposed sharp or cutting edge. Approval is on a game-to-game basis.
Women's basketball	NCAA	The referee shall not permit any player to wear equipment that in his or her judgment is dangerous to other players. Elbow, hand, finger, wrist or forearm guards, casts or braces made of fiberglass, plaster, metal or any other nonpliable substance, shall be prohibited. Pliable (flexible or easily bent) material, covered on all exterior sides and edges with no less than $1/2$-inch thickness of a slow-rebounding foam, may be used to immobilize and/or protect an injury. Equipment that could cut or cause an injury to another player is prohibited, without respect to whether the equipment is hard.
	WNBA	The officials shall not permit any player to wear equipment which, in his or her judgment, is dangerous to other players. Any equipment that is of hard substance (casts, splints, guards, and braces) must be

(continued on next page)

Table 1
(continued)

Sport		Rules Governing Special Protective Equipment
		padded or foam covered and has no exposed sharp or cutting edge. Approval is on a game-to-game basis
Field hockey	NCAA	Players shall not wear anything that is dangerous to other players.
	USA Field Hockey/FIH	Players must not wear anything that is dangerous to other players.
Football	NCAA	Illegal equipment includes the following: • Equipment worn by a player, including artificial limbs, that would endanger other players. • Hard, abrasive, or unyielding substances on the hand, wrist, forearm, or elbow of any player, unless covered on all exterior sides and edges with closed-cell, slow-recovery foam padding no less than $1/2$-inch thick, or an alternate material of the same minimum thickness and similar physical properties. Hard or unyielding substances are permitted, if covered, only to protect an injury. Hand and arm protectors (covered casts or splints) are permitted only to protect a fracture or dislocation. • Projection of metal or other hard substance from a player's person or clothing
	NFL	Prohibited: Hard objects and substances, including but not limited to casts, guards or braces for hand, wrist, forearm, elbow, hip, thigh, knee, and shin, unless such items are appropriately covered on all edges and surfaces by a minimum of $3/8$-inch foam rubber or similar soft material. Any such item worn to protect an injury must be reported by the applicable coaching staff to the umpire in advance of the game, and a description of the injury must be provided.
Ice hockey	NCAA	The use of pads or protectors made of metal or any other material likely to cause injury to a player is prohibited. The use of any protective equipment that is not injurious to the player wearing it or other players is recommended.
	NHL	The use of pads or protectors made of metal or of any other material likely to cause injury to an opposing player is prohibited. Referees have the authority to prohibit any equipment they feel may cause injury to any participants in the game. Failure to comply with the referees' instructions shall result in the assessment of a minor penalty for delay of game. In the first instance, the injured player shall be entitled to wear any protective device prescribed by the Club doctor. If any opposing Club objects to the device, the Club may record its objection with the Commissioner.
Women's lacrosse	NCAA	Protective devices necessitated on genuine medical grounds must be approved by the umpires. No equipment, including protective devices, may be used unless it complies with the rules or manufacturers' specification and is deemed not dangerous to other players by the officials. Hard and unyielding items (guards, casts, braces, splints) on the hand, wrist, forearm, elbow, upper arm, or shoulder are prohibited unless padded with a closed cell, slow-recovery foam padding no less than $1/2$" thick.
	US Lacrosse	Hard and unyielding items (guards, casts, braces, splints) on the hand, wrist, forearm, elbow, upper arm, or shoulder are prohibited unless padded with a closed-cell, slow-recovery foam padding no <1/2" thick.
Men's lacrosse	NCAA	A player shall not wear any equipment that, in the opinion of the official, endangers the individual or others.
	NLL	No restrictions listed.
	US Lacrosse	No restrictions listed.

(continued on next page)

Table 1 (continued)		
Sport		**Rules Governing Special Protective Equipment**
Soccer	NCAA	A player shall not wear anything that is dangerous to another player. Casts are permitted if they are covered and the referee does not consider them dangerous.
Softball	NCAA	Casts, braces, splints and prostheses may be worn by players as long as the equipment is well-padded to protect not only the affected player, but also her opponents. Any such device with exposed rivets, pins, sharp edges or any form of exterior fastener that would present a hazard, must be properly padded. Casts, braces, splints, and prostheses on a pitcher's nonpitching arm shall not be distracting as determined by the umpire. Pitchers may wear casts, braces, splints, or prostheses on their pitching arms, provided such devices do not cause safety risks or create unfair competitive advantages. In addition, any such device must be neutral in color so as not to be distracting and must function in such a way that it does not alter the natural motion of the pitching arm.
Track and field	NCAA	No taping of any part of the hand, thumb, or fingers will be permitted in the discus and javelin throws, and the shotput, except to cover or protect an open wound. In the hammer throw, taping of individual fingers is permissible. Any taping must be shown to the head event judge before the event starts. In the pole vault, the use of a forearm cover to prevent injuries is permissible.
	USA Track & Field	The following shall be considered assistance and are therefore not allowed in throwing events: • The taping of 2 or more fingers together. If taping is used on the hands and fingers, it may be continuous provided that as a result no 2 or more fingers are taped together in such a way that the fingers cannot move individually. The taping should be shown to the Chief Judge before the event starts.
Volleyball	NCAA	It is forbidden to wear any object that may cause an injury or give an artificial advantage to the player, including but not limited to unsafe casts or braces. Hard splints or other potentially dangerous protective devices worn on the arms or hands are prohibited, unless padded on all sides with slow-rebounding foam at least 1.25 cm ($\frac{1}{2}$-inch) thick. Padding or covering may be necessary for casts or braces on other parts of the body. A soft bandage to cover a wound or protect an injury on the arms or hands is permissible.
Wrestling	NCAA	Anything that does not allow normal movement of the joints and prevents one's opponent from applying normal holds shall be barred. Any protective device that is hard and abrasive must be covered properly and padded with high-density foam. Loose pads are prohibited.

Abbreviations: FIH, International Hockey Federation; MLB, Major League Baseball; NCAA, National Collegiate Athletic Association; NHL, National Hockey League; NLL, National Lacrosse League; WNBA, Women's National Basketball Association.

before the athlete may RTP. Minimally displaced waist fractures heal routinely and players can often RTP quickly, whereas proximal pole fractures and scaphoid nonunions may need to be followed closer and protected longer given the impaired healing potential that is related to the retrograde vascular supply of the scaphoid. The specific sport can also influence timing of RTP. Hockey players can return early (as early as 2 weeks after surgery) because they wear stiff, protective gloves and can often handle a stick while wearing a splint or cast.[44] Return to unprotected play in basketball is generally at 4 to 6 weeks postoperatively when the athlete has regained wrist range of motion, and there is evidence of osseous bridging on postoperative computed tomography scan.[42,44] RTP for football players with scaphoid fractures is somewhat more variable and depends heavily on the specific position and demands on the player. If the position allows, a player may resume protected play as early as 2 weeks postoperatively and resume unprotected play at 6 to 12 weeks depending on the individual circumstances.[43] A survey of professional team physicians reported that 51% allowed athletes to return to protected play 4 to 6 weeks after ORIF of a nondisplaced scaphoid fracture, and 32% allowed immediate return to protected play.[24] The same survey found that recommendations for return to unprotected play after ORIF of a nondisplaced scaphoid fracture were more variable with 24% recommending RTP at 4 to 6 weeks, 49% at 6 to 12 weeks, and 27% greater than 12 weeks.

Return to Play Rules

Each professional and elite athletic organization has its own rules regarding RTP and specific regulations regarding the types of protective equipment that may be worn during play. Knowledge of such regulations is helpful to the team physician when considering the multiple factors involved in RTP decisions. A summary of rules and regulations for RTP and protective equipment can be found in **Table 1**.

SUMMARY

RTP decisions often represent a challenge to physicians caring for athletes. The multifaceted and unique nature of each RTP decision makes standardization of the decision-making process impossible and demands of the physician thoughtful consideration of all competing interests and variables. Such difficult medical decisions are further complicated by unique ethical and legal considerations that often represent shades of gray rather than clear black or white. However, as the field of sports medicine continues to mature and grow, so does the collective experience of the medical community responsible for caring for athletes, which will continue to promote as safe and expeditious RTP for elite athletes as possible.

REFERENCES

1. Drakos MC, Domb B, Starkey C, et al. Injury in the National Basketball Association: a 17-year overview. Sports Health 2010;2(4):284–90.
2. Conte S, Camp CL, Dines JS. Injury trends in Major League Baseball over 18 seasons: 1998-2015. Am J Orthop 2016;45(3):116–23.
3. Lawrence DW, Hutchison MG, Comper P. Descriptive epidemiology of musculoskeletal injuries and concussions in the National Football League, 2012-2014. Orthop J Sports Med 2015;3(5). 2325967115583653.
4. Fuller CW. Managing the risk of injury in sport. Clin J Sport Med 2007;17(3):182–7.
5. Matheson GO, Shultz R, Bido J, et al. Return-to-play decisions: are they the team physician's responsibility? Clin J Sport Med 2011;21:25–30.
6. Creighton DW, Shrier I, Shultz R, et al. Return-to-play in sport: a decision-based model. Clin J Sport Med 2010;20:379–85.
7. The team physician and return-to-lay issues: a consensus statement. Med Sci Sports Exerc 2002;34:1212–4.
8. Dunn WR, George MS, Churchill L, et al. Ethics in sports medicine. Am J Sports Med 2007;35(5):840–4.
9. American Medical Association: Code of medical ethics. E-3.06 Sports Medicine. Issued June 1983, updated June 1994. Available at: http://www.ama-assn.org/ama/pub/physician-resources/medical-ethics/code-medical-ethics/opinion306.page. Accessed May 23, 2016.
10. American Medical Association: Code of medical ethics. E-5.05 Confidentiality. Issued June 1983, updated June 1994. Available at: http://www.ama-assn.org/ama/pub/physician-resources/medical-ethics/code-medical-ethics/opinion505.page. Accessed May 23, 2016.
11. American Academy of Orthopaedic Surgeons: Code of medical ethics and professionalism for orthopaedic surgeons. Adopted 1988, revised 2011. Available at: http://www.aaos.org/uploadedFiles/PreProduction/About/Opinion_Statements/ethics/Code%20of%20Ethics%202013%20color%20logo.pdf. Accessed May 23, 2016.
12. Bernstein J, Perlis C, Bartolozzi AR. Ethics in sports medicine. Clin Orthop Relat Res 2000;(378):50–60.
13. Tucker AM. Ethics and the professional team physician. Clin Sports Med 2004;23:227–41.
14. Magee JT, Almekinders LC, Taft TN. HIPAA and the team physician. Sports Med Update 2003;4–8.
15. Mitten MJ. Emerging legal issues in sports medicine: a synthesis, summary, and analysis. St Johns Law Rev 2002;76(1):5–86.
16. Jenkins S, Maese R. NFL medical standards, practices are different than almost anywhere else. Washington Post. 2013. Available at: https://www.washingtonpost.com/sports/redskins/nfl-medical-standards-practices-are-different-than-almost-anywhere-else/2013/03/16/b8c170bc-8be8-11e2-9f54-f3fdd70acad2_story.html. Accessed June 2, 2016.
17. Hike JB. An athlete's right to privacy regarding sport-related injuries: HIPAA and the creation of the mysterious injury. Ind Health L Rev 2009;6(47):48–76.
18. Graham TJ. Care of phalangeal fractures in the elite athlete's hand. In: Carlson MG, Goldfarb CA,

editors. The athlete's hand and wrist: a master skills publication. Chicago: ASSH; 2014. p. 95–105.

19. Gaston RG, Chadderdon C. Phalangeal fractures: displaced/nondisplaced. Hand Clin 2012;28:395–401.

20. Gaston RG. Football commentary: phalangeal fractures – displaced/nondisplaced. Hand Clin 2012; 28:407–8.

21. Shin SS. Phalangeal fractures in baseball: commentary. Hand Clin 2012;28:403.

22. Evans P. Sports specific commentary: phalangeal fractures in basketball. Hand Clin 2012;28:405.

23. Rossenwasser MP. Proximal interphalangeal joint fracture dislocations in professional baseball players. Hand Clin 2012;28:417–20.

24. Dy CJ, Khmelnitskaya E, Hearns KA, et al. Opinions regarding the management of hand and wrist injuries in elite athletes. Orthopedics 2013;36(6):815–9.

25. Clinkscales C. Sports-specific commentary on PIP joint fracture dislocations in professional basketball players. Hand Clin 2012;28:421–2.

26. Williams CS 4th. Football commentary: PIP fracture. Hand Clin 2012;28:423–4.

27. Fufa DT, Goldfarb CA. Fractures of the thumb and finger metacarpals in athletes. Hand Clin 2012;28: 379–88.

28. Goldfarb CA. Commentary metacarpal fracture in the professional baseball player. Hand Clin 2012; 28:389.

29. Singletary S, Freeland AE. Metacarpal fractures in athletes: treatment, rehabilitation, and safe early return to play. J Hand Ther 2003;16(2):171–9.

30. Rettig AC, Ryan R, Shelbourne KD, et al. Metacarpal fractures in the athletes. Am J Sports Med 1989;17: 567–72.

31. Johnson JW, Culp RW. Acute ulnar collateral ligament injury in the athlete. Hand Clin 2009;25(3):437–42.

32. Lee AT, Carlson MG. Thumb metacarpophalangeal joint collateral ligament injury management. Hand Clin 2012;28:361–70.

33. Werner BC, Hadeed MM, Lyons ML, et al. Return to football and long-term clinical outcomes after thumb ulnar collateral ligament suture anchor repair in collegiate athletes. J Hand Surg Am 2014;39(10):1992–8.

34. Lutsky K, Goldfarb CA. Thumb collateral ligament injuries in the athlete. In: Carlson MG, Goldfarb CA, editors. The athlete's hand and wrist: a master skills publication. Chicago: ASSH; 2014. p. 45–54.

35. Hove LM. Epidemiology of scaphoid fractures in Bergen, Norway. Scand J Plast Reconstr Surg 1999;33:423–6.

36. Singh HP, Taub N, Dias JJ. Management of displaced fractures of the waist of the scaphoid: meta-analyses of comparative studies. Injury 2012; 43(6):933–9.

37. Yin ZG, Zhang JB, Kan SL, et al. Treatment of acute scaphoid fractures: systematic review and meta-analysis. Clin Orthop Relat Res 2007;460:142–51.

38. Symes TH, Stothard J. A systematic review of the treatment of acute fractures of the scaphoid. J Hand Surg Eur Vol 2011;36(9):802–10.

39. Suh N, Benson EC, Faber KJ, et al. Treatment of acute scaphoid fractures: a systematic review and meta-analysis. Hand (N Y) 2010;5(4):345–53.

40. Ibrahim T, Qureshi A, Sutton AJ, et al. Surgical versus nonsurgical treatment of acute minimally displaced and undisplaced scaphoid waist fractures: pairwise and network meta-analyses of randomized controlled trials. J Hand Surg Am 2011;36(11): 1759–68.

41. Belsky MR. Commentary: scaphoid fracture in an elite or professional baseball player. Hand Clin 2012;28:279–80.

42. Carlson MG. Commentary on scaphoid fractures in basketball. Hand Clin 2012;28:281–2.

43. Gaston RG. Scaphoid fractures in professional football players. Hand Clin 2012;28:283–4.

44. Husband JB. Return to play after scaphoid fractures in hockey players. Hand Clin 2012;28(3):285.

Shoulder Injuries in the Overhead Throwing Athlete

Ryan A. Mlynarek, MD[a], Simon Lee, MD[a],
Asheesh Bedi, MD[b],*

KEYWORDS

- Shoulder anatomy • Shoulder abnormality • Kinetic chain • Throwing mechanics
- Glenohumeral internal rotation deficit • Microinstability • Labrum • Labral tear

KEY POINTS

- The glenohumeral joint provides greater range of motion than any other joint in the human body and is dependent on the complex interplay of static and dynamic stabilizers to maintain its congruence.
- Repetitive overhead throwing may cause adaptive and/or pathologic changes to the osseous, capsuloligamentous, and muscular structures about the shoulder.
- The overhead throwing mechanism involves the entire kinetic chain, requiring activation from the lower extremities through the core/trunk and culminating in power transfer to the upper extremity.
- Properly directed stretching, interval throwing programs, and sound mechanics may prevent shoulder injuries, but surgical intervention may be indicated in the elite thrower presenting with structural abnormality.

INTRODUCTION

Overhead throwing imposes the shoulder to extreme multidirectional forces and high-tensile loads. Injuries are most commonly described in baseball pitchers, but similar injuries may be observed in softball, tennis, football, and even javelin throwers.[1,2]

Repetitive throwing motion can cause adaptive bony, capsuloligamentous, and muscular changes to increase glenohumeral external rotation and thus limit glenohumeral internal rotation. Over time, these adaptive changes may lead to pathologic kinematics and glenohumeral internal rotation deficit (GIRD), internal impingement, rotator cuff tears, superior labrum anterior to posterior (SLAP) tears, and scapular dyskinesia.[3–8]

ANATOMY

The glenohumeral joint provides more freedom of motion than any other joint, with the sacrifice of decreased stability. The balance between stability and mobility in the shoulder is balanced with a complex network involving both static and dynamic elements. Bony elements in the joint include the humerus, glenoid, and scapula. Dynamic stabilizers include the functional muscular groups, whereas passive stabilizers include the glenoid labrum, articular cartilage, glenohumeral ligaments, and the shoulder joint capsule.

Labrum

The labrum is a triangular fibrocartilaginous structure encircling the glenoid rim and functions to

The authors have nothing to disclose.
[a] Department of Orthopaedic Surgery, University of Michigan, 2912 Taubman Center, Ann Arbor, MI 48109-5328, USA; [b] Department of Orthopaedic Surgery, Shoulder and Sports Medicine, University of Michigan, 24 Frank Lloyd Wright Drive, Lobby A, Suite 1000, Ann Arbor, MI 48106, USA
* Corresponding author.
E-mail address: abedi@med.umich.edu

Hand Clin 33 (2017) 19–34
http://dx.doi.org/10.1016/j.hcl.2016.08.014
0749-0712/17/© 2016 Elsevier Inc. All rights reserved.

increase the articulating surface area for the humeral head as well as deepening the glenoid socket to provide improved glenohumeral stability. This structural configuration helps maintain the negative intra-articular pressure environment of the joint and centers the humeral head on the glenoid. The labrum is therefore an important shoulder stabilizer and provides up to 10% of glenohumeral stability.[9–11] The superior labrum blends onto the proximal long head of the biceps tendon immediately distal to its insertion on the supraglenoid tubercle and is the commonly injured structure in overhead throwers.[12] A fibrocartilaginous transition zone bridges the labrum to the hyaline articular cartilage.[13] The capsular attachments of the labrum further contribute to shoulder stability. Vascular supply to the labrum consists of multiple vessels, including the posterior humeral circumflex, and the suprascapular and circumflex scapular arteries. However, vascular penetration of the labrum is limited to the periphery, predisposing the superior labrum to injury and impaired healing.[13]

Long Head of the Biceps Tendon

The long head of the biceps tendon primarily originates from superior glenoid tubercle, incorporating anteriorly and posteriorly into the superior labrum. The structure is located within the rotator interval and traverses inferiorly within the bicipital groove to the distal extremity. Because of its origin and function, the long head of the biceps tendon limits translation of the humeral head and contributes to anterior shoulder stability, reducing the overall stress placed on the inferior glenohumeral ligament during the late cocking phase of overhead throwing.[14]

Scapula

The scapula serves as a mobile connection between the thorax and the upper extremity, with the serratus anterior, trapezius, rhomboids, and levator scapulae providing scapulothoracic stabilization. The scapula is a critical structure for coordinated upper extremity movement and serves as an origin or insertion for 17 periscapular muscles. The acromioclavicular and coracoclavicular ligaments are the only other indirect attachments to the thorax, thus enabling the shoulder to have the most extensive range of motion of any joint in the body. The scapula is therefore a platform that provides both the power and the flexibility required for efficient throwing biomechanics.[15]

SHOULDER HISTORY AND PHYSICAL EXAMINATION

The history and physical examination are crucial in the initial evaluation of the symptomatic overhead throwing shoulder. Even though most athletes present with pain, an unexplained loss of throwing velocity and pitch control reported by the athlete hints at potential abnormality. Identification of the throwing phase that best reproduces symptoms is particularly helpful because various abnormalities present more frequently during different phases. It is important to delineate whether the symptoms are acute or insidious onset. Recent alterations in throwing mechanics should be explored because shoulder abnormality frequently occurs when athletes modify their throwing motion too rapidly. Evaluation of the athlete's preinjury level of competition as well as their career goals is appropriate at this point, because different treatment modalities may be more appropriate depending on each athlete's desired outcome.

Physical examination begins with direct observation of the undressed shoulder girdles, comparing the symptomatic shoulder to the contralateral side. Appropriate alignment of the glenohumeral, acromioclavicular joint, and scapulothoracic joint should be evaluated. Muscular hypertrophy may be noted in the dominant arm as a result of progressive adaptive changes. Active and passive shoulder range of motion should be performed. Overhead athletes often exhibit increased external rotation and concomitantly decreased internal rotation as a result of adaptive changes due to repetitive throwing. However, limited internal rotation may also reflect posterior capsule tightness secondary to abnormality. Palpation and visualization of the scapula are important to evaluate for abnormal or asymmetric motion concerning for scapula dyskinesia. Strength testing should be performed to the various functional muscle groupings. Shoulders that are painful with both active and passive motion are concerning for true shoulder stiffness, whereas restricted active motion and relatively pain-free passive motion may be the result of pain or weakness of muscular origin. Direct observation of the athlete's throwing motion for any obvious abnormalities should be performed if the patient's clinical condition allows. A thorough evaluation of the neurovascular status as well as a complete cervical spine examination should be performed. Multiple provocative tests exist for evaluation of the symptomatic shoulder and are discussed later in relation to each relevant condition.

A conventional shoulder radiograph series is the initial imaging of choice in the evaluation of a symptomatic shoulder. This radiograph series typically includes an anteroposterior view with the shoulder internally rotated, the Grashey view (an anteroposterior view with the shoulder externally rotated), the axillary view, and the scapular-Y view. If equivocal and the clinical picture warrants further evaluation, MRI is often the next study of choice. Specifically, MR arthrography with gadolinium is useful because of its higher sensitivity and specificity for partial rotator cuff tears and labral injury.[16,17] Ultrasound is a useful imaging modality, specifically to evaluate the rotator cuff, but its limited depth of penetration prohibits its use to evaluate for labral abnormality.[18,19] Imaging strategies specific to each shoulder abnormality are explored in more detail in the following sections.

THROWING MECHANICS

The overhead throwing athlete's objective is to generate the most speed, accuracy, and efficiency for each pitch thrown. In order to achieve this, pitchers use their entire body to coordinate a kinetic chain of motion to maximize the power released through the shoulder. The kinetic energy is transferred from the lower extremities to the trunk and finally to the upper extremity. Analysis of throwers' kinetic chain mechanics has become increasingly important to maximize power and efficiency as well as decrease the rate of injury. In fact, several authors[20–23] have shown that deficits within the proximal segments of the kinetic chain (legs, hips, core/trunk, and scapula) have been associated with 50% to 67% of athletes presenting with shoulder injuries. Knowledge about proper throwing mechanics and the kinematics of the pitching motion is paramount for a clinician to properly diagnose and treat throwing injuries of the shoulder. Although the baseball pitch provides the prototypical structure, the 6 classic phases described by Dillman and colleagues[24] can be extrapolated to similar throwing motions found in softball, football, tennis, and javelin throwers. A single pitching motion takes less than 2 seconds and is divided into 6 phases: wind-up, stride, late-cocking, acceleration, deceleration, and follow-through (**Fig. 1**).

Phase 1: Wind-up

This phase begins in the dual-leg stance and ends with the thrower in a balanced single-leg stance as the baseball is removed from the glove (see **Fig. 1**A). During this phase, the lower extremities prepare a stable base for energy transfer. It requires isometric contraction of hip abductors, hip flexors/extensors, and quadriceps to control pelvic tilt and knee flexion to maintain balance and control the thrower's center of gravity.[25] Although the risk of injury to the shoulder is low during this phase, weakness in the aforementioned muscle groups may lead to an unstable base of support and imbalance during the single-leg stance phase, which can lead to a "catch-up" phenomenon and associated injury to the distal throwing segments.[26] For example, Burkhart and colleagues[27] reported an association of decreased hip rotation flexibility and hip abduction strength in 49% of throwers with arthroscopic-proven posterior superior labral tears. Core weakness may lead to poor trunk control, allowing the thrower to prematurely lean toward the target during the single-leg stance phase. This alteration in mechanical form can alter the critical timing of the kinetic chain, thus increasing forces on the distal components, promoting further risk of injury to the throwing shoulder and elbow.

Phase 2: Stride (Early Cocking)

This phase begins at the peak knee height of the single-leg stance and ends when the lead throwing foot impacts the ground (see **Fig. 1**B). The stride phase is responsible for core and lower extremity positioning to optimize energy transfer to the upper extremity. In doing so, the thrower's center of gravity is lowered; and the hip of the single-stance leg internally rotates to uncoil and rotate the pelvis, thus facilitating the stride leg to extend toward the target. Proper rotation and trunk control are necessary to optimize stride length, stride angle, knee flexion angle, and rotational foot position, because all of these factors can impact subsequent shoulder throwing mechanics.[28–31] As the stride phase progresses, the upper extremity musculature begins to activate, as the serratus anterior and upper trapezius muscles position the scapula in protraction, forward tilt, and lateral rotation. This positioning maximizes the subacromial space and prevents outlet impingement, as the deltoid and supraspinatus initiate horizontal abduction and external rotation of the humerus relative to the glenoid.[15,32]

Phase 3: Late Cocking

The late cocking phase begins as the lead foot impacts the ground and ends with maximum external rotation of the glenohumeral joint (see **Fig. 1**C). The goal of this phase is to transfer the elastic stored energy from the lower extremities and core to the shoulder. As the stride foot lands, the pelvis and lower trunk rotate toward the target, the lumbar spine hyperextends, and the upper abdominal and oblique musculature stretch to maximize the potential energy of the shoulder.[28]

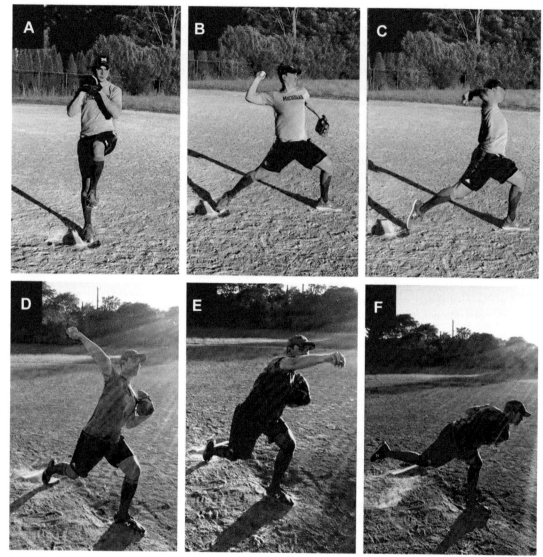

Fig. 1. The 6 phases of throwing: (*A*) wind-up, (*B*) stride (early-cocking), (*C*) late-cocking, (*D*) acceleration, (*E*) deceleration, (*F*) follow-through.

Simultaneously, the shoulder abducts to 90° and achieves maximal external rotation to 165° to 180°, and thus, is positioned to begin acceleration toward the target.

Phase 4: Acceleration

The acceleration phase begins with maximal glenohumeral external rotation and concludes with ball release (see **Fig. 1**D). This phase is initiated by concentric contraction of the triceps, pectoralis major, latissimus dorsi, and serratus anterior, as the humerus accelerates forward (horizontal adduction) and internally rotates approximately 80° before ball release. Dillman and colleagues[24] studied 29 elite pitchers and found that this motion

occurs in approximately 29 milliseconds, generating a mean maximum angular velocity of 6940°/s ± 1080°/s, making this one of the fastest human movements recorded in any physical skill.

Phase 5: Deceleration

The deceleration phase begins with ball release and ends with maximal shoulder internal rotation and 35° of horizontal adduction (see **Fig. 1**E). This phase causes the greatest amount of glenohumeral joint loading and potential for shear injury.[25] Large eccentric contraction forces are required to decelerate the throwing arm and limit the anterior humeral translation relative to the glenoid. This deceleration is accomplished by contraction of the posterior deltoid, the rotator cuff (primarily infraspinatus and teres minor), the anterior labrum, and the posterior capsule. The periscapular musculature also contributes to decelerate the shoulder and return the scapula to an anteriorly tilted position.

Phase 6: Follow-Through

During the final throwing phase, the thrower's body weight is transferred to the planted stride leg (see **Fig. 1**F). The stride leg absorbs the thrower's momentum and body weight as the trunk decelerates and moves into a flexed position over the planted leg for stability. The throwing arm continues to adduct to approximately 60°, the trail leg knee and hip flex to clear the mound, and the phase ends with the pitcher in the fielding position.

MICROINSTABILITY, INTERNAL IMPINGEMENT, AND GLENOHUMERAL INTERNAL ROTATION DEFICIT

In the late-cocking and early acceleration phase of throwing, the overhead athlete's shoulder exhibits maximal abduction and external rotation. In this position, there is normal physiologic contact between the posterosuperior glenoid and the greater tuberosity. With repetitive throwing motions, the shoulder can undergo adaptive changes to bony, capsuloligamentous, and muscular structures for increased glenohumeral external rotation.[33,34] Thus, Walch and colleagues[8] first proposed that with increased external rotation and repetitive loading, the physiologic contact between the posterosuperior glenoid rim and the greater tuberosity may cause pathologic internal impingement of the posterosuperior labrum and rotator cuff. Burkhart and colleagues[35] proposed that posterior capsular contracture caused a relative posterosuperior shift in the humeral center of rotation, thus leading to posterosuperior microinstability. Jobe and colleagues[36] further theorized that anterior capsuloligamentous laxity is a contributing factor to the development of internal impingement. Currently, differing opinions exist regarding the implications of anterior capsular laxity being a contributing factor in the development of this condition, but regardless, it is clear that glenohumeral microinstability secondary to adaptive changes in static and dynamic stabilizers of the glenohumeral joint induces supraphysiologic posterosuperior microinstability of the glenohumeral joint, which may result in pathologic internal impingement.

Symptomatic throwing athletes presenting with microinstability and internal impingement often report pain in the late-cocking position located in the posterior aspect of the shoulder as well as subjective feelings of subluxation in repetitive positioning of abduction and external rotation.[37] A thorough throwing history and shoulder physical examination should be performed, with special consideration to any limits in range of motion (ie, internal rotation seen in GIRD), posterior glenohumeral joint line pain, and instability provocation (apprehension-relocation testing). Meister and colleagues[38] also describes the "posterior impingement sign," which is performed with the examiner palpating the posterior glenohumeral joint line with the thrower's shoulder in the late-cocking position (90°–110° of abduction, slight extension, and maximal external rotation). Reproduction of pain is indicative of a positive test, which demonstrates an overall sensitivity of 75% and specificity of 85% to identify partial-thickness rotator cuff tears and/or posterior labral injuries.[39] Secondary to aforementioned adaptive changes, throwing shoulders will often exhibit increased external rotation and decreased internal rotation compared with the contralateral shoulder. However, Ruotolo and colleagues[40] reported an average 10° decrease in total arc of motion of symptomatic throwing shoulders compared with asymptomatic throwing shoulders. Internal rotation deficit is most common in throwers, and when there is greater than 18° loss of internal rotation compared with the contralateral shoulder, this is consistent with GIRD and may lead to altered shoulder mechanics, thus increased stress on the dynamic stabilizers (labrum, biceps tendon, and rotator cuff).[23,41]

Radiographic evaluation of the shoulder begins with plain radiographs, which can identify mineralization of the inferior glenohumeral ligament (Bennett lesion), cystic changes of the posterosuperior humeral head, sclerosis of the greater tuberosity, and/or erosions of the posterosuperior glenoid rim.[42–45] MRI is considered the diagnostic standard for throwers with persistent posterior shoulder pain. Abnormal findings most commonly demonstrate thickened inferior glenohumeral ligaments, partial-thickness articular-sided rotator cuff tears, and/or posterosuperior labral tears.[46–48]

The most efficacious approach to prevent posterior capsular contracture, internal impingement, and asymmetric range of motion deficits is by means of structured stretching programs, dynamic stabilizer strengthening, and neuromuscular stimulation.[49–52] Aldridge and colleagues[53] implemented a 12-week posterior capsule stretching program for asymptomatic National Collegiate Athletic Association Division 1 pitchers and found a significant increase in internal rotation and total arc of motion after completion of the program. However, there are no studies to date comparing a stretching program to control group to evaluate effectiveness in prevention of posterior capsular contracture, internal impingement, or GIRD. When throwers present with symptoms of GIRD and internal impingement, nonoperative management begins with rest, ice, anti-inflammatory medications, and physical therapy targeted at posterior capsular stretching and strengthening of the rotator cuff periscapular musculature. When symptoms improve, throwers are to follow an interval throwing program before return to play. Tyler and colleagues[54] studied 22 athletes with internal impingement undergoing a stretching and mobilization protocol of the posterior shoulder and found a statistically significant improvement in internal rotation deficit, SST outcome, and pain scores.

Operative intervention is reserved for those athletes with refractory symptoms despite adequate nonoperative treatment for 4 to 6 months. The patient's examination and imaging will guide treatment options, which often include arthroscopic posterior labral debridement versus repair (**Fig. 2**), anterior capsular plication, and/or posteroinferior capsular release. Payne and Altchek[55] colleagues demonstrated a 25% return to play and 37% satisfaction rate in athletes with anterior microinstability and internal impingement who underwent arthroscopic labral or partial rotator cuff tear debridement alone. Sonnery-Cottet and colleagues[56] reported similar outcomes with 50% return to sport with 91% of the treated athletes reporting persistent shoulder pain. Poor outcomes associated with this approach are thought to be secondary to the anterior capsular laxity and microinstability.[57,58] Chambers and Altchek[37] and Jones and colleagues,[59] among others, now prefer anterior capsule-to-labrum plication and report 90% return to sport at a mean follow-up of 3.6 years, with an average Kerlan-Jobe

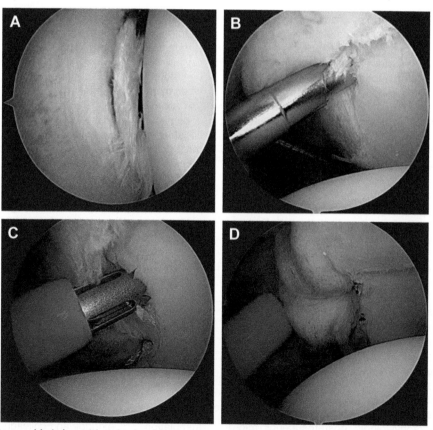

Fig. 2. A 16-year-old pitcher with right shoulder recurrent posterior instability underwent arthroscopic posteroinferior labral repair. (*A*) Posterior labral tear is identified, extending from 7 o'clock to 11 o'clock. (*B*) The posterior glenoid margin was freshened with a motorized shaver to healthy bleeding cancellous bone and the posterior labral tear was fully mobilized. (*C*) Using the pinch-tuck technique, the posterior band of the inferior glenohumeral ligament and labrum is captured to re-tension the posterior band and posterior capsule. (*D*) Suture anchors are placed at the 7:00 o'clock, 9:00 o'clock, and 10:30 o'clock to complete restoration of the posterior labral bumper.

Orthopaedic Clinic score of 82 without appreciable loss in external rotation. Burkhart and colleagues[35,60,61] advocate for posteroinferior capsular release to address the posterior capsular contracture, and Codding and colleagues[62] reported 6 overhead athletes with internal impingement who underwent this procedure alone, and 7 athletes in combination with anterior capsular plication. Limited by lack of control group and small sample size, no difference was noted between the groups, but they reported an overall 77% return to play, suggesting that this procedure may have a role in a select population with predominantly posterior capsular contracture.[62] Concomitant abnormalities may be addressed at the same time, but rarely indicated (Bennett lesions, osteochondral lesions of humeral head or glenoid, and glenoid retroversion).[63–66]

ROTATOR CUFF TEARS

Rotator cuff tears can be categorized as full or partial thickness, and the latter can be further classified as bursal, articular, or intrasubstance partial-thickness tears. Partial-thickness tears are significantly more common in overhead athletes than full-thickness tears.[67,68] Three mechanisms of rotator cuff tear development have been proposed in overhead throwing athletes: tensile overload, primary extrinsic impingement, and the aforementioned internal impingement.[8,69,70] During the deceleration phase, the rotator cuff must impart well-coordinated eccentric contraction to maintain glenohumeral compression, thus exposing the rotator cuff to extreme tensile and shear forces during this phase. Repetitive throwing can cause changes in vascularity patterns within the tendon fibers, thus weakening the tendon structure and facilitating attritional wear.[70] The most common location for this to occur is in the posterior half of the supraspinatus and anterior half of the infraspinatus.

Although less common than attritional tensile overload, extrinsic impingement can occur as the throwing shoulder is exposed to supraphysiologic ranges of motion during throwing. Subacromial impingement may occur in the overhead athlete, but this is less common than impingement secondary to the coracoacromial ligament or against the coracoacromial arch secondary to scapular dyskinesis.[71,72] This impingement may lead primarily to bursal-sided tearing of the rotator cuff. Rotator cuff tears in the throwing athlete are most commonly caused by internal impingement. As the cascade of posterior capsule contracture occurs, the center of rotation of the glenohumeral joint shifts relatively posterosuperiorly, resulting in increased shear force on the adjacent rotator cuff tendon with repetitive throwing, leading primarily to articular-sided tears of the posterior supraspinatus and anterior half of the infraspinatus.

Diagnosis of rotator cuff tears begins with a thorough history and physical examination of the shoulder. Special attention must be given to rotator cuff strength testing, provocative stability and impingement testing, and scapular and shoulder range of motion. Complete evaluation includes diagnostic imaging, which should include plain radiographs. Ultrasonography has been shown repeatedly to be an effective tool in diagnosing partial- and full-thickness rotator cuff tears. Although operator dependence is often cited as being a potential drawback, its utility in dynamic assessment is useful. Wiener and Seitz[73] reported sensitivity of 94% and specificity of 93% when diagnosing partial-thickness rotator cuff tears. Magnetic resonance remains the standard imaging modality to evaluate athletes for suspected rotator cuff abnormality. Intra-articular contrast may be used to increase the sensitivity and specificity when detecting partial-thickness tears, which Meister and colleagues[74] reported as 84% and 96%, respectively.

Nonoperative treatment begins with rest, ice, anti-inflammatory medication, and evaluation of the thrower's throwing mechanics. Dedicated physical therapy is targeted to a stretching program if associated with internal impingement and/or strengthening of the rotator cuff and periscapular musculature. Like any patient, these modalities should be maximized before considering operative intervention, but especially in a throwing athlete. A thorough understanding of the athlete's timing within the season as well as career goals and expectations is necessary when contemplating surgical intervention.

Full-thickness tears of the rotator cuff in the overhead athlete are treated much like the nonathletic population. The goal is to restore the anatomic footprint and optimize the healing environment. The authors' preferred technique is to perform a linked and self-reinforcing, transosseous-equivalent double-row repair, because this has been shown to decrease the amount of gap formation and thus improve the biomechanical strength of the repair and allow for accelerated rehabilitation to prevent stiffness.[75,76]

Surgical approach to partial-thickness tears is dependent on the tear character, depth, and location. In the general population, if a tear is less than 50%, it is debrided; if it is 50% or greater, it is repaired. Historically, this approach was extrapolated to throwing athletes as well; however, more recent data suggested that the overhead throwing population must repeatedly endure greater tensile forces in exaggerated positions; thus, the authors advocate repair of partial-thickness tears greater than 25% in this population.[77] Some investigators choose to complete a partial-thickness tear and then proceed with repair; however, the authors' preference is to use the transtendon repair technique to avoid length-tension mismatch of the repaired tendon, as described by Lo and colleagues.[78] For partial-thickness tears with significant intratendinous delamination, the authors prefer an intratendinous repair technique described by Conway and Brockmeier colleagues.[79,80]

There is a paucity of literature reporting outcomes of arthroscopic repair of full-thickness rotator cuff tears in the overhead athlete secondary to its rarity. Dines and colleagues[81] evaluated 6 professional pitchers who underwent full-thickness rotator cuff repair using the lateralized footprint technique.[81] They reported 5/6 (86%) of the pitchers had returned to their preinjury level of competition for at least one full season. Payne and colleagues[82] evaluated 29 overhead throwing athletes who underwent arthroscopic debridement and subacromial decompression for treatment of partial-thickness rotator cuff tears. They reported 66% of patients with satisfactory results and 45% return to preinjury level of competition. Conway[79] evaluated 14 overhead athletes with partial-thickness, articular-sided intrasubstance delamination. Using the intratendinous repair technique, 8/9 (89%) patients available for follow-up were able to return to play at the same level postoperatively.

SUPERIOR LABRUM ANTERIOR-POSTERIOR LESIONS

Labral injuries are common in overhead athletes, and disruption of the superior labrum and biceps anchor may be particularly debilitating. Injuries of the anterosuperior labrum in proximity to the origin of the long head of the biceps tendon was first described by Andrews and colleagues[83] in 1985, but the term SLAP lesion and its subsequent 4-type classification system was not introduced until 1990 by Snyder and colleagues.[84] Type I lesions are characterized by localized tissue degeneration and fraying at the free edge of the superior labrum with a stable biceps anchor. Type II lesions are the most common subtype, accounting for 55% of SLAP injuries in a series of 140 cases by Snyder and colleagues[85] and represents a frequent cause of shoulder pain in overhead athletes. The type II lesion is characterized by the detachment of both the superior labrum and the biceps anchor

from the supraglenoid tubercle, often with significant displacement of the biceps-superior labrum complex. Type II lesions are further divided into 3 subtypes based on the extension of the injury, with IIA being anterior, IIB being posterior, and IIC being anterior and posterior. Significant glenohumeral instability may result from IIB and IIC lesions, causing disabling dysfunction for overhead athletes. Type III lesions are characterized by the presence of a bucket handle injury with an intact biceps tendon anchor. Type IV lesions also involve bucket handle abnormality in addition to injury extending to the biceps tendon anchor. The original 4-type classification system of SLAP lesions by Snyder and colleagues[86] has since been expanded to 10 types by various investigators.[87]

There are several proposed pathophysiologic processes attributed to the SLAP lesion with significant controversy among surgeons in the literature. Overhead athletes repetitively stress the shoulder at extremes of motion, particularly in the late-cocking phase.[87] Some clinicians argue that this position predisposes the labrum to be physiologically impinged between the glenoid and humeral head, causing a type of internal impingement.[69] Biomechanical and arthroscopic evaluations support that these supraphysiologic motions may cause SLAP tears, caused by the compressive and shear forces at the glenohumeral joint and the strain at the capsulolabral junction.[7,35,88,89] Andrews and colleagues[83] proposed that a deceleration traction force from the pull of the biceps tendon during the follow-through phase of overhead throwing may result in injury to the superior labrum.[90] Burkhart and colleagues[35] alternatively suggested that posterior capsule contracture may be a primary instigator to labral injuries due to the subsequent posterosuperior migration of the humeral head in the joint. Burkhart and Morgan[89] also suggested a "peel-back" mechanism of injury in which increased strain at the biceps anchor during the late-cocking phase at maximum external rotation leads to excessive tension and eventual injury at the superior labrum.[89] Kuhn and colleagues[91] demonstrated that the long head of the biceps tendon functions as an important dynamic restraint to shoulder external rotation, supporting the "peel-back" theory.

The diagnosis of SLAP lesions can be difficult, despite advances in imaging technique as well as recognition of the high incidence in overhead athletes. It is important to realize that SLAP lesions frequently present with concomitant shoulder injuries, as Kim and colleagues[92] has demonstrated that 88% of SLAP injuries in a series of 193 patients had evidence of other intra-articular abnormalities. Pain is usually localized at the posterior superior glenohumeral joint line and is exacerbated by throwing motions, frequently experienced during the late-cocking phase.[93] Gradual functional limitations in overhead activities usually develop with subsequent decrease in throwing velocity.[94,95] The patient may experience varying degrees of mechanical symptoms, including catching, locking, snapping, or shoulder instability, depending on the type and size of the lesion. Patients may also experience the so-called vague dead arm sensation often reported by baseball pitchers with chronic cases.[27]

Provocative examination of the superior labrum is most commonly conducted with the O'Brien's active compression test.[96] The athlete's shoulder is positioned in 90° of forward flexion, 20° of horizontal abduction, and maximum internal rotation. The examiner applies a downward force, asking the athlete to resist. The extremity is then externally rotated with the palm facing upward and the maneuver is repeated. Reproduction of pain during internal rotation with decreased pain during external rotation represents a positive test. The maneuver is based pon re-creating the impingement of the anterosuperior labrum between the humeral head and the glenoid. A meta-analysis by Meserve and colleagues[97] showed that a positive O'Brien's active compression test was most predictive test for SLAP injury. Other commonly used examination maneuvers include the Biceps Load II test, Dynamic Labral Shear test (O'Driscoll's test), Speed's test, and Labral Tension test.[96,98] However, Cook and colleagues[99] have shown that these tests individually and in combination demonstrated poor utility in the diagnosis of SLAP lesions, necessitating radiographic workup.

Radiographic evaluation should begin with the standard conventional radiograph shoulder series. Although radiographs do not directly visualize labral integrity, it is useful to evaluate for other potential or coexisting shoulder abnormality. The use of coronal oblique sequenced magnetic resonance arthrography is therefore paramount and stands as the standard for diagnosis of SLAP tears.[100–102]

Overhead athletes with SLAP lesions are typically managed with an initial trial of nonoperative treatment, which includes rehabilitation, posterior capsular stretching, rest, ice, and anti-inflammatory medications. Strength training exercises are only initiated following the resolution of pain. The goals of rehabilitation are to restore glenohumeral and scapular thoracic motion as well as regain strength and endurance. Neuromuscular control, proprioception, and stability must also be emphasized. In a series of athletes with SLAP injuries managed nonoperatively, Edwards and colleagues[103] demonstrated that patients achieved improved pain relief, functional outcomes, and quality of life. However, only 66% returned to sport at a similar or higher level of play, and 51% eventually elected to pursue operative intervention.

SLAP type I lesions are degenerative in nature and are uncommon in overhead athletes. These injuries do not result in instability of the superior labrum or the biceps anchor and are therefore amenable to arthroscopic debridement of the damaged tissue. SLAP type II, III, and IV lesions typically require surgical intervention. Several operative strategies have been described for refixation of the labrum, including transosseous sutures, staples, screws, arthroscopic sutures, and bioabsorbable tacks. Type II lesions in younger athletes should be repaired with proper refixation of the labrum for adequate healing (**Fig. 3**). Recent studies have supported the growing trend of using biceps tenodesis for older throwing athletes as an alternative to labral refixation for improved outcomes. In a comparative study examining older patients undergoing SLAP repair (mean age of 37 years) and biceps tenodesis (mean age 52 years), Boileau and colleagues[104] found that the tenodesis group achieved superior activity subscores, return to play (86% vs 20%), and satisfaction scores (93% vs 40%) compared with the SLAP repair group. The investigators concluded that arthroscopic biceps tenodesis may be an effective alternative to SLAP repair in an older patient population. The bucket handle portion of an SLAP type III lesion is frequently excised while the remainder of the labrum is evaluated for stability, particularly if there is involvement of the middle glenohumeral ligament. For type IV lesions, the extent of biceps anchor involvement as well as patient demographics guides management decisions. Isolated arthroscopic debridement of the labrum and biceps anchor is recommended when less than 30% of the biceps anchor is involved in the injury, whereas labral repair with biceps tenodesis has been recommended for young active patients with greater than 30% of biceps anchor involvement.[105]

Initial reports found that up to 87% of athletes with repair of a type II SLAP lesion return to play.[87,106] Better fixation techniques and advances in the understanding of the role of the labrum in throwing biomechanics have led to continually improved outcomes. Ide and colleagues[107] reported 90% good to excellent results and 75% return to preinjury level of play in a cohort of 40 overhead athletes undergoing SLAP repair. In a review of 30 overhead athletes undergoing

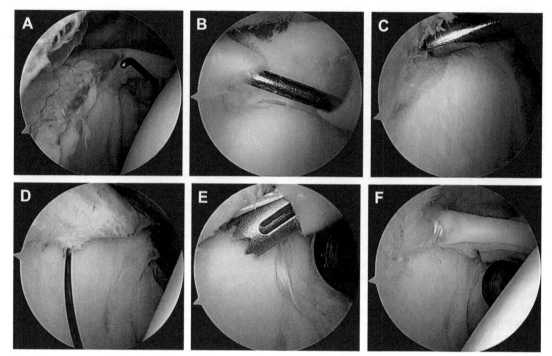

Fig. 3. A 22-year-old pitcher with refractory shoulder pain and loss of velocity and control underwent arthroscopic SLAP repair. (*A, B*) An unstable type II SLAP tear is identified with exposed bone just posterior to the biceps anchor, extending to the 10 o'clock position. (*C*) A motorized shaver is used to freshen the glenoid to healthy bleeding cancellous bone. (*D*) A 45° passer was used to perform pinch-tuck technique to capture the superior labral complex, taking care to stay well posterior to the biceps anchor to avoid incarceration. (*E, F*) Knotless suture anchors (2.9-mm) were placed to mitigate likelihood of knot irritation, achieving an anatomic reduction and repair of the superior labrum to the glenoid.

type II SLAP repair, Neuman and colleagues[108] also reported a high overall satisfaction rate of 93% and improved functional outcomes scores, but concluded that outcomes are less reliable in throwers as they returned to approximately 84.1% of their pre-injury level of function. These results were mirrored in a systematic review by Sayde and colleagues,[109] which showed that 83% of those patients who underwent type II SLAP repair exhibited "good to excellent" patient satisfaction, and 63% returned to their previous level of play.

SCAPULAR MALPOSITION, INFERIOR MEDIAL BORDER PROMINENCE, CORACOID PAIN AND MALPOSITION, AND DYSKINESIA OF SCAPULAR MOVEMENT SCAPULA/SCAPULA DYSKINESIA

Scapular dyskinesia is becoming a more commonly recognized cause for shoulder pain and dysfunction, particularly in overhead athletes. This abnormality is present in as many as 67% to 100% of athletes with shoulder injuries, and a systematic review by Burn and colleagues[110,111]

found that scapular dyskinesia had a greater reported prevalence in overhead athletes (61%) compared with non-overhead athletes (33%). Priest and Nagel[112] were the first to describe this abnormality and originally coined it "tennis shoulder" in 1976. Burkhart and colleagues[60] subsequently described the SICK scapula (scapular malposition, inferior medial border prominence, coracoid pain and malposition, and dyskinesia of scapular movement) syndrome, which incorporates several positional and muscular abnormalities in symptomatic shoulder motion. The altered kinematics has 3 recognizable patterns of dyskinesia with type 1: inferior medial scapular border prominence; type 2: medial scapular border prominence, more commonly associated with labral abnormality; and type 3: prominence of the superomedial border of the scapula, more commonly associated with rotator cuff abnormality.[60] It is currently unclear whether SICK scapula/scapular dyskinesia is a primary disorder or secondary to preexisting abnormality altering shoulder biomechanics and leading to scapular malfunction. Previous studies have shown that shoulder pain may result in functional tightening of the upper trapezius and pectoralis minor as well as inhibition of the lower trapezius and serratus anterior.[113–115]

In overhead athletes, these biomechanical alterations may lead to scapular impingement onto the thorax during the late-cocking phase of throwing.[116–118] Overuse, fatigue, direct trauma, or nerve injury may result in asynchrony of the periscapular muscles and lead to significant dysfunction. The scapula acts as a critical link in the kinetic chain between the energy-producing lower extremities/trunk and the throwing arm. Therefore, scapular destabilization disrupts efficient energy transfer, leads to dysfunctional throwing mechanics, and results in elevated stress at the glenohumeral and scapulothoracic joints.[119] In order for overhead athletes to achieve the extremes of motion required for high release velocities, coordinated function of the serratus anterior, trapezius, and rhomboid muscles is required for optimal scapular motion. Counterclockwise rotation of the scapula in the sagittal plane must occur for the acromion to elevate and avoid impingement. Scapular retraction is also necessary to maintain the humeral head centered onto the glenoid fossa. Failure of these motions may lead to humeral hyperangulation relative to the glenoid during throwing, thus resulting in increased strain at the anterior aspect of the shoulder capsule. Progressive damage to the anterior shoulder structures may lead to increasing instability and impingement.[120,121] In addition, athletes often overcompensate for the loss of velocity due to scapular dyskinesia with increased force placed by the shoulder musculature, thus creating elevated strain at the glenohumeral articulation.[122]

Symptomatic scapular dyskinesia may present with any combination of nonspecific anterior or superior shoulder pain, posterosuperior scapular pain, or proximal lateral arm pain. Athletes with anterior shoulder complaints and an SICK scapula are commonly found to have marked coracoid tenderness, because the coracoid tilts inferiorly due to tightening of the pectoralis minor, distracting the bone laterally and causing pain. The surgeon should observe the athlete's exposed upper back and shoulders from behind, noting any asymmetry of the scapulae. The inferior medial scapular border appears prominent, whereas the superior medial border and acromion are more subtle in appearance. However, it is important to note that muscular hypertrophy and chronic adaptive changes in the overhead athlete may result in mild scapular asymmetry that should not be mistaken for dyskinesia. A 4 part classification system for scapular dyskinesia by Kibler and colleagues[123] is available, but has exhibited only moderate reliability in symptomatic patients and low reliability in healthy patients.[124] The athlete may perform a wall pushup, active forward flexion, or abduction to elicit any asymmetrical motion of the scapula. Serratus anterior weakness may be evaluated with the athlete's arms initially at their sides and then performing resisted forward flexion. The stability of the sternal clavicular and acromial clavicular joints should be assessed. Efforts to distinguish true scapular muscular dysfunction from secondary dysfunction due to pain must be made. If scapular dyskinesia is present, improvement in active range of motion with assisted protraction and posterior tilt of the scapula may be diagnostic of true muscular dysfunction.[125]

Because there is a high prevalence of scapular dyskinesia in overhead athletes, clinicians should be vigilant in recognizing the "shoulder at risk" in this population. Scapular dyskinesia is a prodromal condition that begins with glenohumeral internal rotation tightness as well as a degree of scapular dyskinesia. Athletes often describe the inability to "get loose." Continued competitive overhead play results in worsening stiffness due to progressive posterosuperior capsular tightening. Progression of this contracture increases the risk of other intra-articular distraction type injuries. Athletes with "shoulders at risk" in the setting of SICK scapula and GIRD have a particularly high predisposition for intra-articular damage as they lead the thrower to overly abduct in extension and hyperangulate in external rotation during the late-cocking phase of throwing. Early recognition and management of this condition involve shoulder internal rotation stretching as well as periscapular musculature strengthening with the goal of mitigating the risk of glenohumeral internal derangement and potential subsequent injuries to superior labrum and rotator cuff tendons.

Conservative management focusing on perimuscular rehabilitation is typically first line for the treatment of SICK scapula/scapular dyskinesia regardless of the degree of scapular malposition or presenting symptoms. However, any coabnormality amenable to surgical management should be treated before scapular rehabilitation in order to minimize any anatomic or physiologic limitations to normal scapular function. Although most scapular dysfunction may be successfully managed with rehabilitation programs, conditions such as scapular bursitis or snapping scapula may indicate surgical intervention. Excision of the offending tissues at the inferior margin of the scapula has demonstrated excellent outcomes with the appropriate patient population.[117,118,126] Athletes demonstrating scapular dyskinesia often do poorly in rehabilitation programs because of the relatively small emphasis placed on scapular stabilization; therefore, specific guidance for rehabilitation may be crucial for success.

The rehabilitation program should initially focus on acquiring flexibility and mobility, particularly with stretching exercises for pectoralis minor tightness anteriorly and posteriorly inferior capsular tightness with GIRDs. Once adequate range of motion and flexibility is achieved, focus is turned to core and periscapular muscular strengthening to optimize scapular control and subsequently kinetic chain energy transfer. Initially, closed-chain exercises improve overall scapular control, followed by open-chain exercises with progressive weights for strengthening. In addition to strengthening, emphasis must be placed on scapular neuromuscular control and proprioception for optimal outcomes.

SUMMARY

The overhead athlete subjects their shoulder to a tremendous amount of stress during the act of throwing. The shoulder is an inherently unstable joint that relies on many static and dynamic stabilizers to function. Repetitive throwing stresses these stabilizers to the maximum to allow the overhead athlete to throw with optimal velocity and control. Thus, injuries of the throwing shoulder in the overhead athlete are common and can be challenging to treat.

REFERENCES

1. Dines JS, Bedi A, Williams PN, et al. Tennis injuries: epidemiology, pathophysiology, and treatment. J Am Acad Orthop Surg 2015;23(3):181–9.
2. Schmitt H, Hansmann HJ, Brocai DR, et al. Long term changes of the throwing arm of former elite javelin throwers. Int J Sports Med 2001;22(4):275–9.
3. Ryu RK, Dunbar WH, Kuhn JE, et al. Comprehensive evaluation and treatment of the shoulder in the throwing athlete. Arthroscopy 2002;18(9 Suppl 2):70–89.
4. Dines JS, Frank JB, Akerman M, et al. Glenohumeral internal rotation deficits in baseball players with ulnar collateral ligament insufficiency. Am J Sports Med 2009;37(3):566–70.
5. Grossman MG, Tibone JE, McGarry MH, et al. A cadaveric model of the throwing shoulder: a possible etiology of superior labrum anterior-to-posterior lesions. J Bone Joint Surg Am 2005;87(4):824–31.
6. Wilk KE, Macrina LC, Fleisig GS, et al. Correlation of glenohumeral internal rotation deficit and total rotational motion to shoulder injuries in professional baseball pitchers. Am J Sports Med 2011;39(2):329–35.
7. Kuhn JE, Lindholm SR, Huston LJ, et al. Failure of the biceps superior labral complex: a cadaveric biomechanical investigation comparing the late cocking and early deceleration positions of throwing. Arthroscopy 2003;19(4):373–9.
8. Walch G, Boileau P, Noel E, et al. Impingement of the deep surface of the supraspinatus tendon on the posterosuperior glenoid rim: an arthroscopic study. J Shoulder Elbow Surg 1992;1(5):238–45.
9. Habermeyer P, Schuller U, Wiedemann E. The intra-articular pressure of the shoulder: an experimental study on the role of the glenoid labrum in stabilizing the joint. Arthroscopy 1992;8(2):166–72.
10. Fehringer EV, Schmidt GR, Boorman RS, et al. The anteroinferior labrum helps center the humeral head on the glenoid. J Shoulder Elbow Surg 2003;12(1):53–8.
11. Halder AM, Kuhl SG, Zobitz ME, et al. Effects of the glenoid labrum and glenohumeral abduction on stability of the shoulder joint through concavity-compression: an in vitro study. J Bone Joint Surg Am 2001;83-A(7):1062–9.
12. Vangsness CT Jr, Jorgenson SS, Watson T, et al. The origin of the long head of the biceps from the scapula and glenoid labrum. An anatomical study of 100 shoulders. J Bone Joint Surg Br 1994;76(6):951–4.
13. Sidana A, Sarkar S, Balasundaram S, et al. Increased sensitivity to atypical antipsychotics in a patient with Dandy-Walker variant with schizophrenia. J Neuropsychiatry Clin Neurosci 2013;25(3):E31–2.
14. Rodosky MW, Harner CD, Fu FH. The role of the long head of the biceps muscle and superior glenoid labrum in anterior stability of the shoulder. Am J Sports Med 1994;22(1):121–30.
15. Meyer KE, Saether EE, Soiney EK, et al. Three-dimensional scapular kinematics during the throwing motion. J Appl Biomech 2008;24(1):24–34.
16. Flannigan B, Kursunoglu-Brahme S, Snyder S, et al. MR arthrography of the shoulder: comparison with conventional MR imaging. AJR Am J Roentgenol 1990;155(4):829–32.
17. Magee T, Williams D, Mani N. Shoulder MR arthrography: which patient group benefits most? AJR Am J Roentgenol 2004;183(4):969–74.
18. Teefey SA, Rubin DA, Middleton WD, et al. Detection and quantification of rotator cuff tears. Comparison of ultrasonographic, magnetic resonance imaging, and arthroscopic findings in seventy-one consecutive cases. J Bone Joint Surg Am 2004;86-A(4):708–16.
19. Taljanovic MS, Carlson KL, Kuhn JE, et al. Sonography of the glenoid labrum: a cadaveric study with

19. arthroscopic correlation. AJR Am J Roentgenol 2000;174(6):1717–22.

20. Vad VB, Bhat AL, Basrai D, et al. Low back pain in professional golfers: the role of associated hip and low back range-of-motion deficits. Am J Sports Med 2004;32(2):494–7.

21. Young JL, Herring SA, Press JM, et al. The influence of the spine on the shoulder in the throwing athlete. J Back Musculoskeletal Rehabil 1996; 7(1):5–17.

22. Kibler WB, Press J, Sciascia A. The role of core stability in athletic function. Sports Med 2006;36(3): 189–98.

23. Myers JB, Laudner KG, Pasquale MR, et al. Glenohumeral range of motion deficits and posterior shoulder tightness in throwers with pathologic internal impingement. Am J Sports Med 2006;34(3): 385–91.

24. Dillman CJ, Fleisig GS, Andrews JR. Biomechanics of pitching with emphasis upon shoulder kinematics. J Orthop Sports Phys Ther 1993;18(2): 402–8.

25. Seroyer ST, Nho SJ, Bach BR Jr, et al. Shoulder pain in the overhead throwing athlete. Sports Health 2009;1(2):108–20.

26. Eckenrode BJ, Kelley MJ, Kelly JD 4th. Anatomic and biomechanical fundamentals of the thrower shoulder. Sports Med Arthrosc 2012;20(1): 2–10.

27. Burkhart SS, Morgan CD, Kibler WB. Shoulder injuries in overhead athletes. The "dead arm" revisited. Clin Sports Med 2000;19(1):125–58.

28. Fleisig GS, Barrentine SW, Escamilla RF, et al. Biomechanics of overhand throwing with implications for injuries. Sports Med 1996;21(6):421–37.

29. Calabrese GJ. Pitching mechanics, revisited. Int J Sports Phys Ther 2013;8(5):652–60.

30. Ramsey DK, Crotin RL. Effect of stride length on overarm throwing delivery: Part II: An angular momentum response. Hum Mov Sci 2016;46:30–8.

31. Escamilla RF, Andrews JR. Shoulder muscle recruitment patterns and related biomechanics during upper extremity sports. Sports Med 2009; 39(7):569–90.

32. De Wilde L, Plasschaert F, Berghs B, et al. Quantified measurement of subacromial impingement. J Shoulder Elbow Surg 2003;12(4):346–9.

33. Crockett HC, Gross LB, Wilk KE, et al. Osseous adaptation and range of motion at the glenohumeral joint in professional baseball pitchers. Am J Sports Med 2002;30(1):20–6.

34. Thomas SJ, Swanik CB, Higginson JS, et al. A bilateral comparison of posterior capsule thickness and its correlation with glenohumeral range of motion and scapular upward rotation in collegiate baseball players. J Shoulder Elbow Surg 2011;20(5):708–16.

35. Burkhart SS, Morgan CD, Kibler WB. The disabled throwing shoulder: spectrum of pathology Part I: pathoanatomy and biomechanics. Arthroscopy 2003;19(4):404–20.

36. Jobe FW, Kvitne RS, Giangarra CE. Shoulder pain in the overhand or throwing athlete. The relationship of anterior instability and rotator cuff impingement. Orthop Rev 1989;18(9):963–75.

37. Chambers L, Altchek DW. Microinstability and internal impingement in overhead athletes. Clin Sports Med 2013;32(4):697–707.

38. Meister K. Internal impingement in the shoulder of the overhand athlete: pathophysiology, diagnosis, and treatment. Am J Orthop 2000;29(6):433–8.

39. Meister K, Buckley B, Batts J. The posterior impingement sign: diagnosis of rotator cuff and posterior labral tears secondary to internal impingement in overhand athletes. Am J Orthop 2004;33(8):412–5.

40. Ruotolo C, Price E, Panchal A. Loss of total arc of motion in collegiate baseball players. J Shoulder Elbow Surg 2006;15(1):67–71.

41. Kibler WB, Kuhn JE, Wilk K, et al. The disabled throwing shoulder: spectrum of pathology-10-year update. Arthroscopy 2013;29(1):141–61.e26.

42. Bennett GE. Elbow and shoulder lesions of baseball players. Am J Surg 1959;98:484–92.

43. Walch G, Liotard JP, Boileau P, et al. Postero-superior glenoid impingement. Another impingement of the shoulder. J Radiol 1993;74(1):47–50 [in French].

44. Wright RW, Paletta GA Jr. Prevalence of the Bennett lesion of the shoulder in major league pitchers. Am J Sports Med 2004;32(1):121–4.

45. Levigne C, Garret J, Grosclaude S, et al. Surgical technique arthroscopic posterior glenoidplasty for posterosuperior glenoid impingement in throwing athletes. Clin Orthop Relat Res 2012;470(6): 1571–8.

46. Davidson PA, Elattrache NS, Jobe CM, et al. Rotator cuff and posterior-superior glenoid labrum injury associated with increased glenohumeral motion: a new site of impingement. J Shoulder Elbow Surg 1995;4(5):384–90.

47. Connell DA, Potter HG. Magnetic resonance evaluation of the labral capsular ligamentous complex: a pictorial review. Australas Radiol 1999;43(4): 419–26.

48. Connell DA, Potter HG, Wickiewicz TL, et al. Noncontrast magnetic resonance imaging of superior labral lesions. 102 cases confirmed at arthroscopic surgery. Am J Sports Med 1999;27(2): 208–13.

49. Reinold MM, Macrina LC, Wilk KE, et al. Electromyographic analysis of the supraspinatus and deltoid muscles during 3 common rehabilitation exercises. J Athl Train 2007;42(4):464–9.

50. Reinold MM, Gill TJ, Wilk KE, et al. Current concepts in the evaluation and treatment of the shoulder in overhead throwing athletes, part 2: injury prevention and treatment. Sports Health 2010; 2(2):101–15.

51. Townsend H, Jobe FW, Pink M, et al. Electromyographic analysis of the glenohumeral muscles during a baseball rehabilitation program. Am J Sports Med 1991;19(3):264–72.

52. Davies GJ, Dickoff-Hoffman S. Neuromuscular testing and rehabilitation of the shoulder complex. J Orthop Sports Phys Ther 1993;18(2):449–58.

53. Aldridge R, Stephen Guffey J, Whitehead MT, et al. The effects of a daily stretching protocol on passive glenohumeral internal rotation in overhead throwing collegiate athletes. Int J Sports Phys Ther 2012; 7(4):365–71.

54. Tyler TF, Nicholas SJ, Lee SJ, et al. Correction of posterior shoulder tightness is associated with symptom resolution in patients with internal impingement. Am J Sports Med 2010;38(1):114–9.

55. Payne LZ, Altchek DW. The surgical treatment of anterior shoulder instability. Clin Sports Med 1995;14(4):863–83.

56. Sonnery-Cottet B, Edwards TB, Noel E, et al. Results of arthroscopic treatment of posterosuperior glenoid impingement in tennis players. Am J Sports Med 2002;30(2):227–32.

57. Jobe FW, Giangarra CE, Kvitne RS, et al. Anterior capsulolabral reconstruction of the shoulder in athletes in overhand sports. Am J Sports Med 1991; 19(5):428–34.

58. Paley KJ, Jobe FW, Pink MM, et al. Arthroscopic findings in the overhand throwing athlete: evidence for posterior internal impingement of the rotator cuff. Arthroscopy 2000;16(1):35–40.

59. Jones KJ, Kahlenberg CA, Dodson CC, et al. Arthroscopic capsular plication for microtraumatic anterior shoulder instability in overhead athletes. Am J Sports Med 2012;40(9):2009–14.

60. Burkhart SS, Morgan CD, Kibler WB. The disabled throwing shoulder: spectrum of pathology Part III: the SICK scapula, scapular dyskinesis, the kinetic chain, and rehabilitation. Arthroscopy 2003;19(6): 641–61.

61. Burkhart SS, Morgan CD, Kibler WB. The disabled throwing shoulder: spectrum of pathology. Part II: evaluation and treatment of SLAP lesions in throwers. Arthroscopy 2003;19(5):531–9.

62. Codding J, Dahm DL, McCarty LP 3rd, et al. Arthroscopic posterior-inferior capsular release in the treatment of overhead athletes. Am J Orthop 2015;44(5):223–7.

63. Ferrari JD, Ferrari DA, Coumas J, et al. Posterior ossification of the shoulder: the Bennett lesion. Etiology, diagnosis, and treatment. Am J Sports Med 1994;22(2):171–5 [discussion: 175–6].

64. Meister K, Andrews JR, Batts J, et al. Symptomatic thrower's exostosis. Arthroscopic evaluation and treatment. Am J Sports Med 1999;27(2):133–6.

65. Yoneda M, Nakagawa S, Hayashida K, et al. Arthroscopic removal of symptomatic Bennett lesions in the shoulders of baseball players: arthroscopic Bennett-plasty. Am J Sports Med 2002; 30(5):728–36.

66. Riand N, Levigne C, Renaud E, et al. Results of derotational humeral osteotomy in posterosuperior glenoid impingement. Am J Sports Med 1998; 26(3):453–9.

67. Reynolds SB, Dugas JR, Cain EL, et al. Debridement of small partial-thickness rotator cuff tears in elite overhead throwers. Clin Orthop Relat Res 2008;466(3):614–21.

68. Tibone JE, Elrod B, Jobe FW, et al. Surgical treatment of tears of the rotator cuff in athletes. J Bone Joint Surg Am 1986;68(6):887–91.

69. Halbrecht JL, Tirman P, Atkin D. Internal impingement of the shoulder: comparison of findings between the throwing and nonthrowing shoulders of college baseball players. Arthroscopy 1999;15(3): 253–8.

70. Economopoulos KJ, Brockmeier SF. Rotator cuff tears in overhead athletes. Clin Sports Med 2012; 31(4):675–92.

71. Williams GR, Kelley M. Management of rotator cuff and impingement injuries in the athlete. J Athl Train 2000;35(3):300–15.

72. Warner JJ, Micheli LJ, Arslanian LE, et al. Patterns of flexibility, laxity, and strength in normal shoulders and shoulders with instability and impingement. Am J Sports Med 1990;18(4):366–75.

73. Wiener SN, Seitz WH Jr. Sonography of the shoulder in patients with tears of the rotator cuff: accuracy and value for selecting surgical options. AJR Am J Roentgenol 1993;160(1):103–7 [discussion: 109–10].

74. Meister K, Thesing J, Montgomery WJ, et al. MR arthrography of partial thickness tears of the undersurface of the rotator cuff: an arthroscopic correlation. Skeletal Radiol 2004;33(3):136–41.

75. Burkhart SS, Diaz Pagan JL, Wirth MA, et al. Cyclic loading of anchor-based rotator cuff repairs: confirmation of the tension overload phenomenon and comparison of suture anchor fixation with transosseous fixation. Arthroscopy 1997;13(6): 720–4.

76. Franceschi F, Papalia R, Franceschetti E, et al. Double-row repair lowers the retear risk after accelerated rehabilitation. Am J Sports Med 2016;44(4): 948–56.

77. Rudzki JR, Shaffer B. New approaches to diagnosis and arthroscopic management of partial-thickness cuff tears. Clin Sports Med 2008;27(4): 691–717.

78. Lo IK, Burkhart SS. Transtendon arthroscopic repair of partial-thickness, articular surface tears of the rotator cuff. Arthroscopy 2004;20(2):214–20.

79. Conway JE. Arthroscopic repair of partial-thickness rotator cuff tears and SLAP lesions in professional baseball players. Orthop Clin North Am 2001; 32(3):443–56.

80. Brockmeier SF, Dodson CC, Gamradt SC, et al. Arthroscopic intratendinous repair of the delaminated partial-thickness rotator cuff tear in overhead athletes. Arthroscopy 2008;24(8):961–5.

81. Dines JS, Jones K, Maher P, et al. Arthroscopic management of full-thickness rotator cuff tears in major league baseball pitchers: the lateralized footprint repair technique. Am J Orthop 2016;45(3): 128–33.

82. Payne LZ, Altchek DW, Craig EV, et al. Arthroscopic treatment of partial rotator cuff tears in young athletes. A preliminary report. Am J Sports Med 1997;25(3):299–305.

83. Andrews JR, Carson WG Jr, McLeod WD. Glenoid labrum tears related to the long head of the biceps. Am J Sports Med 1985;13(5):337–41.

84. Snyder SJ, Karzel RP, Del Pizzo W, et al. SLAP lesions of the shoulder. Arthroscopy 1990;6(4): 274–9.

85. Snyder SJ, Banas MP, Karzel RP. An analysis of 140 injuries to the superior glenoid labrum. J Shoulder Elbow Surg 1995;4(4):243–8.

86. Maffet MW, Gartsman GM, Moseley B. Superior labrum-biceps tendon complex lesions of the shoulder. Am J Sports Med 1995;23(1):93–8.

87. Morgan CD, Burkhart SS, Palmeri M, et al. Type II SLAP lesions: three subtypes and their relationships to superior instability and rotator cuff tears. Arthroscopy 1998;14(6):553–65.

88. Pradhan RL, Itoi E, Hatakeyama Y, et al. Superior labral strain during the throwing motion. A cadaveric study. Am J Sports Med 2001;29(4): 488–92.

89. Burkhart SS, Morgan CD. The peel-back mechanism: its role in producing and extending posterior type II SLAP lesions and its effect on SLAP repair rehabilitation. Arthroscopy 1998;14(6): 637–40.

90. Yeh ML, Lintner D, Luo ZP. Stress distribution in the superior labrum during throwing motion. Am J Sports Med 2005;33(3):395–401.

91. Kuhn JE, Huston LJ, Soslowsky LJ, et al. External rotation of the glenohumeral joint: ligament restraints and muscle effects in the neutral and abducted positions. J Shoulder Elbow Surg 2005; 14(1 Suppl S):39S–48S.

92. Kim TK, Queale WS, Cosgarea AJ, et al. Clinical features of the different types of SLAP lesions: an analysis of one hundred and thirty-nine cases. J Bone Joint Surg Am 2003;85-A(1):66–71.

93. Braun S, Kokmeyer D, Millett PJ. Shoulder injuries in the throwing athlete. J Bone Joint Surg Am 2009;91(4):966–78.

94. Barber A, Field LD, Ryu R. Biceps tendon and superior labrum injuries: decision-marking. J Bone Joint Surg Am 2007;89(8):1844–55.

95. Bedi A, Allen AA. Superior labral lesions anterior to posterior-evaluation and arthroscopic management. Clin Sports Med 2008;27(4):607–30.

96. O'Brien SJ, Pagnani MJ, Fealy S, et al. The active compression test: a new and effective test for diagnosing labral tears and acromioclavicular joint abnormality. Am J Sports Med 1998;26(5):610–3.

97. Meserve BB, Cleland JA, Boucher TR. A meta-analysis examining clinical test utility for assessing superior labral anterior posterior lesions. Am J Sports Med 2009;37(11):2252–8.

98. Bennett WF. Specificity of the Speed's test: arthroscopic technique for evaluating the biceps tendon at the level of the bicipital groove. Arthroscopy 1998;14(8):789–96.

99. Cook C, Beaty S, Kissenberth MJ, et al. Diagnostic accuracy of five orthopedic clinical tests for diagnosis of superior labrum anterior posterior (SLAP) lesions. J Shoulder Elbow Surg 2012;21(1):13–22.

100. Jee WH, McCauley TR, Katz LD, et al. Superior labral anterior posterior (SLAP) lesions of the glenoid labrum: reliability and accuracy of MR arthrography for diagnosis. Radiology 2001;218(1):127–32.

101. Ohshima M, Yamazoe M, Tamura Y, et al. Immediate effects of percutaneous transvenous mitral commissurotomy on pulmonary hemodynamics at rest and during exercise in mitral stenosis. Am J Cardiol 1992;70(6):641–4.

102. Waldt S, Burkart A, Lange P, et al. Diagnostic performance of MR arthrography in the assessment of superior labral anteroposterior lesions of the shoulder. AJR Am J Roentgenol 2004;182(5): 1271–8.

103. Edwards SL, Lee JA, Bell JE, et al. Nonoperative treatment of superior labrum anterior posterior tears: improvements in pain, function, and quality of life. Am J Sports Med 2010;38(7):1456–61.

104. Boileau P, Parratte S, Chuinard C, et al. Arthroscopic treatment of isolated type II SLAP lesions: biceps tenodesis as an alternative to reinsertion. Am J Sports Med 2009;37(5):929–36.

105. Keener JD, Brophy RH. Superior labral tears of the shoulder: pathogenesis, evaluation, and treatment. J Am Acad Orthop Surg 2009;17(10):627–37.

106. Burkhart SS, Morgan C. SLAP lesions in the overhead athlete. Orthop Clin North Am 2001;32(3): 431–41, viii.

107. Ide J, Maeda S, Takagi K. Sports activity after arthroscopic superior labral repair using suture anchors in overhead-throwing athletes. Am J Sports Med 2005;33(4):507–14.

108. Neuman BJ, Boisvert CB, Reiter B, et al. Results of arthroscopic repair of type II superior labral anterior posterior lesions in overhead athletes: assessment of return to preinjury playing level and satisfaction. Am J Sports Med 2011;39(9): 1883–8.

109. Sayde WM, Cohen SB, Ciccotti MG, et al. Return to play after type II superior labral anterior-posterior lesion repairs in athletes: a systematic review. Clin Orthop Relat Res 2012;470(6):1595–600.

110. Pluim BM. Scapular dyskinesis: practical applications. Br J Sports Med 2013;47(14):875–6.

111. Burn MB, McCulloch PC, Lintner DM, et al. Prevalence of scapular dyskinesis in overhead and non-overhead athletes: a systematic review. Orthop J Sports Med 2016;4(2).

112. Priest JD, Nagel DA. Tennis shoulder. Am J Sports Med 1976;4(1):28–42.

113. Kibler WB, McMullen J. Scapular dyskinesis and its relation to shoulder pain. J Am Acad Orthop Surg 2003;11(2):142–51.

114. McClure PW, Michener LA, Sennett BJ, et al. Direct 3-dimensional measurement of scapular kinematics during dynamic movements in vivo. J Shoulder Elbow Surg 2001;10(3):269–77.

115. McQuade KJ, Dawson J, Smidt GL. Scapulothoracic muscle fatigue associated with alterations in scapulohumeral rhythm kinematics during maximum resistive shoulder elevation. J Orthop Sports Phys Ther 1998;28(2):74–80.

116. Sethi PM, Tibone JE, Lee TQ. Quantitative assessment of glenohumeral translation in baseball players: a comparison of pitchers versus non-pitching athletes. Am J Sports Med 2004;32(7): 1711–5.

117. Lehtinen JT, Tetreault P, Warner JJ. Arthroscopic management of painful and stiff scapulothoracic articulation. Arthroscopy 2003;19(4):E28.

118. Sisto DJ, Jobe FW. The operative treatment of scapulothoracic bursitis in professional pitchers. Am J Sports Med 1986;14(3):192–4.

119. Struyf F, Nijs J, Meeus M, et al. Does scapular positioning predict shoulder pain in recreational overhead athletes? Int J Sports Med 2014;35(1):75–82.

120. Warner JJ, Micheli LJ, Arslanian LE, et al. Scapulothoracic motion in normal shoulders and shoulders with glenohumeral instability and impingement syndrome. A study using Moire topographic analysis. Clin Orthop Relat Res 1992;(285):191–9.

121. McMahon PJ, Jobe FW, Pink MM, et al. Comparative electromyographic analysis of shoulder muscles during planar motions: anterior glenohumeral instability versus normal. J Shoulder Elbow Surg 1996;5(2 Pt 1):118–23.

122. Kibler WB. The role of the scapula in athletic shoulder function. Am J Sports Med 1998;26(2):325–37.

123. Kibler WB, Uhl TL, Maddux JW, et al. Qualitative clinical evaluation of scapular dysfunction: a reliability study. J Shoulder Elbow Surg 2002;11(6):550–6.

124. Ellenbecker TS, Kibler WB, Bailie DS, et al. Reliability of scapular classification in examination of professional baseball players. Clin Orthop Relat Res 2012;470(6):1540–4.

125. Tate AR, McClure P, Kareha S, et al. A clinical method for identifying scapular dyskinesis, part 2: validity. J Athl Train 2009;44(2):165–73.

126. Nicholson GP, Duckworth MA. Scapulothoracic bursectomy for snapping scapula syndrome. J Shoulder Elbow Surg 2002;11(1):80–5.

Biceps and Triceps Ruptures in Athletes

Jared R. Thomas, MD[a], Jeffrey Nathan Lawton, MD[b],*

KEYWORDS

- Distal biceps tendon rupture • Triceps tendon rupture • Tendon injuries • Athletes elbow

KEY POINTS

- Operative management of complete distal biceps and triceps tendon ruptures is required in most cases, especially for active patients, laborers, and athletes wishing to return to competition.
- Full range of motion and strength can be achieved following anatomic, stable repair and appropriate rehabilitation of distal biceps tendon rupture; return to play after triceps tendon rupture repair can be expected, although rehabilitation may be considerably longer.
- Surgical approach and fixation method for repair of distal biceps tendon ruptures should be determined based on the experience and comfort level of the treating surgeon; however, the chosen technique should focus on anatomic reinsertion of the tendon with a construct that can tolerate early range of motion.

INTRODUCTION

Most commonly the result of a traumatic forceful eccentric load on a contracting muscle, rupture of the distal biceps or triceps tendons occurs infrequently even in athletes. Together, these injuries represent the most (biceps) and least (triceps) common tendon injuries about the elbow. Rupture of the distal biceps tendon results in weakness in flexion and more noticeably supination, whereas triceps tendon rupture results in profound weakness or inability to actively extend the elbow. Early diagnosis and prompt intervention are essential for a successful outcome for both injuries, especially in athletes. Acute anatomic surgical repair of complete ruptures of either tendon has been shown to provide good and predictable outcomes.[1–4] Nonoperative management is best suited for patients with partial injuries and minimal functional loss who experience resolution of both pain and weakness with appropriate rest and rehabilitation.

Nonoperative management is most likely to be considered only in the nondominant arms of self-employed tradespersons for whom the economic impact of the recovery from surgery would be a hardship.

BICEPS TENDON RUPTURES

The reported incidence of distal biceps tendon ruptures is 1.2 per 100,000 people, making it a rare injury. Accounting for 3% of all biceps tendon injuries, ruptures of the distal biceps tendon affect the dominant arm in 86% of individuals.[5] This injury occurs almost entirely in men, although there have been reported cases in female athletes. An average age of 50 years has been cited in the literature, with a reported age range of 19 to 72 years. Common risk factors other than male gender include smoking, anabolic steroid use, and body building.[5–7] Distal biceps tendon ruptures are seldom encountered in overhead athletes and

Disclosures: J.N. Lawton has been a consultant for Innomed, Savannah, GA, and has received research support from Depuy/Synthes, Paoli, PA. J. Thomas has no disclosures.
[a] Department of Orthopaedic Surgery, University of Michigan, 2098 South Main Street, Ann Arbor, MI 48103-5827, USA; [b] Hand and Upper Extremity, Department of Orthopaedic Surgery, University of Michigan, 2098 South Main Street, Ann Arbor, MI 48103-5827, USA
* Corresponding author.
E-mail address: jeflawto@med.umich.edu

Hand Clin 33 (2017) 35–46
http://dx.doi.org/10.1016/j.hcl.2016.08.019

are most common in weight lifters and body builders.

Ruptures of the distal biceps tendon are classified as complete or partial. Complete ruptures are further classified as acute or chronic, with the distinction drawn at 4 weeks; partial ruptures are not further classified. Descriptively, the anatomic location of the rupture is classified as tendinous/insertional, musculotendinous junction, and intramuscular. The anatomic location as well as the distinctions between partial and complete rupture and acute versus chronic injuries play important roles in management. Intratendinous ruptures and insertional avulsion are amenable to surgical repair, and should be surgically repaired, whereas intramuscular rupture is typically not repairable. Partial tears may be amenable to nonoperative management, whereas complete tears require repair if anatomically conducive. Chronic injuries may require reconstruction with tendon grafts.[8]

In athletes, this injury can occur during strength training or competition. In this population, the injury most commonly presents after a single traumatic event; however, there is evidence that predisposition to injury may be the result of both hypovascularity at the tendon insertion and possible mechanical impingement during forearm rotation. The mechanism of distal biceps tendon rupture is that of forced extension of the elbow held in 90° flexion while the forearm is supinated, a position commonly encountered in both weight training and athletic competition.

Presentation and Examination

Classically, patients describe a painful audible or palpable pop in their elbow during an activity involving the mechanism described earlier. Occasionally a prodromal ache localized to the antecubital fossa is described by the patient. There is often immediate onset of ecchymosis and swelling in the antecubital region. In addition, patients may complain of asymmetry of their arms, a palpable mass or lump, or pain and weakness with elbow flexion and/or supination.

Physical examination findings often confirm the presenting complaints with antecubital and medial elbow swelling and ecchymosis, a palpable mass in the proximal arm, or the so-called Popeye deformity. The absence of a palpable biceps tendon at the elbow crease is also often appreciated. An intact lacertus fibrosis may confound physical examination findings by confining the hematoma or restraining proximal migration of the ruptured tendon, leading to the absence of both ecchymosis and significant deformity on physical examination. Further findings of objective weakness

with elbow flexion and supination can be combined with provocative maneuvers to verify the clinical diagnosis of distal biceps tendon rupture. Complete distal biceps tendon rupture can be further confirmed on physical examination with the hook test, which in some studies has been shown to be both 100% sensitive and specific.[9] The hook test is performed with the patient's elbow held in 90° of flexion with the forearm supinated. The examiner then attempts to hook the distal biceps tendon by pushing a flexed finger across the antecubital region from lateral to medial, thereby hooking an intact tendon (**Fig. 1**). Lack of resistance or absence of a palpable tendinous cord is considered a positive test. If the test is done in reverse; that is from medial to lateral, the examiner may be misled by the presence of an intact lacertus fibrosis. Pain with hook test can be a sign of partial tear.

Imaging

Despite the seemingly straightforward clinical diagnosis of distal biceps tendon rupture, the use of imaging is often indicated and beneficial. Devereaux and ElMaraghy[10] found that, in patients with surgically confirmed complete tendon rupture, as few as 33% described an audible or palpable pop, and only 38% had visible deformity on examination preoperatively. The evaluation of a

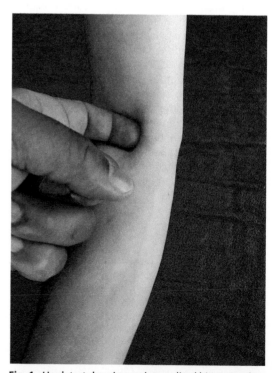

Fig. 1. Hook test showing an intact distal biceps tendon.

traumatic elbow injury requires the use of routine elbow radiographs; however, these are rarely helpful in making the diagnosis of distal biceps tendon rupture. In situations in which imaging is needed to assist with diagnosis, both MRI and ultrasonography have been found to be reliable.

Although costly and not available in all settings, MRI has the benefit of reliably and reproducibly evaluating the tendon in multiple planes. Early use of MRI for the evaluation of the biceps tendon relied primarily on the axial plane with the patient's arm extended. More recently, the flexion, abduction, supination (FABS) view has been shown to be a reliable way to assess the distal biceps tendon from the musculotendinous junction to its insertion on the radial tuberosity. Described by Giuffre and Moss,[11] the FABS view is used in conjunction with conventional elbow MRI (**Fig. 2**) views and is obtained by positioning the patient prone in the scanner with the affected shoulder abducted 180° so the arm is beside the head and then flexing the elbow 90° with the forearm supinated.

Ultrasonography performed by an experienced operator is reliable and cost-effective. In addition to being more widely available and less expensive than MRI, ultrasonography provides dynamic imaging that may be helpful in distinguishing between complete and partial tears. However, ultrasonography is limited by thicker soft tissue envelopes, which may be relevant in muscular athletes. In addition, ultrasonography relies on having a well-trained operator to be useful for the diagnosis of biceps tendon rupture. Beyond determining the presence or absence of a rupture, advanced imaging can give additional information about the degree of degeneration and overall quality of the tendon, as well as the degree of retraction.

Nonoperative Management

- Not a reasonable option for most athletes wishing to return to competition.
- Some investigators suggest a cutoff of 50% tendon involvement for surgical versus nonoperative management.[12,13]
- Treated nonoperatively, patients with complete rupture may see up to a 40% loss of supination strength, 20% loss of flexion power,[1,14] 86% decrease in supination endurance, and 15% decrease in grip strength.
- Despite residual weakness, long-term pain should not be expected in cases of complete rupture.
- Rehabilitation of partial tears should be focused on pain relief and restoration of full range of motion and strength.

Operative Management

Located in the anterior compartment of the arm, the biceps brachii consists of a long head and a short head. The long head of the biceps originates from the superior rim of the glenoid, and the short head originates from the coracoid process. The 2 heads are interconnected to varying degrees starting at the level of the deltoid tuberosity but continue their course separately down the arm with the short head running ulnar to the long head.[15] At the level of the lacertus fibrosis, the 2 tendons may continue to separate or coalesce into a single tendinous structure within a common tendon sheath. The lacertus fibrosis or bicipital aponeurosis arises medially at the musculotendinous junction and courses laterally, crossing the roof of the antecubital fossa obliquely, eventually blending with the pronator-flexor mass fascia and inserting onto the dorsal ulna. The tendon of the long head inserts proximally on the most prominent portion of the radial tuberosity, whereas the short head inserts just distally.

Several neurovascular structures are contained in and about the surgical field. The antecubital fossa is defined by the pronator teres ulnarly, the brachioradialis radially, and the brachialis and supinator deep. This triangular anatomic space contains the biceps tendon, brachial artery, and median nerve in that order from radial to ulnar.

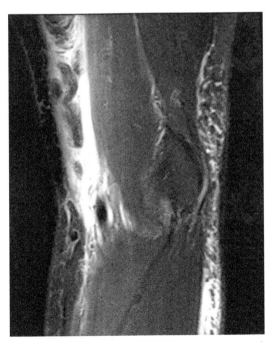

Fig. 2. Sagittal T2-weighted MRI showing a ruptured, retracted distal biceps tendon.

The brachial artery may bifurcate into the ulnar and radial arteries before entering the fossa; however, the radial artery consistently gives rise to its recurrent branches, which cross the antecubital fossa laterally within the surgical field and may require ligation. As the terminal branch of the musculocutaneous nerve, the lateral antebrachial cutaneous nerve travels radial to the biceps tendon and at the level of the antecubital fossa to lie within the superficial fascia, where it is susceptible to iatrogenic injury during biceps tendon repair.[16] The posterior interosseous nerve arises as the deep branch of the radial nerve and is at risk during tendon reattachment, which involves fixation to the dorsal radial cortex after it courses around the radial neck as it passes into the substance of the supinator muscle.[17] The potential complications associated with distal biceps tendon repair are listed in **Box 1**.

Approach

Several options exist for the surgical management of distal biceps tendon ruptures, with most decisions being appropriately guided by surgeon preference, because differences in the outcomes and complication rates of modern techniques have been shown to be minimal.[3,18] In the past, single-incision techniques were linked to higher rates of nerve injury, whereas 2-incision techniques were associated with higher rates of heterotopic ossification. However, a recent systematic review showed only minor differences, with increased transient lateral antebrachial cutaneous nerve neuropraxia with the single-incision technique and higher rates of postoperative stiffness with the 2-incision technique.[19] The same systematic

Box 1
Potential complications of repair
Distal biceps tendon repair
Radioulnar synostosis
Posterior interosseous neuropraxia
Lateral antebrachial nerve injury
Superficial radial nerve injury
Heterotopic ossification
Rerupture
Infection
Triceps tendon repair
Rerupture
Poor wound healing
Ulnar nerve neuropraxia

review also examined complication rates with varying fixation methods. A significantly lower rate of complications was found for bone tunnel and suture button techniques compared with suture anchors and transosseous screws.[19] Regardless of fixation method or surgical approach, it is generally accepted that repair of acute ruptures within 2 to 3 weeks is recommended to prevent musculotendinous adhesions, which may limit the surgeon's ability to mobilize the tendon back to its anatomic insertion.

Two-incision technique

First described by Boyd and Anderson,[20] this approach has seen many modifications over the years. In its current form the steps are as follows:

- Anterior incision (transverse or longitudinal) is made 2 to 3 finger breadths distal to the elbow flexion crease. Superficial dissection is designed to identify and protect of the lateral antebrachial cutaneous nerve.
- Blunt finger dissection is used to locate the tendon stump, which is debrided and secured via whip stitch with heavy nonabsorbable suture.
- Blunt finger dissection is used to develop the interval between brachioradialis and the pronator teres, with care taken to ligate recurrent branches of the radial artery.
- The radial tuberosity is palpated in the developed interval and a curved clamp is passed just ulnar through the interosseous ligament and advanced until it lies in the subcutaneous tissue of the dorsolateral forearm.
- An incision is made over the subcutaneous clamp and, with the forearm maximally pronated, the radial tuberosity is exposed by splitting the extensor carpi ulnaris.
- An oval trough is then created on the ulnar aspect of the tuberosity, followed by three 2.0-mm drill holes in the base of the trough through the dorsal cortex of the radius.
- The sutures securing the biceps tendon stump are then passed through the trough and out of the drill holes to dock the tendon.
- The anterior wound is then closed and the sutures tightened securely over bony bridges through the dorsal wound, which is then closed after thorough irrigation of any bony debris.

Single-incision technique

Much like the 2-incision technique, this approach has undergone several modifications since it was first described as an S-shaped extended Henry approach crossing the antecubital fossa. This traditional approach was associated with higher rates of neurologic complication.[20] In its current form, the choice of incision remains variable but should proceed in a similar fashion to the following:

- A transverse or longitudinal incision (**Fig. 3**) is made just distal to the elbow flexion crease. Again the lateral antebrachial cutaneous nerve is identified and protected. Alternatively, a longitudinal incision can be made, which allows for proximal extension if needed.
- Blunt finger dissection is used to locate the tendon stump, which is debrided and secured via whip stitch with heavy nonabsorbable suture (**Fig. 4**).
- Blunt finger dissection is used to develop the interval between brachioradialis and the pronator teres, with care taken to ligate recurrent branches of the radial artery.
- The radial tuberosity is then palpated, visualized and cleared of any soft tissue.
- Before proceeding with bone tunnel preparation, the forearm should be brought into full supination to protect the posterior interosseous nerve, which lies deep to the dorsal cortex of the radius within the supinator.
- Bone is prepared for preferred fixation method.

Fixation Methods

Suture button
Gaining popularity for its low learning curve, strong construct, and good outcomes, this method proceeds as follows:

- A bicortical guidewire is placed at the midpoint of the radial tuberosity with a 30° ulnar trajectory to maximize the distance from the posterior interosseous nerve. Fluoroscopy can be used to assist with placement of the guidewire.

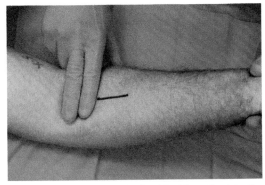

Fig. 3. Marked-out longitudinal incision distal to the elbow flexion crease.

- The near cortex is then reamed with an 8.0-mm bit, creating a bone socket. Extreme care is taken to avoid bicortical reaming (**Fig. 5**).
- Bony debris is thoroughly irrigated.
- Suture from the previously secured tendon stump is fed through the button, and an introducer is used to deliver the button through the near and far cortex.
- The button is then flipped by toggling the sutures. Using the same toggling motion, the tendon is advanced by sliding and tightening the sutures until the tendon stump is docked within the bone socket, coming to lie interosseously (**Fig. 6**).
- This fixation can be further secured with an interference screw placed radial to the tendon, thereby displacing the tendon ulnarly to recreate a more anatomic position. In addition, the free suture limbs can be introduced back through the tendon using a free suture needle and secured with a surgeon's knot.
- Fluoroscopy should be used to confirm that the button is both flipped and directly on bone (**Fig. 7**).
- Alternatively, a similar technique can be used with only an interference screw.

Suture anchor
The tendon can be secured to bone by placing a suture anchor on the ulnar aspect of the radial tuberosity. This technique has the advantage of avoiding drilling of the far cortex, thereby reducing the risk of posterior interosseous nerve injury. However, this method has been shown to have a significantly lower load to failure than the suture button method, which may make it a less suitable choice of fixation in the high-demand athletic population.[21]

Recovery and Postoperative Care

Postoperatively, patients are splinted in 90° of elbow flexion with the forearm supinated for comfort. Within the first week the splint is discontinued and active, active-assisted, and gentle passive range of motion are allowed. Initiation of progressive strengthening is allowed 6 to 8 weeks after surgery. Return to sport should be expected 3 to 6 months after repair when normal strength, range of motion, and resolution of pain have been achieved.

Outcomes

D'Alessandro and colleagues[6] examined the outcomes of 10 athletes who underwent distal biceps tendon repair via a 2-incision bone tunnel

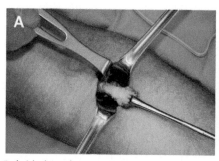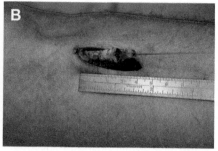

Fig. 4. (*A*) Debrided tendon stump. (*B*) Whip-stitched tendon stump.

technique. They reported all patients graded their result as excellent, with an average rating of 9.75 on a 10-point scale. All 10 patients, 8 of whom were weight lifters or body builders, were able to return to full, unrestricted activities without pain. In addition, dynamometer strength and endurance testing showed near or complete recovery of supination and flexion strength after repair.[6]

In a prospective randomized clinical trial, Grewal and colleagues[3] found no significant differences in outcomes as measured by the American Shoulder and Elbow Surgeons score, the Disabilities of the Arm, Shoulder, and Hand score, and Patient-Rated Elbow Evaluation score between single-incision and 2-incision techniques. Strength testing revealed a 10% advantage in final flexion strength in the 2-incision group. Complication rate was higher in the single-incision group, almost entirely because of a significantly higher rate of transient lateral antebrachial cutaneous nerve neuropraxia.[3]

A recent systematic review seeking to determine a consensus on both approaches and repair techniques found no difference in complication rate between single-incision and 2-incision techniques. Because of a lack of uniformity, the investigators chose not to analyze clinical outcomes scores. Moreover, the data suggested that bone tunnel and suture button methods were safer than suture

anchors or transosseous screws.[19] In addition, biomechanical studies have shown cortical buttons to have superior strength with higher load to failure and pullout strength than other methods of fixation.[21,22]

TRICEPS TENDON RUPTURES

Constituting one of the rarest reported tendon injuries,[23] rupture of the triceps tendon typically occurs in young men as the result of a forceful eccentric load against a contracting triceps muscle. Triceps ruptures have also been reported after a direct impact to the triceps insertion or via direct laceration. In the athletic population, this injury has been most commonly reported in football players, body builders, and power lifters.[24–26] Several studies have investigated distal triceps tendon ruptures in professional football players. Mair and colleagues[25] identified 21 triceps tendon tears in 19 National Football League players over a 6-year period, with 11 of them being complete ruptures. Finstein and colleagues[24] reported on 37 triceps tendon ruptures that required surgery over 10 seasons, and identified positions that involve blocking as most at risk in addition to concluding that football players have a higher risk of triceps tendon rupture than the general population. There is thought to be a predisposing association

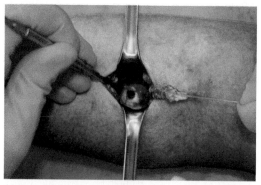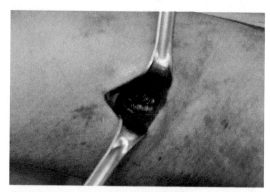

Fig. 5. Reamed bone socket.

Fig. 6. Tendon docked in bone socket.

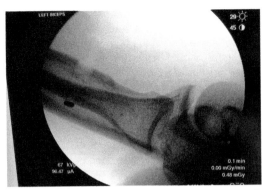

Fig. 7. Intraoperative fluoroscopy image of a well-placed and flipped cortical button.

between rupture and local corticosteroid injection as well as systemic anabolic steroid use. Other identified risk factors include a history of chronic olecranon bursitis,[27] chronic renal failure, and hyperparathyroidism.

Although there is no specific classification system for triceps tendon ruptures, decision making parallels that in the management of other tendon injuries.

Presentation and Examination

Much like with biceps tendon rupture, patients with rupture of the triceps present with a history of an audible or palpable pop. Mechanisms of injury include a fall onto an outstretch hand, a direct blow to the triceps tendon, or most commonly a sudden forced flexion of an extended elbow. In contradistinction to the complaints of patients with biceps injuries, triceps ruptures are localized to the posterior aspect of the elbow, where swelling and ecchymosis can be seen about the olecranon. Patients may report pain with elbow motion or only in terminal flexion. In addition, patients report marked weakness with, or complete absence of, active elbow extension.

Physical examination shows swelling and ecchymosis posteriorly near or proximal to the olecranon. A palpable defect in the triceps tendon can confirm the diagnosis if not masked by swelling or the patient's soft tissue envelope (**Fig. 8**). Resisted elbow extension may accentuate the palpable defect and/or elicit pain. Range of motion may be full against gravity even in cases of complete central tendon rupture if the lateral expansion remains intact, which has been shown to lead to misdiagnosis in up to half of acute tendon ruptures.[4] Absence of extension against gravity is considered a classic finding and should confirm complete rupture in the absence of neurologic injury. A modification of the Thompson test described by Viegas[28] may also be helpful in diagnosing complete rupture. This test is performed by placing the elbow in 90° of flexion with the arm supported and forearm allowed to hang free over the edge of the examiner's table. The triceps muscle belly is then squeezed, with failure to induce elbow extension interpreted as positive for complete rupture.

Imaging

Routine elbow radiographs should be obtained. A flake sign may be appreciated on lateral projections indicating an avulsion of the distal triceps from its insertion on the olecranon and is considered pathognomonic for triceps rupture (**Fig. 9**). Even when near clinical certainty can be had with physical examination and radiograph, advance imaging is typically still useful. Both ultrasonography and sagittal MRI have proved particularly useful at showing the extent of tendon injury,[29,30] with MRI being the imaging modality of choice. MRI can distinguish complete from partial injuries in addition to localizing the tear to the insertion, myotendinous junction, or intramuscular region.

Anatomy and Biomechanics

The 3 heads of the triceps occupy the entirety of the posterior compartment of the arm. Innervated by the radial nerve, the medial and lateral heads

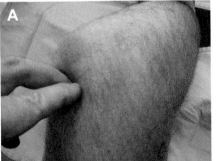
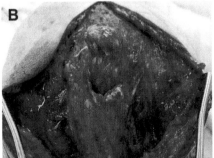

Fig. 8. (A) Palpable triceps tendon defect. (B) Central triceps tendon defect.

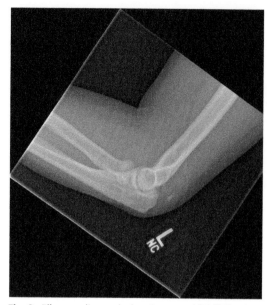

Fig. 9. Elbow radiograph showing a positive flake sign.

originate from the posterior humerus and intermuscular septum and serve only as elbow extensors, whereas the long head, which originates from the infraglenoid tubercle, is thought to contribute to shoulder adduction and extension. Distally the 3 heads of the triceps insert via a broad attachment that can be divided into a proper attachment beginning at the medial border of the olecranon and a lateral expansion that extends beyond the olecranon laterally to blend with the anconeus and antebrachial fascia before inserting distally on the radial aspect of the proximal ulna. This lateral expansion in some ways is similar to the lacertus fibrosis of the biceps tendon in that the presence of a tear in this portion of the tendon dictates the amount of tendon retraction. The broad footprint as defined by Keener and colleagues[31] extends distal to the olecranon by 12 mm and has an overall footprint of 466 mm², which may be important when considering repair techniques.

Operative Management

Athletes with acute complete or partial ruptures of greater than 50% of the tendon should undergo direct repair of the tendon back to the native olecranon insertion. Indications for operative management of triceps tendon rupture include:

- Partial tears in athletes and laborers
- Partial tears in elderly patients still active enough for activities of daily living
- Partial tears in patients who have failed nonoperative management
- Complete tears

Many techniques have been described; however, the technique used is determined by the acuity and completeness of the tear. Whenever possible the tendon should be reattached to the olecranon but, when this is not possible, techniques involving graft augmentation or rotation flaps have been described.[32] As with biceps tendon injuries, triceps ruptures are best addressed within 2 to 3 weeks, especially when there is significant tendon retraction, although primary repair as late as 8 months after injury has been described.[33]

Approach

A posterior approach is used. The skin incision can be placed midline or more advisably just radial to the midline to avoid incising the thin soft tissue envelope directly over the olecranon as well as to avoid the ulnar nerve medially. Full-thickness flaps are developed and the olecranon, triceps, and proximal ulna are exposed. The ulnar nerve is identified and protected. The central tendon stump is rarely retracted and should be readily identified, freed of any adhesions, and debrided in preparation for repair (**Fig. 10**). The tendon is typically secured with heavy nonabsorbable sutures using a Krackow or Bunnell suture configuration and any of several methods used to secure the tendon back to bone. Before securing the tendon back to bone, thorough soft tissue debridement should be performed to prepare a bony bed. Regardless of the preferred

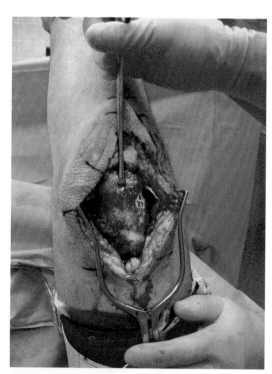

Fig. 10. Debrided distal triceps tendon.

fixation method, special attention must be paid to the position of the elbow during repair. Two common techniques are described here.

Bone tunnels

- Using a 2.5-mm drill, 2 crossing or 3 parallel bone tunnels are made through the olecranon starting from the native triceps footprint and exiting dorsal (**Fig. 11**).
- With the elbow in 90° of flexion, the sutures are shuttled through the bone tunnels and the tendon appropriately attached. The sutures are then tied over a bone bridge.

- Care is taken to avoid leaving these large knots from the nonabsorbable sutures in a subcutaneous position.

Transosseous equivalent (anatomic double row)

- A Krackow stitch is used to secure the central tendon (**Fig. 12**).
- Two anchors are placed approximately 12 mm distal to the tip of the olecranon within the triceps anatomic footprint.
- The sutures from the anchors are then passed through the tendon in a horizontal mattress fashion.

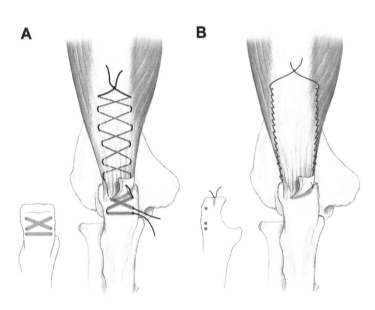

A   B

Fig. 11. (*A*) Bone tunnel construct. (*B*) Transosseous equivalent technique. (*C*) Bone tunnel construct and transosseous equivalent technique shown together.

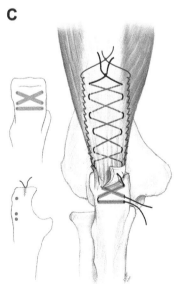

C

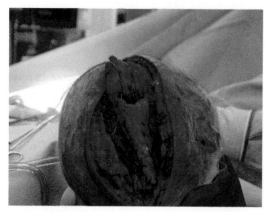

Fig. 12. Central triceps tendon secured with a Krackow stitch.

- The free ends of the Krackow stitch then join the anchor sutures and are then secured to 2 additional suture anchors that are placed distal to the anatomic footprint, thereby compressing the width of the tendon to the prepared bony bed beneath (see **Fig. 11**).
- This construct has been shown to have significantly greater repair strength than suture anchors or the traditional bone tunnel technique in addition to more accurately recreating the native anatomic footprint.[34]
- Other methods using alternative means of bony fixation back to the anatomic footprint, such as suture anchors or knotless systems, have also been described.

Recovery and Postoperative Care

Although widely variable postoperative rehabilitation protocols have been reviewed in the literature, the following regimen has been recommended[35]:

- Immobilization for 2 weeks at 30° elbow flexion with full-extension splint at night if passive extension is difficult.
- Progressive flexion block at 30°, 45°, 60°, and 90° by week 5. Full flexion by week 6.
- Active extension by week 6.
- Strengthening initiated by 12 weeks.
- Unrestricted activity at 5 months.

In the athletic population, the question of return to sport is always a concern. Athletes who sustain partial tears that are amenable to nonoperative management may be able to return to play after several weeks of rest and progressive rehabilitation if pain has resolved and normal strength returned. One study of professional football players who had partial injuries treated nonoperatively reported an average time until return to full competition of 5 weeks with the use of a brace.[25]

Residual pain and weakness may persist despite appropriate rest, warranting continued rest or surgical consideration. There have been documented cases of progression to complete rupture and chronic triceps dysfunction in athletes who return to participation immediately.[25,26,36,37]

The literature regarding return to sport after operative repair is not robust. The published literature suggests a lengthy recovery with some investigators delaying initiation of strengthening until 3 months postoperatively. One study of professional football players had 1 patient who returned to full competition 7 weeks postoperatively without rerupture; however, the remaining athletes took considerably longer. Currently available guidance suggests allowing 4 to 6 months for recovery and rehabilitation before return to sports.[4,38] There are reports of rerupture occurring in patients who return sooner.[26] Potential complications after triceps tendon repair include rerupture, poor wound healing, and ulnar nerve neuropraxia (see **Box 1**). Clearly, further studies would be helpful in determining recommendations regarding return to play after triceps tendon repair.

SUMMARY

Although rare, biceps and triceps ruptures in athletes are debilitating injuries, with weight lifting, body building, and football identified as high-risk athletic activities. Almost without exception these injuries require surgical repair in this population. Occasionally, partial injuries can be treated nonoperatively when they involve less than 50% of the tendon or occur intramuscularly or at the musculotendinous junction. Even though several surgical techniques have been described, treating surgeons should focus on principles of a robust repair that restores preinjury anatomy to permit early and aggressive rehabilitation. Postoperative care should be focused on adequate healing time followed by physical therapy that restores range of motion and strength. With appropriate treatment and rehabilitation, athletes should expect near full return of strength in addition to unrestricted return to competition within 4 to 6 months after surgery and sooner in partial injuries treated nonoperatively.

REFERENCES

1. Baker BE, Bierwagen D. Rupture of the distal tendon of the biceps brachii. Operative versus non-operative treatment. J Bone Joint Surg Am 1985; 67(3):414–7.
2. Bava ED, Barber FA, Lund ER. Clinical outcome after suture anchor repair for complete traumatic

rupture of the distal triceps tendon. Arthroscopy 2012;28(8):1058–63.

3. Grewal R, Athwal GS, MacDermid JC, et al. Single versus double-incision technique for the repair of acute distal biceps tendon ruptures: a randomized clinical trial. J Bone Joint Surg Am 2012;94(13):1166–74.

4. van Riet RP, Morrey BF, Ho E, et al. Surgical treatment of distal triceps ruptures. J Bone Joint Surg Am 2003;85-A(10):1961–7.

5. Safran MR, Graham SM. Distal biceps tendon ruptures: incidence, demographics, and the effect of smoking. Clin Orthop Relat Res 2002;(404):275–83.

6. D'Alessandro DF, Shields CL Jr, Tibone JE, et al. Repair of distal biceps tendon ruptures in athletes. Am J Sports Med 1993;21(1):114–9.

7. Visuri T, Lindholm H. Bilateral distal biceps tendon avulsions with use of anabolic steroids. Med Sci Sports Exerc 1994;26(8):941–4.

8. Patterson RW, Sharma J, Lawton JN, et al. Distal biceps tendon reconstruction with tendoachilles allograft: a modification of the endobutton technique utilizing an ACL reconstruction system. J Hand Surg Am 2009;34(3):545–52.

9. O'Driscoll SW, Goncalves LB, Dietz P. The hook test for distal biceps tendon avulsion. Am J Sports Med 2007;35(11):1865–9.

10. Devereaux MW, ElMaraghy AW. Improving the rapid and reliable diagnosis of complete distal biceps tendon rupture: a nuanced approach to the clinical examination. Am J Sports Med 2013;41(9):1998–2004.

11. Giuffre BM, Moss MJ. Optimal positioning for MRI of the distal biceps brachii tendon: flexed abducted supinated view. AJR Am J Roentgenol 2004; 182(4):944–6.

12. Durr HR, Stabler A, Pfahler M, et al. Partial rupture of the distal biceps tendon. Clin Orthop Relat Res 2000;(374):195–200.

13. Vardakas DG, Musgrave DS, Varitimidis SE, et al. Partial rupture of the distal biceps tendon. J Shoulder Elbow Surg 2001;10:377–9.

14. Morrey BF, Askew LJ, An KN, et al. Rupture of the distal tendon of the biceps brachii. A biomechanical study. J Bone Joint Surg Am 1985;67(3):418–21.

15. Eames MH, Bain GI, Fogg QA, et al. Distal biceps tendon anatomy: a cadaveric study. J Bone Joint Surg Am 2007;89(5):1044–9.

16. Chiavaras MM, Jacobson JA, Billone L, et al. Sonography of the lateral antebrachial cutaneous nerve with magnetic resonance imaging and anatomic correlation. J Ultrasound Med 2014;33(8):1475–83.

17. Lawton JN, Cameron-Donaldson M, Blazar PE, et al. Anatomic considerations regarding the posterior interosseous nerve at the elbow. J Shoulder Elbow Surg 2007;16(4):502–7.

18. El-Hawary R, Macdermid JC, Faber KJ, et al. Distal biceps tendon repair: comparison of surgical techniques. J Hand Surg Am 2003;28(3):496–502.

19. Watson JN, Moretti VM, Schwindel L, et al. Repair techniques for acute distal biceps tendon ruptures: a systematic review. J Bone Joint Surg Am 2014; 96(24):2086–90.

20. Boyd HB, Anderson LD. A method for reinsertion of the distal biceps brachii tendon. J Bone Joint Surg Am 1961;43(7):1041–3.

21. Mazzocca AD, Burton KJ, Romeo AA, et al. Biomechanical evaluation of 4 techniques of distal biceps brachii tendon repair. Am J Sports Med 2007;35(2): 252–8.

22. Greenberg JA, Fernandez JJ, Wang T, et al. EndoButton-assisted repair of distal biceps tendon ruptures. J Shoulder Elbow Surg 2003;12(5):484–90.

23. Anzel SH, Covey KW, Weiner AD, et al. Disruption of muscles and tendons; an analysis of 1, 014 cases. Surgery 1959;45(3):406–14.

24. Finstein JL, Cohen SB, Dodson CC, et al. Triceps tendon ruptures requiring surgical repair in National Football League players. Orthop J Sports Med 2015; 3(8). 2325967115601021.

25. Mair SD, Isbell WM, Gill TJ, et al. Triceps tendon ruptures in professional football players. Am J Sports Med 2004;32(2):431–4.

26. Sollender JL, Rayan GM, Barden GA. Triceps tendon rupture in weight lifters. J Shoulder Elbow Surg 1998;7(2):151–3.

27. Clayton ML, Thirupathi RG. Rupture of the triceps tendon with olecranon bursitis. A case report with a new method of repair. Clin Orthop Relat Res 1984;(184):183–5.

28. Viegas SF. Avulsion of the triceps tendon. Orthop Rev 1990;19(6):533–6.

29. Kaempffe FA, Lerner RM. Ultrasound diagnosis of triceps tendon rupture. A report of 2 cases. Clin Orthop Relat Res 1996;(332):138–42.

30. Kijowski R, Tuite M, Sanford M. Magnetic resonance imaging of the elbow. Part II: Abnormalities of the ligaments, tendons, and nerves. Skeletal Radiol 2005; 34(1):1–18.

31. Keener JD, Chafik D, Kim HM, et al. Insertional anatomy of the triceps brachii tendon. J Shoulder Elbow Surg 2010;19(3):399–405.

32. Sanchez-Sotelo J, Morrey BF. Surgical techniques for reconstruction of chronic insufficiency of the triceps. Rotation flap using anconeus and tendo Achillis allograft. J Bone Joint Surg Br 2002;84(8):1116–20.

33. Inhofe PD, Moneim MS. Late presentation of triceps rupture. A case report and review of the literature. Am J Orthop (Belle Mead NJ) 1996;25(11):790–2.

34. Yeh PC, Stephens KT, Solovyova O, et al. The distal triceps tendon footprint and a biomechanical analysis of 3 repair techniques. Am J Sports Med 2010;38(5):1025–33.

35. Blackmore SM, Jander RM, Culp RW. Management of distal biceps and triceps ruptures. J Hand Ther 2006;19(2):154–68.

36. Duchow J, Kelm J, Kohn D. Acute ulnar nerve compression syndrome in a powerlifter with triceps tendon rupture–a case report. Int J Sports Med 2000;21(4):308–10.

37. Kokkalis ZT, Sotereanos DG. Biceps tendon injuries in athletes. Hand Clin 2009;25(3):347–57.

38. Singh RK, Pooley J. Complete rupture of the triceps brachii muscle. Br J Sports Med 2002;36(6):467–9.

Medial Elbow Injuries in the Throwing Athlete

 CrossMark

Jimmy H. Daruwalla, MD[a], Charles A. Daly, MD[a], John G. Seiler III, MD[b],*

KEYWORDS

- Ulnar collateral ligament • UCL reconstruction • Throwing elbow injuries
- Adolescent sports injuries • Tommy John surgery

KEY POINTS

- The anterior bundle of the ulnar collateral ligament (UCL) is the primary restraint to valgus stress in the elbow.
- The incidence of athletes undergoing UCL reconstruction has been increasing substantially.
- Advances in the surgical technique of UCL reconstruction have minimized postoperative complications.
- Most athletes are able to return to a high level of competition following both nonoperative and surgical treatment of medial elbow injuries.

INTRODUCTION

Since its first description in 1946, ulnar collateral ligament (UCL) and other medial elbow injuries have been observed with increasing frequency in the overhead athlete.[1] Presumably due to increased participation in throwing sports as well as an enhanced awareness of this injury constellation, there has also been a significant increase in the incidence diagnosis and treatments required for these injuries.[2,3] Fortunately, a concomitant awareness to the issue within the orthopedic community has lead to the development of a substantial body of research on the pathophysiology and treatment of medial elbow abnormality. Jobe and colleagues[4] pioneered UCL reconstruction (colloquially known as Tommy John surgery) in 1974, and since then, multiple technical multiple alterations in both technique and the scope of the procedure have been proposed.[5] In addition, research has led to advances in measures designed to limit injury risk and postoperative rehabilitation methods to facilitate safe return to play.[6,7]

Owing to a discrete pattern of supraphysiologic and pathologic forces acting on the elbow during the throwing motion, medial elbow injuries are most commonly observed in the overhead-throwing athlete. Although most classically and frequently described in baseball players (>95% in one study of 1266 patients[8]), UCL injury and other medial elbow abnormality have been reported in a variety of overhead athletes, including gymnasts, javelin throwers, cheerleaders, and tennis and football players.[7,8] Although the overall rate of elbow injuries is low, the total number of these injuries is significant because of an increasing participation nationally in overhead athletics.[2] Even though no national database of these injuries is available to determine the exact rate of medial elbow injury in the throwing athlete, the incidence of these injuries has reportedly been increasing.[2,9,10] For example, the number

Disclosures: The authors have no commercial or financial conflicts of interest to disclose. There was no external funding source used for this article.
[a] Department of Orthopaedic Surgery, Emory University School of Medicine, 59 Executive Park South, Atlanta, GA 30329, USA; [b] Georgia Hand, Shoulder & Elbow, 2061 Peachtree Road, Northeast, Suite 500, Atlanta, GA 30309, USA
* Corresponding author.
E-mail address: jgseiler@gahand.org

Hand Clin 33 (2017) 47–62
http://dx.doi.org/10.1016/j.hcl.2016.08.013

hand.theclinics.com

of UCL reconstruction procedures has increased 193% in New York State from 2002 to 2011.[11] Fleisig and Andrews[2] reported a 22-fold increase in the incidence of UCL reconstruction from 1994 to 2010 at their institution. The purpose of this article is to review current concepts related to medial elbow injury and reconstruction in the overhead athlete.

RELEVANT ANATOMY OF THE MEDIAL ELBOW

The osseous structures of the medial elbow consist of the ulnohumeral articulation between the trochlea of the humerus and the sigmoid notch of the olecranon (**Fig. 1**), which normally features a valgus carrying angle of 11° to 16°. This bony articulation contributes to valgus stability of the elbow from full extension to ~30° flexion. In greater degrees of flexion, stability is mainly determined by UCL function.[12]

The UCL comprises 3 different bundles of fibers: the anterior, posterior, and transverse bundles. The posterior bundle of the UCL is a fan-shaped thickening of the posteromedial joint capsule. It provides minimal stability to the medial elbow. Its average length and width are 16.5 and 9.9 mm, respectively.[13] The transverse, or oblique, bundle originates and inserts on the ulna and thus does not contribute to elbow joint stability.

The anterior bundle of the UCL is the primary restraint to valgus stress at the elbow during range of motion (ROM) between 20° and 120°.[14] As the strongest and stiffest ligament of all the elbow stabilizers, the anterior bundle is well defined and easily discernible from, although still intimately associated with, the medial joint capsule underneath. It originates from anterior-inferior edge of the medial epicondyle and inserts on the sublime tubercle of the proximal ulna. The ulnar insertion begins an average of 2.8 mm distal to the ulnar articular surface and extends distally an average of 29 mm along a bony prominence known as the medial ulnar collateral ridge (**Fig. 2**).[15] The anterior bundle has an average length reported between 21 and 59 mm and average width of 7.6 mm.[13,15] The anterior bundle itself separates into an anterior and posterior band at its insertion. The anterior band provides the major source of valgus stability, whereas the posterior band becomes a significant restraint at flexion past 90°.[16]

The ulnar nerve passes posterior to the medial epicondyle of the humerus through the cubital tunnel, in which the floor is made up of the posterior and transverse bundles of the UCL. The nerve leaves the elbow as it passes between the 2 heads of the flexor carpi ulnaris (FCU). Around the elbow, the nerve may be compressed by medial epicondyle osteophytes, Osborne ligament (roof of the cubital tunnel), or the arcuate ligament (aponeurosis of the 2 heads of the FCU).

Originating from the medial epicondyle, the flexor-pronator muscle group includes the pronator teres (PT), flexor carpi radialis (FCR), palmaris longus, flexor digitorum superficialis (FDS), and the FCU. From this group, the PT, FDS, and FCU contribute to dynamic valgus elbow stability. The FCU, in particular, overlies the UCL in nearly the entire ROM of the elbow.[17]

In the skeletally immature patient, the developing growth plates (physes) are relatively weak compared with the other surrounding structures, predisposing to unique injury patterns in this population. The medial epicondyle apophysis begins its ossification at ~5 years of age and completes ossification at ~15 years of age, a time at which

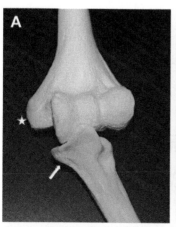 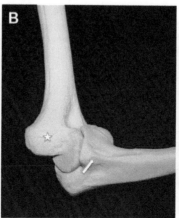 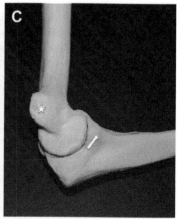

Fig. 1. AP (*A*), oblique (*B*), and lateral (*C*) views of a model detailing the osseous anatomy of the medial epicondyle (*star*) and sublime tubercle (*arrow*).

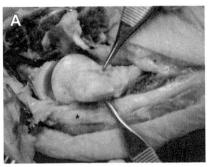
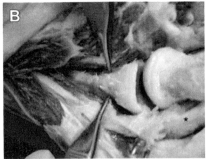

Fig. 2. Cadaveric dissection detailing the UCL's origin from the medial epicondyle of the humerus (*A*) and insertion onto the sublime tubercle of the ulna (*B*), indicated by the forceps. The ulnar nerve is seen coursing posterior to the medial epicondyle (*star*).

the apophysis is particularly susceptible to traction injury.

NORMAL BIOMECHANICS OF OVERHEAD THROWING

The throwing motion is a kinetic chain involving the whole body that efficiently transfers energy from the lower extremities, through the abdominal core and trunk, and into the upper extremity. There are 6 phases of the overhead throwing motion, classically described in relation to the baseball pitch (**Fig. 3**).

1. Wind-up: In this initial phase, the thrower stands in an athletic starting position. Minimal elbow or shoulder motion occurs at this time.
2. Stride: This phase begins while the front leg is moving forward in the direction of the throw and ends once the front foot contacts the ground. During this time, the shoulder begins to abduct and externally rotate, and elbow flexion begins.
3. Arm Cocking: This phase begins at the time of front foot contact. The throwing shoulder abducts to ~90° and rotates toward maximal external rotation. At the end of the cocking phase, an eccentric internal rotation torque is

created at the shoulder to prevent overrotation externally. Similarly, a varus torque at the elbow is produced to prevent valgus extension as the arm begins to derotate from the cocked position.[18] This torque is produced via tension through the UCL and contraction flexor-pronator muscles.[2]
4. Acceleration: From the cocked position, internal rotation of the shoulder is initiated to begin the acceleration phase. The elbow then begins to extend from its maximal degree of flexion. As the acceleration phase occurs, the elbow extends rapidly with peak angular velocity reaching 2000–2300°/s just before ball release.[18]
5. Deceleration: Deceleration of the arm begins after ball release and ends when the arm reaches maximal internal rotation. The elbow is decelerated by a flexion torque via eccentric biceps contraction before full extension is reached. This force helps to dynamically stabilize the elbow by providing a compression force across the joint to prevent distraction.[18]
6. Follow-through: In this phase, the pitcher returns to a balanced fielding position. During this time, motion of other parts of the body besides the arm, such as the trunk and legs, helps to dissipate energy from the throwing arm.

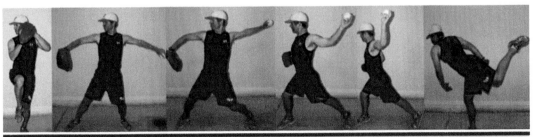

Windup   Stride   Early Cocking   Late Cocking   Acceleration   Deceleration/Follow-through

Fig. 3. The phases of throwing.

PATHOPHYSIOLOGY OF MEDIAL ELBOW INJURIES

During overhead throwing, 3 discrete pathologic forces are imparted on the elbow by the valgus moment: (1) tensile force on the medial stabilizing structures, including the UCL; (2) compressive force on the radiocapitellar joint; and (3) shear forces directed medially in the posteromedial compartment.[19] During the acceleration phase, large tensile forces are transmitted through the medial elbow, estimated at up to 290 N in one study.[18] Although this force may exceed the tensile strength of the anterior bundle of the UCL (which, based on biomechanical study, has an average load to failure of 260N),[13] the entirety of forces on the medial elbow are fortunately dissipated through multiple structures, including osseous articulations and dynamic stabilization from the flexor-pronator muscles, anconeus, and triceps.[18] Nonetheless, the UCL still absorbs at least half of the stress through the medial elbow and, as dynamic stabilizers such as the flexor-pronator muscles start to show fatigue, an increasing amount of force is transmitted to the UCL.[20] Thus, through chronic and repeated stress with throwing, the ligament eventually becomes attenuated and valgus elbow instability develops.

Once the UCL becomes incompetent, pathologic contact within the elbow occurs during repetitive valgus stress, resulting in a spectrum of secondary abnormalities to the ulnohumeral and radiocapitellar joints.[20–23] For example, the ulnohumeral joint becomes slightly subluxated in a valgus position, leading to impingement of the posteromedial tip of the olecranon on the medial olecranon fossa. Over time, this may result in olecranon chondromalacia, osteophytes at the posteromedial tip of the olecranon, and/or loose bodies, a syndrome known as valgus extension overload (VEO). On the lateral side of the elbow, pathologic compressive forces may result in osteochondritis dissecans (OCD) of the radiocapitellar joint, osteochondral chip fractures, or avascular necrosis.[8,9,21]

Additional pathophysiology unique to the pediatric population is also important to acknowledge. Although younger pitchers produce less torque than adults during a throw, skeletally immature athletes have more compliant connective tissue, open physes, and underdeveloped muscles that are susceptible to injury. Moreover, pitchers at the youth level have greater inconsistency in their throwing biomechanics,[24] which may lead to increased elbow varus torque and increased risk of injury.[2]

Medial epicondylar apophysitis or apophyseal avulsion, known colloquially as "Little League elbow," may result from repetitive valgus and tensile forces imparted to the medial epicondyle.[23,25] Even in asymptomatic youth throwers, apophyseal hypertrophy and delayed closure of the epicondylar growth plate are extremely common.[26] In more severe cases, apophyseal separation/fracture can occur. Microtraumatic vascular insufficiency secondary to repetitive trauma from throwing may also lead to OCD, although the complete cause of this disease process is unknown. These lesions are seen mostly in adolescents older than 13 years and usually involve the lateral compartment, specifically the capitellum.[27]

Risk Factors for Elbow Injury

Several studies in baseball pitchers have demonstrated that pitch count, within a game and over the course of a season, is significantly associated with medial elbow injuries.[10,28] A 10-year prospective study of 481 youth pitchers demonstrated that those who pitched more than 100 innings a year were 3.5 times more likely to be injured.[28] In a retrospective study of 140 pitchers 14 to 20 years old, pitch count and inadequate rest were the most salient risk factors for injury. Specifically, multivariable logistic regression demonstrated that averaging more than 80 pitches per game and pitching for more than 8 months per year increased the odds of surgery substantially (odds ratio 3.83 and 5.05, respectively).[10] Similarly, among Little League and high school pitchers, those who also pitch for travel and club teams are at an increased risk for elbow injury.[2]

Pitch type has also been studied as a risk factor for elbow injury. Sports medicine experts have traditionally warned that throwing curveballs, especially at a young age, may lead to elbow injury because the arm must be placed in a position that increases strain on the medial elbow.[29] However, biomechanical studies comparing the curveball to the fastball have not supported this theory, showing equivalent or even less elbow torque with the curveball.[30–32] Clinical studies have likewise demonstrated no increased risk of injury in pitchers who started throwing curveballs at an early age.[10,28] A systematic review by Grantham and colleagues[33] of 15 studies regarding the curveball echoed the above findings, concluding that, despite the debate in the baseball community, the available data do not support an increased risk of injury when compared with the fastball. The authors believe that, while attempting to throw a curveball, younger athletes are really throwing a "slider," which puts significantly increased strain on the medial elbow structures.

Injury Prevention Strategies

On the basis of data demonstrating the strong correlation between overuse and injury, prevention programs have been developed in order to reduce the incidence of medial elbow abnormality in the overhead athlete. The foremost strategy is based on preventing overuse by limiting pitch counts in pitchers. In 2007, Little League Baseball replaced their inning limits with pitch count limits, and numerous other youth baseball organizations have followed suit. Pitchers are also discouraged from pitching for multiple teams and pitching year round. In addition, coaching efforts to correct errors in throwing mechanics have also been instituted.[2] In the authors' experience, education has been an important tool in injury prevention. They have emphasized the importance of stretching, improved pitching mechanics, limiting pitch selection by age, and actively improving core strength as a mainstay of their program. However, despite the understanding of the risk factors that predict medial elbow injury, no studies currently exist to prove that prevention programs have lowered the incidence of these injuries.

CLINICAL EVALUATION OF MEDIAL ELBOW INJURIES
History and Physical Examination

Appropriate evaluation of the overhead-throwing athlete begins with a thorough history, including a full review of past medical and surgical history. Documentation of sport and position played, level of competition, and timing in the season is important. For pitchers, the average pitch count, number of innings pitched, and type of pitches thrown should also be documented. Throwers with instability will report pain particularly during late cocking and acceleration phases, whereas those with VEO will report pain at ball release when the elbow nears full extension.[21] Pitchers with instability or other medial elbow abnormalities may also relay a history of decreased velocity and accuracy.[34] Only up to half of patients are typically able to identify an acute, inciting episode.[8,34] About one-quarter of patients will present with neurologic symptoms, most commonly paresthesias in the ulnar nerve distribution, aggravated by throwing.[8] Younger pitchers presenting with OCD lesions or adults with fragmented olecranon osteophytes may report mechanical symptoms, from intra-articular loose bodies.[21]

Physical examination begins with inspection, palpation, and assessment of ROM of the elbow and basic neurovascular examination of the extremity. The average overhead athlete patient will have a subtle flexion contracture.[8,34] Palpation of the UCL may or may not elicit tenderness depending on the chronicity of injury. A Tinel test at the medial elbow tests for ulnar nerve sensitivity. The nerve should also be examined for stability by feeling for subluxation during elbow ROM, especially with flexion beyond 90°. Palpation of the flexor-pronator origin and medial epicondyle is used to examine for flexor-pronator injury and medial epicondylitis. Pain with resisted wrist flexion can also indicate flexor-pronator wad abnormality. Skeletally immature patients with apophysitis or apophyseal avulsion may exhibit focal swelling over the medial epicondyle.

To elicit UCL incompetency and valgus instability, the examiner places the elbow in 30° of flexion to eliminate bony support and stabilizes the distal humerus with one hand and applies a valgus force to the elbow, inducing tension through the medial elbow. The test, specific for the anterior band of the anterior bundle, is considered positive when there is laxity greater than 2 mm and/or a significantly softer end point when compared with the contralateral elbow.[8] Medial-sided elbow pain elicited with this test may also indicate UCL injury. The milking maneuver specifically tests the posterior band of the anterior UCL bundle. It is performed by abducting the shoulder, flexing the elbow to greater than or equal to 90°, supinating the forearm, and applying a valgus stress to the elbow by pulling on the patient's thumb (**Fig. 4**). It is important to note that the amount of laxity at the elbow may be too small to detect on examination, even in the presence of a complete UCL tear. In a series of 1266 UCL reconstructions, Cain and colleagues[8] reported that only 22% of patients demonstrated valgus instability with manual testing. VEO may be elicited by forcibly extending the elbow from a flexed position while maintaining a valgus stress. Pain at the posteromedial tip of the olecranon with this maneuver is considered pathognomonic for VEO.[21]

Concomitant wrist and shoulder abnormality is not uncommon and thus should be assessed during evaluation of the elbow. Failure to address these issues, such as a glenohumeral internal rotation deficit, may adversely affect outcomes of treatment of medial elbow abnormality. In addition, when conducting a preoperative assessment, the presence of a palmaris longus tendon should be determined.

Imaging

Standard radiographic assessment begins with plain radiographs, which are normal in up to 40% to 50% of patients with a UCL injury.[8] In the study

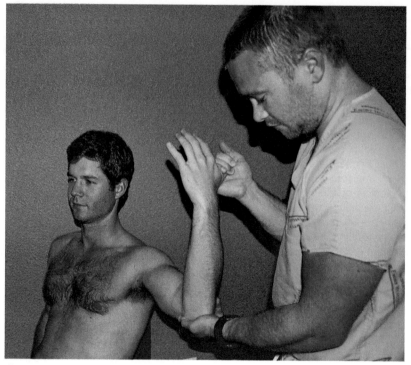

Fig. 4. The milking maneuver, demonstrated here, examines the posterior band of the anterior bundle of the UCL.

by Cain and colleagues,[8] 57% of patients had radiographic abnormalities, of which olecranon osteophytes and calcification within the substance of the UCL were the most common findings. Adolescents with Little League elbow may demonstrate irregular ossification and/or enlargement of the medial epicondyle apophysis. Later in the disease progression, fragmentation and frank avulsion of the medial epicondyle may be observed.[27,35]

Valgus stress anteroposterior (AP) radiographs of the elbow can be obtained to elicit medial instability that may not be evident on physical examination. These radiographs may be performed by transmitting a standardized, sequential series of forces through the elbow using a fixed armholder.[34] Alternatively, gravity valgus stress radiography without specialized equipment may be used. The patient is placed supine with the shoulder in external rotation, the upper arm resting on the table, and the forearm free to hang off the table, imparting a valgus stress moment via gravity. An AP radiograph is taken with the elbow in 20° to 30° flexion.[36] A positive stress radiograph, defined as greater than 2 mm opening between the trochlea and the coronoid compared with the neutral AP radiograph, was reported in 46% of patients in a series of 91 overhead athletes

undergoing surgery.[34] Interestingly, several investigators have noted that even normal elbows can demonstrate medial gapping with valgus stress.[36,37]

Advanced imaging is commonly obtained, with MRI or MRI arthrogram (MRA) being the study of choice for detecting UCL tears (**Fig. 5**). In a study of 25 patients undergoing elbow arthroscopy, MRI successfully identified all patients with complete UCL tears, although its sensitivity decreased to 57% when including patients with partial UCL tears.[38] Other findings that may be visualized on MRI or MRA include flexor-pronator tendinopathy or edema, medial epicondylitis, medial extravasation of contrast out of the joint, OCD lesions, intra-articular loose bodies, and olecranon stress fracture.

NONOPERATIVE TREATMENT OF VALGUS ELBOW INSTABILITY

Once a diagnosis of UCL injury has been established, the demands of the patient, degree of instability, age, and concomitant injuries must be considered when formulating a treatment plan. A trial of nonoperative treatment is appropriate, particularly in the young athlete with an acute injury.[39] Partial tears in young athletes necessitate

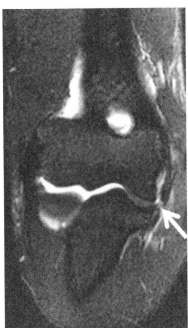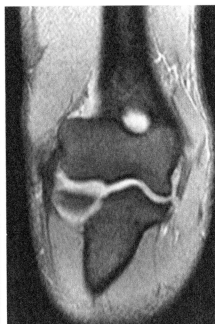

Fig. 5. Coronal MRI images demonstrating a UCL tear. Tear with surrounding edema (*arrow*).

at least 6 weeks of rest from throwing, followed by a structured rehabilitation program and gradual return to sport with a progressive throwing program.[6] Older athletes with similar injuries may require a longer period of rest and rehabilitation. To improve the chance of success, rehabilitation programs should be structured to include core strengthening and focus on throwing mechanics. Shoulder ROM and flexor-pronator muscle group strengthening is emphasized as well.[6,22] The patient, therapist, and physician should also agree on the number and type of pitches to be thrown during recovery. There is little evidence that adjunctive biologic treatments, such as platelet-rich plasma, are useful in the treatment of elbow stability.[39] Corticosteroid injection is not recommended, because it may weaken surrounding structures.

SURGICAL TREATMENT OF VALGUS ELBOW INSTABILITY

Surgical intervention is indicated after a 3- to 6-month course of conservative management has failed in an athlete who wishes to return to overhead throwing at the same level. Amateur athletes may not need UCL reconstruction, given that most activities of daily living do not require medial elbow stability.[40] For example, outcomes after nonoperative treatment of simple elbow dislocation, when the UCL is ruptured, are usually excellent in the general population.

Ulnar Collateral Ligament Repair

Direct repair of the UCL following injury is controversial. In the young athlete, UCL repair may be a good option for acute tears directly off of bone, with or without a bony avulsion. However, in older patients, or in those with chronic, attritional intrasubstance injuries, direct repair leads to unpredictable results. In those patients deemed to be a candidate for direct repair, Savoie and colleagues[41] found 93% good to excellent results. However, Conway and colleagues[42] demonstrated just a 50% return to previous level of sport with direct repair, as compared with 68% with reconstruction. Thus, in light of the reproducible results found with UCL reconstruction and the limited report of successful direct ligament repair, the role of direct repair remains incompletely defined.

Ulnar Collateral Ligament Reconstruction

Graft choice

Although multiple graft sources have been described, most surgeons prefer the ipsilateral palmaris longus tendon. The graft is harvested from the volar forearm through 3 small, transverse incisions: at the volar wrist crease, and 4 and 15 cm proximal to the wrist crease. Typically, a graft greater than or equal to 15 cm can be obtained.[39] If the palmaris is absent, use of the gracilis, plantaris, or toe extensor tendons is possible. No significant difference in outcomes between various graft options has been demonstrated.[6]

For some older adults, the use of tendon allograft may be appropriate.

Graft fixation technique

Multiple techniques have been described for UCL reconstruction since its inception in 1974. They differ in the approach to the ulna and medial epicondyle, use of ulnar nerve transposition, and graft fixation technique.

Jobe technique

As the original method for UCL reconstruction, the Jobe technique approaches the UCL via detachment of the flexor-pronator muscle mass from the medial epicondyle.[4] The ulnar nerve is routinely transposed. Two drill holes in the proximal ulna and 3 in the medial epicondyle are used to pass the graft, which is then sutured to itself in a figure-of-8 fashion. A biomechanical study comparing this reconstruction technique to the native elbow demonstrated similar resistance to valgus stress throughout the flexion arc.[43] Smith and colleagues[44] subsequently described a muscle-splitting approach as a modification to the Jobe technique that does not require detachment of the flexor-pronator mass from the medial epicondyle or obligate ulnar nerve transposition.

American Sports Medicine Institute technique

Described by Andrews and colleagues,[45] the American Sports Medicine Institute technique is a figure-of-8 reconstruction of the ligament. The UCL origin is approached via anterior elevation of the flexor-pronator mass off the deep fascia near the sublime tubercle. In this way, the origin of these muscles is left intact on the medial epicondyle. Subcutaneous transposition of the ulnar nerve is routinely performed.

Docking technique

The docking technique was popularized by Rohrbough and colleagues[46] and uses a muscle-splitting approach without nerve transposition. Ulnar tunnel design is similar to the methods described above. The humeral tunnel design uses a single Y-shaped tunnel created with smaller (1.5 mm) exit holes, through which suture is passed and tied over the intervening bone bridge (Fig. 6).[46] As graft is not passed through the 2 proximal holes in the humerus, this technique uses smaller tunnels and a larger intervening bone bridge, potentially decreasing risk of fracture. The docking technique also needs less handling of the ulnar nerve, avoids detachment of the flexor pronator mass from the medial epicondyle, and allows for appropriate tensioning of the graft.[47]

DANE Tommy John technique

This reconstruction technique, named for Drs David Altchek and Neal ElAttrache, features a humeral approach and fixation technique similar to the docking technique, but uses an interference screw on the ulnar side rather than bone tunnels.[48] This method provides favorable results especially in the revision setting and in cases of sublime tubercle insufficiency. Studies have demonstrated that the interference screw fixation provides favorable biomechanical strength and allows for limited dissection distally.[49]

Biomechanical Comparison of Fixation Techniques

Several biomechanical studies have compared the various UCL reconstructive techniques to each other as well as the native ligament. A cadaveric

A   **B**

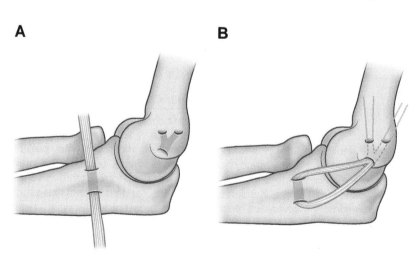

Fig. 6. The bone tunnels for the docking technique for UCL reconstruction (A) and appearance of the graft passed through the humeral tunnels during tensioning (B).

study of 10 pairs by Ciccotti and colleagues[50] demonstrated equivalent stability between the Jobe and Docking techniques. However, Paletta and colleagues[51] also compared the Jobe and Docking techniques biomechanically, determining that the docking technique may have a higher load to failure. The investigators noted that the suture-tendon interface was the most common site of failure with the Jobe technique, whereas suture knot failure was most common with the docking technique.[51] In another biomechanical study comparing the docking, Jobe, interference screw, and ulnar endobutton reconstruction techniques, the docking and endobutton techniques were found to have similar strength and were both superior to the interference screw and Jobe techniques. Failure in the Jobe, endobutton, and docking techniques was most common at the suture-ligament interface, whereas use of an interference screw was associated with graft rupture during screw placement in 2 of 7 specimens.[52]

To date, there is no consensus regarding the ideal reconstruction method. However, the 2 most commonly used methods are the modified Jobe and the docking techniques.[5] Benefits of the docking technique include a lower risk of fracture of the bony bridge between the humeral tunnels and, in some series, a lower rate of ulnar neurapraxia as a result of decreased nerve manipulation.[45,53] As no data currently exist to definitively support one technique over another, the authors recommend that surgeons use the reconstructive technique most familiar to them to maximize outcomes and minimize complications.

Senior Author's Preferred Technique

In the senior author's preferred technique, the patient is placed supine with the shoulder abducted to 90° on a hand table. A sterile tourniquet is used. Regional blocks are typically avoided in order to facilitate examination of ulnar nerve function postoperatively. The presence of valgus instability is confirmed with examination under anesthesia and may also be observed with arthroscopic visualization via a single anterolateral portal. However, the authors do not routinely use arthroscopy unless it is required for another purpose, such as loose body removal.

The skin incision is made over the medial epicondyle and extended about 4 cm proximally and 6 cm distally, forming a 160° angle between the 2 limbs. The medial antebrachial cutaneous nerve is identified within the distal one-third of the incision and mobilized anteriorly along with the medial antebrachial vein. The authors use a muscle-splitting approach to identify the medial

collateral ligament. An incision in line with the ligament fibers allows for inspection of the medial joint line and synovectomy, if necessary. By retracting the triceps, inspection of the posterior joint line can be done, and if necessary, posterior and medial ulnar osteophytes resected. Next, the location for the bone tunnels for ligament reconstruction is determined. A 3.5-mm drill bit is used to develop the ulnar bone tunnel. The holes for the ulnar tunnel are typically placed 7 mm distal to the joint, with the most posterior hole drilled first just below the sublime tubercle. The anterior hole is then drilled just above the sublime tubercle, so that the graft will nicely reconstruct the insertional point of the ligament. The drill holes can be connected with the use of an angled curette. After harvest, the graft is prepared by placing a locking suture of braided Dacron in the end of the graft to facilitate passage of the graft through the bone tunnels. The graft can be passed through the ulnar bone tunnels with a free curved Mayo needle or a suture passer. To ensure a satisfactory bony bridge, the 2 drill holes in the ulna are typically designed to be at least 8 to 10 mm apart. For the humeral tunnel, the authors prefer a Y-shaped tunnel that allows the graft to be easily tensioned. A 4.5-mm drill is used to open the distal humerus at the origin of the UCL. A 3.5-mm drill bit is used to create the 2 posterior bone tunnels that form the Y shape. The graft can then be passed through the Y-shaped tunnel and tensioned. The graft is secured in approximately 30° of flexion with the medial joint line in contact (varus stress). The ulnar nerve is transposed only if there is subluxation identified at the time of the procedure. A layered closure is performed, and the patient is fitted with a well padded posterior fiberglass shell in the operating room.

MANAGEMENT OF OTHER MEDIAL ELBOW ABNORMALITY
Ulnar Neuropathy

Overhead throwing athletes, particularly those with valgus elbow instability, are at increased risk of ulnar neuropathy.[54] In the general population, nonoperative treatment of ulnar neuropathy is highly successful, but overhead athletes have a high recurrence rate on resumption of throwing and thus require surgical intervention at increased frequency.[54] Despite this, an initial treatment course of rest, anti-inflammatory medications, and occasionally a short course of immobilization, should be considered before surgical intervention. Both simple decompression and medial epicondylectomy have demonstrated poor results in throwing athletes, but anterior subcutaneous

Table 1
Postoperative outcomes with relevant treatment variables

Authors	Primary or Revision Reconstruction to UCL	Approach to UCL	Rehabilitation Protocol	Patients at Follow-up	Mean Follow-up (mo)	Return to Sport[a]	Mean Time to Return to Sport (mo)	Complication Rate (%)	Type of Complications
Dodson et al	Primary	Muscle-splitting	ROM at 7 d, strengthening at 6 wk, throwing at 4 mo, return to play at 12 mo	100	36	90% (90/100)	Not reported	3	Ulnar neuropathy requiring reoperation (2%), postoperative stiffness requiring reoperation (1%)
Conway et al	Primary	FPM detachment	ROM at 10 d, strengthening at 4–6 wk, throwing at 4 mo, return to play at 12 mo	68	75.6	68% (38/56)	Not reported	25	Ulnar neuropathy (21%), ulnar neuropathy requiring reoperation (12%), neuroma (2%), hematoma (2%)
Cain Jr et al	Primary	Muscle-splitting	ROM at 7 d, strengthening at 4 wk, throwing at 14 wk	743	38.4	83% (617/743)	11.6	20	Ulnar neurapraxia (16%), superficial wound infection (4%), revision UCL reconstruction (1%)
Thompson et al	Primary	Muscle-splitting	ROM at 7 d, strengthening at 6 wk, throwing at 4 mo, return to play at 12 mo	83	37.2	82% (27/33)	13	10	Transient ulnar neuropathy (5%), flexor-pronator muscle tear (1%), wound hematoma (1%)

Rohrbough et al	Primary	Muscle-splitting	ROM at 7 d, strengthening at 6 wk, throwing at 4 mo, return to play at 9 mo	36	39.6	92% (33/36)	Not reported	5.5	Transient ulnar nerve paresthesia (1%), wound hematoma (1%), reflex sympathetic dystrophy (1%), ulnar tunnel fracture (1%)
Paletta et al	Primary	Muscle-splitting	ROM at 10-14 d, strengthening at 6 wk, throwing at 4 mo, return to play at 10 mo	25	30	92% (23/25)	11.5	8.0	Transient ulnar neuropathy (4%), ulnar tunnel fracture (4%)
Bowers et al	Primary	Muscle-splitting	ROM at 7 d, strengthening at 6 wk, throwing at 4 mo, return to play at 12 mo	21	28	90% (19/21)	Not reported	0	N/A
Dines et al	Revision	FPM detachment (3), muscle-splitting (12)	Not reported	15	40	33% (5/15)	Not reported	40	Postoperative stiffness (13%), postoperative stiffness requiring reoperation (7%), reactive synovitis (7%)
Jones et al	Revision	Not reported	Not reported	18	Not reported	22% (4/18)	18.9	Not reported	Not reported
Marshall et al	Revision	Not reported	Not reported	33	Not reported	65% (19/29)	Not reported	Not reported	Not reported

Abbreviation: FPM, flexor pronator mass.
[a] Defined as Excellent result using the Conway scale (return to preinjury level of play for at least 1 year after reconstruction).

transposition seems to be a reliable procedure for this population.[54]

When the surgeon deems that ulnar nerve transposition is necessary, careful attention must be given to the branches to be ligated. The first (capsular) branch at the elbow may be sacrificed, because it supplies the elbow capsule. However, the subsequent branches are anterior and posterior fibers of the nerve and thus must be protected and preserved. Obligatory ulnar nerve transposition is not performed in the authors' practice, given its association with ulnar neuritis and inferior outcomes.[55] The authors reserve ulnar nerve transposition for throwers with concomitant ulnar neuritis and/or subluxation at the time of elbow stabilization.

Medial Epicondylitis

Initial, nonoperative treatment of medial epicondylitis in the overhead athlete, consisting of rest, anti-inflammatory medications, counterforce bracing, and physical therapy, is highly successful.[56] For individuals who need additional treatment, the authors consider the use of corticosteroid injection. Athletes with recalcitrant symptoms may occasionally require surgical intervention, either in isolation or concomitantly with UCL reconstruction. The goals of surgical interventions are to thoroughly debride all pathologic tissue and provide a secure tendinous repair with as little disruption as possible to the flexor-pronator origin. The origin is incised between the FCR and PT, through which all diseased tissue is sharply excised. The common tendon is then reattached to the medial epicondyle via drill holes or suture anchors.[57]

Valgus Extension Overload

Athletes who have VEO without associated medial elbow instability should undergo a period of conservative treatment with throwing cessation followed by a therapy program to strengthen the flexor-pronator muscle group. Surgical intervention may be considered when symptoms persist and may be performed concomitantly during elbow stabilization.

Anatomic sequelae of VEO are typically addressed arthroscopically. Via the posterolateral and posteromedial portals, a shaver, burr, or small osteotome is used to remove the posteromedial traction spur of the olecranon. A maximum of 8 mm of bone is resected from the tip of the olecranon, because further resection may increase the stress on the UCL during a valgus moment.[58,59] A single lateral radiograph should be obtained to ensure complete excision of the osteophyte. Loose bodies and hypertrophic synovium may

also be removed arthroscopically during this procedure.

Medial Epicondyle Fracture

Management of medial epicondyle fractures is controversial. Typically, treatment is nonsurgical and consists of immobilization in a long arm cast with the elbow flexed to 90°. Outcomes after conservative treatment are generally excellent, with some reporting outcomes similar to surgical treatment even with fractures displaced up to 15 mm.[60] Others, however, argue that displacement greater than 5 mm, especially in overhead-throwing athletes, is a relative indication for surgical fixation to optimize function.[61] Incarcerated fracture fragment within the elbow joint, as can be seen with concurrent elbow dislocation, is the only universally accepted absolute indication for surgical intervention in closed medial epicondyle fractures.

The authors recommend an open reduction with screw fixation when operative intervention is deemed necessary. A posteromedial incision is used just anterior to the medial epicondyle for fracture site exposure and visualization of the ulnar nerve, if needed. Provisional fixation with a K-wire is used after anatomic reduction. A partially threaded, cancellous screw is subsequently placed for compression. Fluoroscopy should be used to confirm reduction.

POSTOPERATIVE REHABILITATION

Rehabilitation protocols vary by institution, and no comprehensive, validated program currently exists. Emphasis should be placed on motion, strength, and neuromuscular control while gradually applying load to the healing tissue. In addition, with the knowledge that the factors extrinsic to the elbow may contribute to UCL injury, abnormality such as glenohumeral internal rotation deficit, scapular dyskinesia, and weak core and lower extremity strength, should be simultaneously addressed during elbow rehabilitation.[62]

Although the protocol used should be tailored to the patient, the sport, and the repair technique used, the rehabilitation process is generally divided into discrete, graduate phases: immediate motion, intermediate phase, advanced strengthening, and return to activity.[50] The immediate motion phase should aim to restore extension to preoperative levels via the use of low-load, long-duration stretches, which produce creep of collagen fibers. The intermediate phase should be initiated when full ROM and at least four-fifths strength in flexion and extension is regained. This phase should focus on improving strength, endurance, and neuromuscular control of the entire upper extremity kinetic chain.[63] The advanced strengthening phase should begin when ~70% of contralateral arm strength has been obtained with painless, full motion.[62] This phase features gradual progression to higher resistance, sport-specific movements, eccentric contraction, and plyometric activities. At about 4 months post-operatively, an interval-throwing program with return to sport is the final phase of rehabilitation. For pitchers, a core strengthening program, mechanics evaluation, and a progressive long toss program are instituted. Pitchers then begin throwing a fastball for velocity on the flat, whereas throwing off the mound is reserved for the end of the program.[64] The authors prefer that pitchers focus on first throwing a fastball and a changeup for location and then progress to breaking pitches. Return to competitive throwing should begin at 9 to 12 months postoperatively.[62] Often, pitchers will comment that although they were able to return to pitching after 1 year, it took an additional year to regain precise control of location for all pitches in their repertoire.

OUTCOMES

UCL reconstruction is successful in returning overhead athletes to sports in most cases (**Table 1**). A meta-analysis of 8 studies and 405 reconstructions over 30 years demonstrated an overall rate of 83% excellent results.[55] Similarly, 83% of 1281 athletes were able to return to their previous level of play in one large series with a minimum 2-year follow-up,[8] and Dodson and colleagues[65] found that 90% of 100 throwers were able to return to the same or higher level than before.

In the revision setting, however, reported rates appear to be more unpredictable, with return to play rates ranging from 33% to 65% in 3 studies.[66–68] In a retrospective review of 15 elite baseball players, Dines and colleagues[66] reported return to play at preinjury level in just 5 (33%) athletes. Six of 15 (40%) had a complication, including one rerupture and one reoperation for lysis of adhesions. Marshall and colleagues[68] reported a 66% return to play in 33 professional pitchers, but only 42% returned to pitch 10 or more games.[69] Moreover, players who did return to play had a significant decline in innings pitched and wins after surgery. Similarly, a study on 18 professional baseball pitchers showed that these athletes were able to pitch in only 50% as many innings as before revision surgery.[67] In light of these data, the authors recommend thoroughly counseling athletes on both the potentially poorer outcomes and the higher complication rates when considering revision UCL reconstruction.

Outcomes appear to also depend in part on the specific reconstructive technique used. Original reports from Jobe reported 63% to 68% return to sport and were associated with relatively high overall complication rates.[4,42] However, with the advent of technique modifications, specifically transitioning from flexor-pronator detachment to a muscle-splitting approach, overall patient outcomes and return to play rates improved significantly.[55] Thompson and colleagues[70] reported excellent outcomes in 93% of their 83-athlete series, with 100% return to play, using their muscle-splitting, modified-Jobe technique without nerve transposition. The docking technique appears to have further improved outcomes over figure-of-8 techniques, with investigators observing rates of return to preinjury level of competition between 90% and 95%.[46,55,71,72]

Multiple studies have demonstrated that the most common complication following UCL reconstruction is ulnar neuropathy/neuropraxia.[5,8,58] Earlier reports using the original Jobe technique were associated with high rates of complications, most commonly related to ulnar neuropathy.[4,42] However, transition to a muscle-splitting approach, which obviates nerve transposition, was associated with improved outcomes and a lower complication rate.[44,55] A systematic review of 8 studies reported a 4% rate of postoperative ulnar neuropathy,[55] whereas Cain and colleagues[8] found a 16% rate of ulnar nerve symptoms in their series of 1281 athletes, all of which were transient. The advent of the docking technique may have led to even lower rates of ulnar neuropathy, reported in 3% in one study of 100 patients.[47,53] Other complications, such as heterotopic ossification, are infrequent. If symptomatic, heterotopic ossification is typically amenable to arthroscopic resection.[58] Medial epicondyle fracture is a rare complication as well, occurring in 0.5% in the series from Cain and colleagues.[8,47]

SUMMARY

A heightened awareness and enhanced diagnostic acumen, combined with refinements in surgical techniques, have led to improved outcomes of medial elbow injuries in the throwing athlete. In particular, transition to muscle-splitting approaches and the use of ulnar nerve transposition only when needed have led to a decrease in surgical morbidity from UCL reconstruction. Continued research into the prevention of and rehabilitation from these injuries will further help to limit the morbidity of the extreme stresses imparted onto the elbow of the throwing athlete.

REFERENCES

1. Waris W. Elbow injuries of javelin-throwers. Acta Chir Scand 1946;93(6):563–75.
2. Fleisig GS, Andrews JR. Prevention of elbow injuries in youth baseball pitchers. Sports Health 2012;4(5):419–24.
3. Wilson AT, Pidgeon TS, Morrell NT, et al. Trends in revision elbow ulnar collateral ligament reconstruction in professional baseball pitchers. J Hand Surg 2015;40(11):2249–54.
4. Jobe FW, Stark H, Lombardo SJ. Reconstruction of the ulnar collateral ligament in athletes. J Bone Joint Surg Am 1986;68(8):1158–63.
5. Chang ES, Dodson CC, Ciccotti MG. Comparison of surgical techniques for ulnar collateral ligament reconstruction in overhead athletes. J Am Acad Orthop Surg 2016;24(3):135–49.
6. Ellenbecker TS, Wilk KE, Altchek DW, et al. Current concepts in rehabilitation following ulnar collateral ligament reconstruction. Sports Health 2009;1(4):301–13.
7. Jones KJ, Dines JS, Rebolledo BJ, et al. Operative management of ulnar collateral ligament insufficiency in adolescent athletes. Am J Sports Med 2014;42(1):117–21.
8. Cain EL Jr, Andrews JR, Dugas JR, et al. Outcome of ulnar collateral ligament reconstruction of the elbow in 1281 athletes: results in 743 athletes with minimum 2-year follow-up. Am J Sports Med 2010;38(12):2426–34.
9. Petty DH, Andrews JR, Fleisig GS, et al. Ulnar collateral ligament reconstruction in high school baseball players: clinical results and injury risk factors. Am J Sports Med 2004;32(5):1158–64.
10. Olsen SJ 2nd, Fleisig GS, Dun S, et al. Risk factors for shoulder and elbow injuries in adolescent baseball pitchers. Am J Sports Med 2006;34(6):905–12.
11. Hodgins JL, Vitale M, Arons RR, et al. Epidemiology of medial ulnar collateral ligament reconstruction: a 10-year study in New York State. Am J Sports Med 2016;44(3):729–34.
12. An KN, Morrey BF, Chao EY. The effect of partial removal of proximal ulna on elbow constraint. Clin Orthop Relat Res 1986;209:270–9.
13. Regan WD, Korinek SL, Morrey BF, et al. Biomechanical study of ligaments around the elbow joint. Clin Orthop Relat Res 1991;271:170–9.
14. Morrey BF, Tanaka S, An KN. Valgus stability of the elbow. A definition of primary and secondary constraints. Clin Orthop Relat Res 1991;265:187–95.
15. Farrow LD, Mahoney AJ, Stefancin JJ, et al. Quantitative analysis of the medial ulnar collateral ligament ulnar footprint and its relationship to the ulnar sublime tubercle. Am J Sports Med 2011;39(9):1936–41.
16. Floris S, Olsen BS, Dalstra M, et al. The medial collateral ligament of the elbow joint: anatomy and kinematics. J Shoulder Elbow Surg 1998;7(4):345–51.
17. Davidson PA, Pink M, Perry J, et al. Functional anatomy of the flexor pronator muscle group in relation to the medial collateral ligament of the elbow. Am J Sports Med 1995;23(2):245–50.
18. Werner SL, Fleisig GS, Dillman CJ, et al. Biomechanics of the elbow during baseball pitching. J Orthop Sports Phys Ther 1993;17(6):274–8.
19. Jones KJ, Osbahr DC, Schrumpf MA, et al. Ulnar collateral ligament reconstruction in throwing athletes: a review of current concepts. AAOS exhibit selection. J Bone Joint Surg Am 2012;94(8):e49.
20. Fleisig GS, Andrews JR, Dillman CJ, et al. Kinetics of baseball pitching with implications about injury mechanisms. Am J Sports Med 1995;23(2):233–9.
21. Dugas JR. Valgus extension overload: diagnosis and treatment. Clin Sports Med 2010;29(4):645–54.
22. Ahmad CS, ElAttrache NS. Valgus extension overload syndrome and stress injury of the olecranon. Clin Sports Med 2004;23(4):665–76, x.
23. Wilson FD, Andrews JR, Blackburn TA, et al. Valgus extension overload in the pitching elbow. Am J Sports Med 1983;11(2):83–8.
24. Fleisig G, Chu Y, Weber A, et al. Variability in baseball pitching biomechanics among various levels of competition. Sports Biomech 2009;8(1):10–21.
25. Hamilton CD, Glousman RE, Jobe FW, et al. Dynamic stability of the elbow: electromyographic analysis of the flexor pronator group and the extensor group in pitchers with valgus instability. J Shoulder Elbow Surg 1996;5(5):347–54.
26. Hang DW, Chao CM, Hang YS. A clinical and roentgenographic study of Little League elbow. Am J Sports Med 2004;32(1):79–84.
27. Chen FS, Diaz VA, Loebenberg M, et al. Shoulder and elbow injuries in the skeletally immature athlete. J Am Acad Orthop Surg 2005;13(3):172–85.
28. Fleisig GS, Andrews JR, Cutter GR, et al. Risk of serious injury for young baseball pitchers: a 10-year prospective study. Am J Sports Med 2011;39(2):253–7.
29. Andrews JR, Fleisig GS. Preventing throwing injuries. J Orthop Sports Phys Ther 1998;27(3):187–8.
30. Dun S, Loftice J, Fleisig GS, et al. A biomechanical comparison of youth baseball pitches: is the curveball potentially harmful? Am J Sports Med 2008;36(4):686–92.
31. Fleisig GS, Kingsley DS, Loftice JW, et al. Kinetic comparison among the fastball, curveball, change-up, and slider in collegiate baseball pitchers. Am J Sports Med 2006;34(3):423–30.
32. Nissen CW, Westwell M, Ounpuu S, et al. A biomechanical comparison of the fastball and curveball in adolescent baseball pitchers. Am J Sports Med 2009;37(8):1492–8.

33. Grantham WJ, Iyengar JJ, Byram IR, et al. The curveball as a risk factor for injury: a systematic review. Sports Health 2015;7(1):19–26.

34. Azar FM, Andrews JR, Wilk KE, et al. Operative treatment of ulnar collateral ligament injuries of the elbow in athletes. Am J Sports Med 2000;28(1):16–23.

35. Kocher MS, Waters PM, Micheli LJ. Upper extremity injuries in the paediatric athlete. Sports Med 2000; 30(2):117–35.

36. Lee GA, Katz SD, Lazarus MD. Elbow valgus stress radiography in an uninjured population. Am J Sports Med 1998;26(3):425–7.

37. Ellenbecker TS, Mattalino AJ, Elam EA, et al. Medial elbow joint laxity in professional baseball pitchers. A bilateral comparison using stress radiography. Am J Sports Med 1998;26(3):420–4.

38. Timmerman LA, Schwartz ML, Andrews JR. Preoperative evaluation of the ulnar collateral ligament by magnetic resonance imaging and computed tomography arthrography. Evaluation in 25 baseball players with surgical confirmation. Am J Sports Med 1994;22(1):26–31 [discussion: 2].

39. Bruce JR, Andrews JR. Ulnar collateral ligament injuries in the throwing athlete. J Am Acad Orthop Surg 2014;22(5):315–25.

40. Miller CD, Savoie FH 3rd. Valgus extension injuries of the elbow in the throwing athlete. J Am Acad Orthop Surg 1994;2(5):261–9.

41. Savoie FH 3rd, Trenhaile SW, Roberts J, et al. Primary repair of ulnar collateral ligament injuries of the elbow in young athletes: a case series of injuries to the proximal and distal ends of the ligament. Am J Sports Med 2008;36(6):1066–72.

42. Conway JE, Jobe FW, Glousman RE, et al. Medial instability of the elbow in throwing athletes. Treatment by repair or reconstruction of the ulnar collateral ligament. J Bone Joint Surg Am 1992;74(1): 67–83.

43. Mullen DJ, Goradia VK, Parks BG, et al. A biomechanical study of stability of the elbow to valgus stress before and after reconstruction of the medial collateral ligament. J Shoulder Elbow Surg 2002;11(3):259–64.

44. Smith GR, Altchek DW, Pagnani MJ, et al. A muscle-splitting approach to the ulnar collateral ligament of the elbow. Neuroanatomy and operative technique. Am J Sports Med 1996;24(5):575–80.

45. Andrews JR, Timmerman LA. Outcome of elbow surgery in professional baseball players. Am J Sports Med 1995;23(4):407–13.

46. Rohrbough JT, Altchek DW, Hyman J, et al. Medial collateral ligament reconstruction of the elbow using the docking technique. Am J Sports Med 2002; 30(4):541–8.

47. Dodson CC, Altchek DW. Ulnar collateral ligament reconstruction revisited: the procedure I use and why. Sports Health 2012;4(5):433–7.

48. Dines JS, ElAttrache NS, Conway JE, et al. Clinical outcomes of the DANE TJ technique to treat ulnar collateral ligament insufficiency of the elbow. Am J Sports Med 2007;35(12):2039–44.

49. Ahmad CS, Lee TQ, ElAttrache NS. Biomechanical evaluation of a new ulnar collateral ligament reconstruction technique with interference screw fixation. Am J Sports Med 2003;31(3):332–7.

50. Ciccotti MG, Siegler S, Kuri JA 2nd, et al. Comparison of the biomechanical profile of the intact ulnar collateral ligament with the modified Jobe and the Docking reconstructed elbow: an in vitro study. Am J Sports Med 2009;37(5):974–81.

51. Paletta GA Jr, Klepps SJ, Difelice GS, et al. Biomechanical evaluation of 2 techniques for ulnar collateral ligament reconstruction of the elbow. Am J Sports Med 2006;34(10):1599–603.

52. Armstrong AD, Dunning CE, Ferreira LM, et al. A biomechanical comparison of four reconstruction techniques for the medial collateral ligament-deficient elbow. J Shoulder Elbow Surg 2005;14(2): 207–15.

53. Watson JN, McQueen P, Hutchinson MR. A systematic review of ulnar collateral ligament reconstruction techniques. Am J Sports Med 2014; 42(10):2510–6.

54. Chen FS, Rokito AS, Jobe FW. Medial elbow problems in the overhead-throwing athlete. J Am Acad Orthop Surg 2001;9(2):99–113.

55. Vitale MA, Ahmad CS. The outcome of elbow ulnar collateral ligament reconstruction in overhead athletes: a systematic review. Am J Sports Med 2008; 36(6):1193–205.

56. Van Hofwegen C, Baker CL 3rd, Baker CL Jr. Epicondylitis in the athlete's elbow. Clin Sports Med 2010;29(4):577–97.

57. Gabel GT, Morrey BF. Operative treatment of medical epicondylitis. Influence of concomitant ulnar neuropathy at the elbow. J Bone Joint Surg Am 1995;77(7):1065–9.

58. Levin JS, Zheng N, Dugas J, et al. Posterior olecranon resection and ulnar collateral ligament strain. J Shoulder Elbow Surg 2004;13(1):66–71.

59. Andrews JR, Heggland EJ, Fleisig GS, et al. Relationship of ulnar collateral ligament strain to amount of medial olecranon osteotomy. Am J Sports Med 2001;29(6):716–21.

60. Farsetti P, Potenza V, Caterini R, et al. Long-term results of treatment of fractures of the medial humeral epicondyle in children. J Bone Joint Surg Am 2001; 83-A(9):1299–305.

61. Gottschalk HP, Eisner E, Hosalkar HS. Medial epicondyle fractures in the pediatric population. J Am Acad Orthop Surg 2012;20(4):223–32.

62. Redler LH, Degen RM, McDonald LS, et al. Elbow ulnar collateral ligament injuries in athletes: can we improve our outcomes? World J Orthop 2016;7(4):229–43.

63. Wilk KE, Yenchak AJ, Arrigo CA, et al. The advanced throwers ten exercise program: a new exercise series for enhanced dynamic shoulder control in the overhead throwing athlete. Phys Sportsmed 2011; 39(4):90–7.

64. Reinold MM, Wilk KE, Reed J, et al. Interval sport programs: guidelines for baseball, tennis, and golf. J Orthop Sports Phys Ther 2002;32(6):293–8.

65. Dodson CC, Thomas A, Dines JS, et al. Medial ulnar collateral ligament reconstruction of the elbow in throwing athletes. Am J Sports Med 2006;34(12): 1926–32.

66. Dines JS, Yocum LA, Frank JB, et al. Revision surgery for failed elbow medial collateral ligament reconstruction. Am J Sports Med 2008;36(6): 1061–5.

67. Jones KJ, Conte S, Patterson N, et al. Functional outcomes following revision ulnar collateral ligament reconstruction in Major League Baseball pitchers. J Shoulder Elbow Surg 2013;22(5):642–6.

68. Marshall NE, Keller RA, Lynch JR, et al. Pitching performance and longevity after revision ulnar collateral ligament reconstruction in Major League Baseball pitchers. Am J Sports Med 2015;43(5): 1051–6.

69. Liu JN, Garcia GH, Conte S, et al. Outcomes in revision Tommy John surgery in Major League Baseball pitchers. J Shoulder Elbow Surg 2016;25(1):90–7.

70. Thompson WH, Jobe FW, Yocum LA, et al. Ulnar collateral ligament reconstruction in athletes: muscle-splitting approach without transposition of the ulnar nerve. J Shoulder Elbow Surg 2001;10(2):152–7.

71. Paletta GA Jr, Wright RW. The modified docking procedure for elbow ulnar collateral ligament reconstruction: 2-year follow-up in elite throwers. Am J Sports Med 2006;34(10):1594–8.

72. Bowers AL, Dines JS, Dines DM, et al. Elbow medial ulnar collateral ligament reconstruction: clinical relevance and the docking technique. J Shoulder Elbow Surg 2010;19(Suppl 2):110–7.

Elbow Dislocations in Contact Sports

CrossMark

Mark S. Morris, MD[a], Kagan Ozer, MD[b],*

KEYWORDS

- Elbow dislocation • Contact sports • Athlete • Lateral ulnar collateral ligament

KEY POINTS

- Elbow dislocations are more common in athletes than in the general population.
- Simple elbow dislocations should be managed with early range of motion. Most simple elbow dislocations do not require surgery.
- Surgical management after simple elbow dislocation is indicated when the elbow remains unstable.
- The lateral ulnar collateral ligament (LUCL) is the most critical structure to repair or reconstruct.
- An athlete can safely return to play if there is no instability and he or she has a painless range of elbow motion.

EPIDEMIOLOGY

The elbow joint is the second most commonly dislocated large joint in the human body after the shoulder. Elbow dislocations occur in 5.1 per 100,000 people in the general population every year in the United States.[1] In a study using the National Electronic Injury Surveillance System database, approximately 44.5% of elbow dislocations were found to be sustained during sports.[1] Elbow dislocations in the National Football League (NFL) are reported to occur in 0.21 per 100,000 athlete exposures,[2] and represent 17.6% of all elbow injuries in NFL players.[3] Adolescent boys are at the highest risk for elbow dislocation (8.91 per 100,000 person-years in boys age 10–19). In high school athletes, 91.3% of dislocations are found in boys, most commonly in wrestling (46.1% of dislocations) and football (37.4% of dislocations).[4] In girls, gymnastics and skating are the most common sports resulting in elbow dislocations. Dislocations are more common in games than in practice in high school and NFL athletes.[3,4] The

mechanism is most commonly contact with another person (46.9%), followed by contact with the ground (46.0%). More than half (52%) of elbow dislocations in high school football players occur on running plays, with running backs being the most frequently the injured player (23.8%).[4]

With the rise in popularity of snowboarding, there has been an increase in elbow injuries. Elbow dislocations are significantly more common in snowboarders than skiers. Twenty-six percent of elbow injuries in snowboarders are dislocations, compared with 5.3% in skiers (P<.001). This is believed to be caused by fixed position of snowboarders' feet, as opposed to skiers who have independent movement of their lower extremities, which in turn results in more impact to upper extremities than lower.[5]

PATHOANATOMY
Osteoarticular and Ligamentous Anatomy

The elbow joint is a ginglymoid (hinged) joint and a trochoid (rotary motion) joint, consisting of the

Disclosures: The authors have no commercial or financial conflicts of interest.
[a] Department of Orthopaedic Surgery, University of Michigan, 1500 East Medical Center Drive TC2912, Ann Arbor, MI 48109-5328, USA; [b] Department of Orthopaedic Surgery, University of Michigan, 2098 South Main Street, Ann Arbor, MI 48103, USA
* Corresponding author.
E-mail address: kozer@med.umich.edu

distal humerus, proximal ulna, and radial head.[6] The olecranon and coronoid processes of the ulna articulate with the trochlea of the humerus. The concave radial head articulates with the convex capitellum of the humerus as an important secondary stabilizer.[7]

The coronoid process is the insertion point for the anterior capsule and the anterior band of the ulnar collateral ligament (UCL), also known as medial collateral ligament complex (MCL). The MCL is composed of anterior, posterior, and transverse bands. The anterior band is the primary static constraint for valgus instability. The anterior band originates from the anteroinferior medial epicondyle and inserts on the sublime tubercle of the coronoid process.[8]

The lateral collateral ligament (LCL) complex is made up of four components: (1) the radial collateral ligament, (2) the lateral ulnar collateral ligament (LUCL), (3) the annular ligament, and (4) the accessory collateral ligament.[9] The LCL complex origin is at the inferior lateral epicondyle. The radial collateral ligament inserts on the annular ligament and stabilizes the radial head. The LUCL inserts on the supinator crest of the ulna. It is a primary static stabilizer of the elbow, providing varus and posterolateral rotatory stability.[10] The annular ligament inserts on the anterior and posterior margins of the lesser sigmoid notch. The radial collateral ligament or the LUCL can be ruptured without resulting in posterolateral rotatory instability when the annular ligament is intact.[11] The accessory collateral ligament inserts on the annular ligament and the on the supinator crest.

The primary stabilizers of the elbow are the ulnotrochlear joint, MCL, and LCL complex. The secondary stabilizers include the radial head, the anterior and posterior joint capsule, and the common flexor and extensor muscle origins. In addition, there are also dynamic stabilizers of the elbow joint. These include the anconeus, biceps, brachialis, and the triceps muscles.

Simple dislocations are defined as dissociation of the ulnohumeral joint without fracture. Complex dislocations are those that are associated with a fracture. Associated fractures include radial head and neck, coronoid, and medial and lateral epicondyles. Most elbow dislocations are simple and posterior in direction.[12]

O'Driscoll and coworkers[10] proposed the term posterolateral rotatory instability to describe the sequence of events that results in an elbow dislocation. Posterolateral rotatory instability results from a fall on an outstretched arm, combined with a rotation of the body on a fixed hand. This results in progressive ligamentous and capsular injury with four consecutive stages:

- Stage I: LUCL disruption, and possible injury to radial collateral ligament and posterolateral capsule.
- Stage II: Ulna (coronoid) perches on the distal humerus. There is disruption of the anterior and posterior capsule. Such an elbow would have a positive lateral pivot-shift test, varus instability, but maintained stability to valgus stress (because the anterior band of the UCL is intact).
- Stage IIIa: Further disruption of the posterior UCL with increased external rotation. Posterior dislocation occurs with axial compression. The coronoid slips under the trochlea and comes to rest posterior to it. The anterior band of the UCL is still intact, so valgus stability is maintained.
- Stage IIIb: Disruption of the anterior band of the UCL.

Although this has historically been the accepted mechanism of posterolateral rotatory instability, others have suggested that at times, dislocation may start medially.[13] Nonetheless, posterior elbow dislocations result in various degrees of ligamentous injuries on the lateral aspect of the elbow. On a much rare form of this injury, the elbow may dislocate posteriorly as a result of an anteriorly directed force. In this rate injury pattern, all anterior structures including anterior portion of the UCL, joint capsule, and brachialis muscle are ruptured (**Figs. 1** and **2**).

EVALUATION OF PATIENT WITH A DISLOCATED ELBOW
Examination

Deformity is usually obvious in the acute setting. Neurovascular examination is important before and after reduction. The ulnar nerve is the most frequently injured nerve; however, both median and radial nerve injuries have been reported.[14–16] Arterial injuries occur in 0.3% to 6% of closed elbow dislocations and in up to 33% of open elbow dislocations.[17–19]

Imaging

Some authors advocate immediate reduction at the sporting event,[20] whereas others argue for radiographs before reduction to identify any associated fractures and to assess the congruency of the joint.[21] We recommend anteroposterior (AP) and lateral radiographs of the elbow before and after reduction. On the lateral radiograph, an ulnohumeral distance (measured from the trochlear sulcus to the olecranon) of greater than or equal to 4 mm is referred to as a positive "drop sign," and

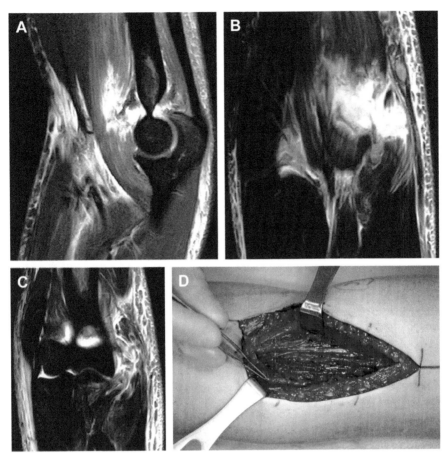

Fig. 1. A 17-year-old football player who got his right elbow caught in extension between two players running in opposite directions at full speed. He had a closed elbow dislocation as a result of an anteriorly directed force resulting in complete disruption of the anterior capsule, near complete disruptions of the brachialis (A), and pronator teres muscles (B). The lateral collateral ligament appears to be intact (C). Intraoperative findings confirmed the injury to the brachialis muscle, which was repaired using 2.0 braided nonabsorbable sutures (D).

suggests instability and may require surgical stabilization.[22] An oblique lateral view (Greenspan view) can provide better visualization of the radial head detect minimally displaced radial head, coronoid, or capitellum fractures.[23]

MRI in the acute setting has limited utility.[24] We do not obtain an MRI in the acute setting. Vascular studies are only required if limb vascularity is compromised. Fluoroscopy can be used during or after reduction to assess stability through the

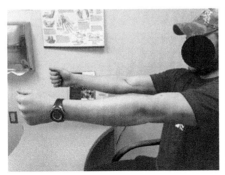 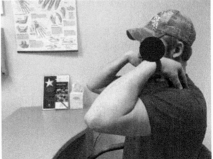

Fig. 2. The patient had full pain-free range of motion 3.5 months following surgery.

arc of motion, and with varus or valgus stress on the elbow joint.

Acute Management of Elbow Dislocation

Reduction of an elbow dislocation should be performed as rapidly as possible. Reduction usually requires conscious sedation or an intra-articular local anesthetic injection. In general, reduction requires correction of medial or lateral displacement followed by longitudinal traction and flexion of the elbow. There are multiple acceptable techniques for reduction of elbow dislocations. The following is a short summary of those methods[24–27]:

- The patient is prone on a table with the affected extremity hanging over the side of the table. Gentle downward traction is applied at the wrist and the necessary time is taken for reduction to occur (usually between 1 and 10 minutes; forceful traction results in spasm and failure). When the olecranon is felt to perch on the humerus, the operator maintains traction on the wrist with one hand while gently lifting the humerus to flex the elbow about 20°, completing the reduction.[25]
- The patient is placed prone, with the humerus supported by the bed and only the forearm hanging free over the table. Gentle downward traction is applied on the wrist with one hand while the operator guides reduction of the olecranon with the opposite hand.[26]
- The elbow is hypersupinated to clear the coronoid from the distal humerus and then extended with a valgus stress applied. Pushing the olecranon distally then reduces the joint. Reduction is often noticed by a palpable clunk.[24]
- The patient is positioned supine and pulled to the edge of the table or stretcher. The patient's elbow is flexed to 90°. For a right elbow dislocation, the operator first places his or her left mid-humerus in the patient's right antecubital fossa with the shoulder flexed to 90°. The operator flexes his or her left elbow while grasping the patient's right wrist or hand with his or her left hand. The operator can now internally or externally rotate his or her shoulder to flex or extend the patient's elbow. The operator's right hand is now placed on the patient's volar forearm to create axial traction. At the same time, the operator extends his or her left forearm in a dart-throwing motion. The left hand can also be used to hypersupinate the forearm to unlock the radius before extension of the elbow.[27]

Regardless of the technique, adequate relaxation is the key to success. At the time of the reduction, a palpable clunk is often felt, and the patient has a feeling of relief. Neurovascular status should be reevaluated after reduction. Under fluoroscopy, the elbow should be visualized in full flexion and extension to ensure its stability.[28]

Operative Versus Nonoperative Management

Next, the most important step is the assessment of stability. Following reduction, the examiner should flex and extend the elbow to assess its stability. If the elbow subluxes or dislocates in extension, stability should then be assessed with the forearm in pronation. In an elbow with an LCL complex injury, pronation hinges the elbow closed on the medial side. If stable in pronation, the elbow should be splinted in 90° of flexion and with the forearm pronated. If the elbow is unstable in less than 30° of flexion with the forearm pronated, it is splinted in 90° of flexion and neutral rotation.[24] If more than 30° to 45° of flexion is required for stability with the forearm pronated, surgical intervention should be considered to address a collateral ligament injury.[21] If the elbow is more stable in supination, however, this suggests that the injury is isolated to the MCL.[21] For a simple elbow dislocation that is stable throughout the arc of motion, splinting may not be necessary and may actually result in elbow contracture.[29] In this case, patients can instead be discharged with a sling for comfort and encouraged to start early motion of the elbow.[21,30]

Nonoperative management

Most simple elbow dislocations are managed nonoperatively with excellent outcomes.[31] Historically, plaster splinting for 3 weeks was accepted as the method of treatment of simple elbow dislocation; however, this is associated with significant limitations in elbow range of motion.[29,32] Protzman[33] studied 49 simple elbow dislocations in US Military Academy cadets (41 caused by sports activities). He found that all patients had normal range of motion in flexion, pronation, and supination at final follow-up (average, 24.5 months; range, 5–54 months). Those that were immobilized for less than 5 days had an average extension loss of 3°, whereas those immobilized for greater than 5 days had an average of 11° extension loss and longer periods of disability. The FuncSIE trial (FUNCtional treatment vs plaster for SImple Elbow dislocations) was a multicenter parallel group randomized trial designed to compare outcomes after early mobilization after 2 days compared with 3 weeks of plaster immobilization in patients with simple elbow dislocations.[30] After 6 weeks, early motion patients had better Quick-DASH and Oxford Elbow Score functional outcome scores, and a larger arc of elbow motion than those treated with immobilization. No differences were found at 1 year.

If there is no instability on postreduction examination, early range of active motion should be started a few days after injury. If instability is present in extension, the elbow is braced with an extension block just before the point in extension where instability occurs. Bracing can usually be discontinued after 3 to 4 weeks, and a stretching program started to regain motion.[24] Postreduction radiographs of the elbow should show a concentrically reduced joint. A positive "drop sign" as discussed previously suggests instability and may indicate a need for surgical stabilization.[22] However, in some patients, muscle activation exercises have been shown to stabilize the joint even when there is joint space widening on postreduction radiographs.[34]

Operative management

After simple elbow dislocation, only 2.3% of patients in the general population require stabilization surgery. Admission to a hospital for reduction independently increases the likelihood of undergoing stabilization surgery (hazard ratio, 2.50; 95% confidence interval, 1.67–3.74; P<.0001) compared with those who are discharged after reduction.[35] Elbow dislocation results in surgical treatment in 13.6% of high school athletes.[4]

Surgical management after simple elbow dislocation is indicated when the elbow remains unstable by physical examination (discussed later). The LUCL is the most critical structure to repair or reconstruct and is therefore addressed first. The LUCL typically avulses from the lateral epicondyle and can usually be repaired in acute cases (<4–6 weeks after injury) but often requires reconstruction in chronic cases (>4–6 weeks after injury).

Patients do well overall after LUCL repair or reconstruction. Olsen and Søjbjerg[36] studied a group of 18 patients after LUCL reconstruction. They found that 17 of 18 (94%) patients were satisfied with their outcome, and 15 of 18 (83%) returned to preaccident activity by the last follow-up visit (average, 44 months). Mayo Elbow Performance scores were excellent or good in 89% of patients at the last follow-up visit. They had one failure requiring revision because of a failed graft. Jones and coworkers[37] studied eight patients who had LUCL reconstruction and found that at a mean of 7.1 years postoperative, six of eight (75%) had resolution of elbow instability, whereas two of eight (25%) had occasional instability with activities of daily living. Mayo Elbow Performance scores at final follow-up (average,

7.1 years) averaged 87.5 (range, 75–100), which is in the good range. In a study of 12 direct LUCL repairs and 33 LUCL reconstructions, Sanchez-Sotelo and coworkers[38] found excellent Mayo Elbow Performance scores in 19, good in 13, fair in seven, and poor in five patients at 6 years after the surgery. Thirty-eight out of 44 patients (86%) were satisfied with their outcome in this study. Five patients in this study had persistent instability, requiring revision in two of the five patients. Four additional patients required further surgery, one because of heterotopic ossification, and the remaining three underwent interposition arthroplasty for posttraumatic arthritis of the elbow. A systematic review calculated the mean elbow range of motion at final follow-up after LUCL repair or reconstruction to be 3° to 138° of flexion.[39]

Return to Sport After Nonoperative Management

Return to play seems to correlate with athletes' ability to regain full or near full, pain-free active range of motion. In a study of NFL athletes, those who sustained injuries resulting in elbow instability (including sprains, dislocation, or subluxation) missed an average of 14 days of practice and play, with no reinjury rate reported.[2] In high school athletes in all sports combined, an elbow dislocation results in removal from play for more than 3 weeks in 23% of athletes, and ends their season in 37%. This is significantly longer than other elbow injuries in this population (P<.0001).[4] Specifically in wrestlers, time off from wrestling is more than 3 weeks in 46.0%, with 42.0% of them being medically disqualified for the remainder of the season.[4]

It is important to remember that these reported rates are based a simple elbow dislocation treated with a sling for a 3 to 4 days followed by early active motion. Otherwise, if the elbow needs to be immobilized longer, overall return to play is also delayed. In Protzman's study[33] of military cadets who sustained simple elbow dislocations, patients who were immobilized for less than 5 days were able to return to full duty after an average of 6 weeks, whereas those who were immobilized for 10 to 15 days did not return to full duty for an average of 19 weeks. Patients who were immobilized for more than 20 days did not return to full duty for an average of 24 weeks. More recent case reports also agree with this finding that longer the immobilization required for treatment, more delayed is the return to play.[40,41]

No clear rules exist for return to sport after an elbow dislocation. Existing publications related to return to play are case series or expert opinions.

Each athlete must be treated individually based on his or her symptoms and examination. Return to sport should be delayed until the elbow is comfortable and has painless near-normal range of motion with symmetric strength to the contralateral upper extremity. Valgus and posterolateral rotatory instability tests should not cause pain or apprehension before return.[21] Most athletes can return to sport in a hinged brace within 2 to 4 weeks of a simple dislocation. In cases that require surgery, the timing of return to sport is variable in the literature, ranging from 3 to 12 months after surgery. Most authors advocate the use of a hinged brace when initiating work on elbow range of motion.[28,36–38,42–44] One study reported a return to preinjury level of activity in 83% of patients after LUCL reconstruction at an average of 44 months postoperative.[36]

EVALUATION OF PATIENTS WITH CHRONIC INSTABILITY
Examination

Chronic elbow instability is defined in various ways in the literature, but generally refers to patients who are more than 4 to 6 weeks out from elbow dislocation with signs of instability on clinical examination.[45,46] They often present with a history of persistent, recurring pain, with clicking, catching, or subluxation during range of motion. Examination may need to be performed under anesthesia depending on the patient's compliance.[47] Several tests are described next for examination of posterolateral rotatory instability:

- Lateral pivot shift: this is performed with the patient supine and the extremity overhead, with the shoulder externally rotated. With the forearm fully supinated, the examiner slowly flexes the elbow while applying valgus stress, supination, and axial compression. At 40°, rotatory displacement is maximized and a dimple is seen in the skin proximal to the radial head and a clunk is felt. If this test is performed with the patient awake, apprehension is also considered a positive test.[10]
- Posterolateral rotatory drawer test: this test is performed by pulling posteriorly on the lateral side of the proximal forearm. A positive test is considered to be when apprehension or a dimple is present.[48]
- Prone push-up test: the patient is instructed to perform a push-up off the floor with the elbows flexed at 90° with the forearms supinated and shoulders abducted. Apprehension or radial head dislocation as the elbow extends are considered a positive test.[49]

- Chair push-up test: the patient is seated with elbows flexed at 90° with forearms supinated and shoulders abducted. The patient pushes down on the chair to rise. The test is positive if there is apprehension or radial head dislocation as the elbow extends.[49]
- Table-top relocation test: the patient performs a press-up on the edge of a table using the affected arm, with the forearm in supination. Apprehension occurs at 40° of elbow flexion and is relieved when the examiner presses on the radial head, which prevents subluxation.[49–51]

Some authors also advocate arthroscopy in the evaluation of elbow instability.[46,52] Arthroscopy can detect even mild forms of instability, cartilage damage, and help evacuate a hemarthrosis.

Imaging of Chronic Elbow Instability
Radiographs
Initial imaging modality is performed, including AP and lateral views. On the lateral radiograph, an ulnohumeral distance (measured from the trochlear sulcus to the olecranon) of greater than or equal to 4 mm is referred to as a positive "drop sign," and suggests instability and may require surgical stabilization.[22] Stress radiographs or examination of posterolateral rotatory instability under fluoroscopy is used and can avoid the cost of an MRI.[53] AP radiographs during posterolateral rotatory stress test may show malalignment of the ulnohumeral joint, and overlap of the radial head and capitellum.[54]

MRI
MRI is considered if a patient has continued instability on examination after 2 to 3 weeks of splinting in a hinged brace, or in patients with recurrent dislocations. MRI should also be considered in a patient who is symptomatic and unable to comply with physical examination. Patients with a stable examination after acute dislocation do not require MRI.

This is performed with the elbow positioned in 20° to 30° of flexion. Collateral ligaments are best visualized on coronal images. In the setting of posterolateral rotatory instability, the LUCL and radial collateral ligament are typically avulsed from their humeral attachments, and there is posterior displacement of the radial head and ulna with respect to the humerus.[23]

Radiocapitellar incongruity greater than 2 mm on the sagittal cuts and ulnohumeral incongruity greater than 1 mm on the axial cuts are highly suggestive of elbow instability.[46] Radiocapitellar incongruity is measured on the sagittal cut through the center of the radial head. A line is drawn at the longitudinal axis of the radius through the center of the radial head and extended through the capitellum. The distance between this line and the rotational center of the capitellum is the radiocapitellar incongruity (**Fig. 3**A). Ulnohumeral incongruity is measured on the axial cuts, through the motion axis of the distal humerus. The distance between the trochlear joint surface and the olecranon joint surface is measured at four points: the ulnar edge, radial edge, and two points in between. The difference between the highest and lowest values represents the ulnohumeral joint space incongruity (see **Fig. 3**B).

Repair Versus Reconstruction

Some authors suggest that primary LUCL repair is no longer possible after as little as 2 weeks postinjury.[52] Lee and Teo[42] retrospectively compared a group of 10 patients who either had repair or reconstruction of the LUCL at an average of 10.4 months postinjury, and concluded that reconstruction was more reliable in achieving an excellent outcome. In a larger study of 44 patients who had either ligament repair or reconstruction at 2.8 years postinjury, Sanchez-Sotelo and coworkers[38] also found that patients who had reconstruction with tendon graft had better results than those who underwent ligament repair when comparing Mayo elbow performance scores.

However, Daluiski and coworkers[45] did show that direct repair was possible in chronic disruptions of the LUCL (average 513 days to surgery), with no significant difference in clinical outcome or range of motion when compared with direct repairs in acute cases (average 9 days to surgery).

Return to Sport After Surgery for Chronic Elbow Instability

In a recent systematic review of seven articles[28,36–38,42,43,45] including 148 patients treated operatively for posterolateral rotatory instability of the elbow, strength training was started between 6 and 8 weeks, and average return to sport varied from 3 to 12 months postoperatively.[55] **Table 1** shows further details of each study included in the systematic review. Although most studies did not mention the level of performance after return, one study reported a return to preinjury level of activity in 83% of their patients.[36]

Studies published in the current literature show a great variation in method of fixation and postoperative rehabilitation. Two studies reported direct repair of the LUCL,[43,45] four reported reconstruction with a free graft,[28,36,37,42] and one had combination of repair and reconstruction.[38] Immobilization in a splint or cast ranges from 1 day to 6 weeks after surgery, and followed by hinged bracing up to 12 weeks.[55] Previous authors have implemented various combinations of limitations of extension or

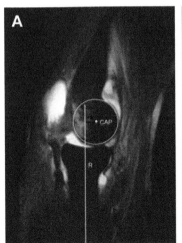 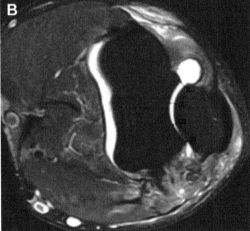

Fig. 3. (*A*) A Measurement of radiocapitellar incongruity (A). Sagittal view through the center of the radial head. The rotational center of the capitulum (CAP) was marked. A line was drawn along the longitudinal axis of the radius (R) through the center of the radial head. The radial head was centered on a coronal (mediolateral) and sagittal (anteroposterior) view. The distance between CAP and R (perpendicular to R) represents the radiocapitellar incongruity (A). (*B*) Measurement of axial ulnohumeral incongruity (D). Axial view through the motion axis of the distal humerus. The distance of the trochlear joint surface to the corresponding joint surface of the olecranon was measured at the ulnar edge (D1) and radial edge (D4), and at two points in between (D2 and D3). (*From* Hackl M, Wegmann K, Ries C, et al. Reliability of magnetic resonance imaging signs of posterolateral rotatory instability of the elbow. J Hand Surg 2015;40(7):1430–1; with permission.)

Table 1
Outcomes after LUCL repair or reconstruction

Study	N	Surgery	Mean Length of Follow-up (mo)	Postoperative Elbow Range of Motion	Mayo Elbow Performance Score	Timing of Return to Sport	Complications
Olsen & Søjbjerg,[36] 2003	18	Reconstruction	44	83% with no reduction in range of motion	92 (60–100)	Return to sport allowed at 6 mo	1 patient with continued instability requiring revision; 1 patient with persistent paralysis of ulnar nerve (sustained at time of dislocation)
Lee & Teo,[42] 2003	10	Reconstruction	24.1	6.5–135		Return to sport allowed at 9 mo	1 postoperative hematoma requiring surgical drainage
Sanchez-Sotelo, et al,[38] 2005	44	12 direct repair 32 reconstruction	72	7–140	85 (60–100)	Full activity allowed at 6 mo, contact sports allowed at 1 y	5 atraumatic recurrent instability, 2 traumatic dislocations, 7 revisions (3 for instability, 1 developed heterotopic ossification, 3 posttraumatic arthritis requiring interposition arthroplasty)
Lin et al,[28] 2012	14	Reconstruction	49	10–132	93 (65–100)	Return to sports allowed at 9 mo	1 revision for persistent instability
Jones et al,[37] 2012	8	Reconstruction	85.2	75% of patients full range of motion, 25% with loss of 5–10° of extension	87.5 (75–100)	Return to full activity allowed at 4–6 mo	No complications or reoperations
Kim et al,[43] 2013	19	Repair	6.6	13–120	86.9 (65–100)	Full activity allowed at 3 mo	1 patient with knot irritation, 5 patients with ectopic ossification
Daluiski et al,[45] 2014	34 (18 acute, 16 delayed)	Direct repair	42	Acute repair group: 18–133 Delayed repair group: 21–137	Acute repair group: 90 Delayed repair group: 89		2 failures of repair requiring intervention

Data from Refs. 28,36–38,42,43,45

flexion range of motion for 6 weeks postoperative.[28,36–38,42,43,45]

There is no consensus regarding rehabilitation and return to sport after operative treatment of posterolateral rotatory instability of the elbow. Each patient should be treated on an individual basis, based on his or her symptoms and athletic demands.

SUMMARY

Elbow dislocations are more common in athletes than in the general population. Simple elbow dislocations should be managed with early range of motion and early return to sport, even with high-level contact athletes. Patients with instability on examination or with complex elbow dislocations may require surgical intervention. Overall, the outcomes after simple elbow dislocations are excellent and athletes should be able to return to play without significant limitations.

REFERENCES

1. Stoneback JW, Owens BD, Sykes J, et al. Incidence of elbow dislocations in the United States population. J Bone Joint Surg Am 2012;94(3):240–5.
2. Carlisle JC, Goldfarb CA, Mall N, et al. Upper extremity injuries in the National Football League: Part II: elbow, forearm, and wrist injuries. Am J Sports Med 2008;36(10):1945–52.
3. Kenter K, Behr CT, Warren RF, et al. Acute elbow injuries in the National Football League. J Shoulder Elbow Surg 2000;9(1):1–5.
4. Dizdarevic I, Low S, Currie DW, et al. Epidemiology of elbow dislocations in high school athletes. Am J Sports Med 2015;44(1):202–8.
5. Takagi M, Sasaki K, Kiyoshige Y, et al. Fracture and dislocation of snowboarder's elbow. J Trauma 1999; 47(1):77–81.
6. Bryce CD, Armstrong AD. Anatomy and biomechanics of the elbow. Orthop Clin North Am 2008; 39(2):141–54.
7. Kovacevic D, Vogel LA, Levine WN. Complex elbow instability. Hand Clin 2015;31(4):547–56.
8. Deutch SR, Olsen BS, Jensen SL, et al. Ligamentous and capsular restraints to experimental posterior elbow joint dislocation. Scand J Med Sci Sports 2003;13(5):311–6.
9. Imatani J, Ogura T, Morito Y, et al. Anatomic and histologic studies of lateral collateral ligament complex of the elbow joint. J Shoulder Elbow Surg 1999;8(6): 625–7.
10. O'Driscoll SW, Bell DF, Morrey BF. Posterolateral rotatory instability of the elbow. J Bone Joint Surg Am 1991;73(3):440–6.
11. Dunning CD, Zarzour ZD, Patterson SD, et al. Ligamentous stabilizers against posterolateral rotatory instability of the elbow. J Bone Joint Surg Am 2001;83(12):1823–8.
12. Rettig AC. Traumatic elbow injuries in the athlete. Orthop Clin North Am 2002;33(3):509–22.
13. Rhyou IH, Kim YS. New mechanism of the posterior elbow dislocation. Knee Surg Sports Traumatol Arthrosc 2012;20(12):2535–41.
14. Galbraith KA, Mccullough CJ. Acute nerve injury as a complication of closed fractures or dislocations of the elbow. Injury 1979;11(2):159–64.
15. Adams JE, Steinmann SP. Nerve injuries about the elbow. J Hand Surg 2006;31(2):303–13.
16. Carter SJ, Germann CA, Dacus AA, et al. Orthopedic pitfalls in the ED: neurovascular injury associated with posterior elbow dislocations. Am J Emerg Med 2010;28(8):960–5.
17. Endea ED, Veldenz HC, Schwarcz TH, et al. Recognition of arterial injury in elbow dislocation. J Vasc Surg 1992;16(3):402–6.
18. Marcheix B, Chaufour X, Ayel J, et al. Transection of the brachial artery after closed posterior elbow dislocation. J Vasc Surg 2005;42(6):1230–2.
19. Ayel JE, Bonnevialle N, Lafosse JM, et al. Acute elbow dislocation with arterial rupture: analysis of nine cases. Orthop Traumatol Surg Res 2009; 95(5):343–51.
20. Skelley NW, Mccormick JJ, Smith MV. In-game management of common joint dislocations. Sports Health 2013;6(3):246–55.
21. Mcguire DT, Bain GI. Management of dislocations of the elbow in the athlete. Sports Med Arthrosc 2014; 22(3):188–93.
22. Coonrad RW, Roush TF, Major NM, et al. The drop sign, a radiographic warning sign of elbow instability. J Shoulder Elbow Surg 2005;14(3):312–7.
23. Beltran L, Bencardino J, Beltran J. Imaging of sports ligamentous injuries of the elbow. Semin Musculoskelet Radiol 2013;17(5):455–65.
24. Parsons BO, Ramsey ML. Acute elbow dislocations in athletes. Clin Sports Med 2010;29(4):599–609.
25. Parvin RW. Closed reduction of common shoulder and elbow dislocations without anesthesia. Arch Surg 1957;75(6):972–5.
26. Meyn MA, Quigley TB. Reduction of posterior dislocation of the elbow by traction on the dangling arm. Clin Orthop Relat Res 1974;(103):106–8.
27. Skelley NW, Chamberlain A. A novel reduction technique for elbow dislocations. Orthopedics 2015; 38(1):42–4.
28. Lin KY, Shen PH, Lee CH, et al. Functional outcomes of surgical reconstruction for posterolateral rotatory instability of the elbow. Injury 2012;43(10):1657–61.
29. Mehlhoff TL, Noble MS, Bennett JB, et al. Simple dislocation of the elbow in the adult. J Bone Joint Surg Am 1988;70(2):244–9.

30. Iordens GT, Van Lieshout EMM, Schep NWL, et al. Early mobilisation versus plaster immobilisation of simple elbow dislocations: results of the FuncSiE multicentre randomised clinical trial. Br J Sports Med 2015;0:1–9.

31. de Haan J, Schep NWL, Zengerink I, et al. Dislocation of the elbow: a retrospective multicentre study of 86 patients. Open Orthop J 2010;4:76–9.

32. Kesmezacar H, Sarikaya IA. The results of conservatively treated simple elbow dislocations. Acta Orthop Traumatol Turc 2010;44(3):199–205.

33. Protzman RR. Dislocation of the elbow joint. J Bone Joint Surg Am 1978;60(4):539–41.

34. Duckworth AD, Kulijdian A, Mckee MD, et al. Residual subluxation of the elbow after dislocation or fracture-dislocation: treatment with active elbow exercises and avoidance of varus stress. J Shoulder Elbow Surg 2008;17(2):276–80.

35. Modi CS, Wasserstein D, Mayne IP, et al. The frequency and risk factors for subsequent surgery after a simple elbow dislocation. Injury 2015;46(6):1156–60.

36. Olsen BS, Søjbjerg JO. The treatment of recurrent posterolateral instability of the elbow. J Bone Joint Surg Am 2003;85(3):342–6.

37. Jones KJ, Dodson CC, Osbahr DC, et al. The docking technique for lateral ulnar collateral ligament reconstruction: surgical technique and clinical outcomes. J Shoulder Elbow Surg 2012;21(3):389–95.

38. Sanchez-Sotelo J, Morrey BF, O'Driscoll SW. Ligamentous repair and reconstruction for posterolateral rotatory instability of the elbow. J Bone Joint Surg Br 2005;87:54–61.

39. Anakwenze OA, Kwon D, O'Donnel E, et al. Surgical treatment of posterolateral rotatory instability of the elbow. Arthroscopy 2014;30(7):866–71.

40. Uhl TL, Gould M, Gieck JH. Rehabilitation after posterolateral dislocation of the elbow in a collegiate football player: a case report. J Athl Train 2000;35(1):108–10.

41. Verrall GM. Return to Australian Rules football after acute elbow dislocation: a report of three cases and review of the literature. J Sci Med Sport 2001; 4(2):245–50.

42. Lee BPH, Teo LHY. Surgical reconstruction for posterolateral rotatory instability of the elbow. J Shoulder Elbow Surg 2003;12(5):476–9.

43. Kim BS, Park KH, Park SY. Ligamentous repair of acute lateral collateral ligament rupture of the elbow. J Shoulder Elbow Surg 2013;22:1469–73.

44. Mccabe MP, Savoie FH. Simple elbow dislocations: evaluation, management, and outcomes. Phys Sportsmed 2012;40(1):62–71.

45. Daluiski A, Schrumpf MA, Schreiber JJ, et al. Direct repair for managing acute and chronic lateral ulnar collateral ligament disruptions. J Hand Surg 2014; 39(6):1125–9.

46. Hackl M, Wegmann K, Ries C, et al. Reliability of magnetic resonance imaging signs of posterolateral rotatory instability of the elbow. J Hand Surg 2015; 40(7):1428–33.

47. Ahmed I, Mistry J. The management of acute and chronic elbow instability. Orthop Clin North Am 2015;46(2):271–80.

48. O'Driscoll SW, Jupiter JB, King GJ, et al. The unstable elbow. Instr Course Lect 2001;50:89–102.

49. Regan W, Lapner PC. Prospective evaluation of two diagnostic apprehension signs for posterolateral instability of the elbow. J Shoulder Elbow Surg 2006;15(3):344–6.

50. Arvind CH, Hargreaves DG. Table top relocation test: new clinical test for posterolateral rotatory instability of the elbow. J Shoulder Elbow Surg 2006; 15(4):500–1.

51. Arvind CH, Hargreaves DG. Tabletop relocation test: a new clinical test for posterolateral rotatory instability of the elbow. J Shoulder Elbow Surg 2006; 15(6):707–8.

52. Dehlinger F, Franke S, Hollinger B. Therapeutic options for acute and chronic elbow instability. Eur J Trauma Emerg Surg 2012;38(6):585–92.

53. Reichel LM, Milam GS, Sitton SE, et al. Elbow lateral collateral ligament injuries. J Hand Surg 2013;38(1): 184–201.

54. O'Driscoll SW. Classification and evaluation of recurrent instability of the elbow. Clin Orthop Relat Res 2000;(370):34–43.

55. Reuter S, Proier P, Imhoff A, et al. Rehabilitation, clinical outcome and return to sporting activities after posterolateral elbow instability: a systematic review. Eur J Phys Rehabil Med 2016. [Epub ahead of print].

Management of Upper Extremity Injury in Divers

Steven C. Haase, MD[a,b,]*

KEYWORDS

- Hand injury • Wrist injury • Divers • Diving

KEY POINTS

- Competitive diving techniques apply repetitive stress to the hands and wrists.
- Injury may be acute or chronic in nature and is often bilateral.
- Many injuries require operative intervention.

INTRODUCTION

Diving is a popular sport around the world, having been a part of the Olympic Games since 1904. In that year, the competitors were all men, and the diving events consisted of 10-m platform diving and a plunge for distance event. Although the latter was quickly dropped from the Games, 10-m platform diving was expanded to include women in 1912 and continues to be an Olympic event in the twenty-first century. Modern Olympic diving events also include 3-m springboard for men and women as well as synchronized diving counterparts for each of these disciplines.[1,2]

Competitive diving requires great strength and flexibility as well as proprioception and kinesthetic sense so that the diver can execute complex acrobatic maneuvers in the course of the dive. In this regard, the diver's skill set closely resembles that of a gymnast. A dive is scored by a panel of judges, with consideration to all 3 parts of the dive: takeoff, flight, and water entry. The basic technical score is then subjected to a multiplier that increases depending on the difficulty of the attempted dive. The difficulty of dives at competitions has steadily increased over the past 30 years.

DIVING PHYSICS

Applying the laws of physics, it is known that a diver falling from a 10-m height accelerates to just about 14.1 m/s (31.5 mph) before impacting the surface of the water. le Viet and colleagues[3] were able to confirm speeds of 14 m/s to 15 m/s with cinematographic analysis. If a diver's launch from the platform adds additional height to the dive, the final speed is even greater. Speeds in excess of 16.4 m/s (36.8 mph) have been postulated.[2] This leads to a significant impact at the surface of the water: between 2.0 g and 2.4 g (1 g = 9.8 m/s^2). With this force of impact comes the risk of serious injury.

During the flight portion of the dive, the diver often spins and/or twists through several complex rotations while airborne. Due to inertia, it is impossible to halt these motions completely at the end of a dive to obtain a smooth, vertical entry into the water. To create the illusion of a more vertical entry, divers time their entry into the water carefully and rely on underwater saves to quickly rotate the body forward or backward, camouflaging any residual rotational motion that might detract from their score. Often, these saves require rapid shoulder and wrist motions to swim out of the dive quickly and minimize splash. These maneuvers can lead to additional upper extremity injury.

WATER ENTRY

Every competitive diver's goal is to enter the water in a vertical position, with as little splash as

Disclosure Statement: The author has nothing to disclose.
[a] Department of Surgery, University of Michigan Health System, Ann Arbor, MI, USA; [b] Department of Orthopaedic Surgery, University of Michigan Health System, Ann Arbor, MI, USA
* 1500 East Medical Center Drive, 2130 Taubman Center, Ann Arbor, MI 48109.
E-mail address: shaase@med.umich.edu

Hand Clin 33 (2017) 73–80
http://dx.doi.org/10.1016/j.hcl.2016.08.017
0749-0712/17/© 2016 Elsevier Inc. All rights reserved.

possible, to maximize the score for the dive. A perfect water entry—vertical position with minimal splash—is termed a *rip entry*. Choices for water entry are feet-first, with arms held against the sides of the body, or hands-first, with the arms raised over the head and elbows extended. Although dives with advanced difficulty, including multiple flips and twists, have been developed for both feet-first and hands-first entries, divers prefer hands-first dives for several reasons. First, hands-first dives are typically more graceful and appealing to both audience and judges. Second, hands-first dives offer better consistency and control. The diver can see the water during the entry for better timing and positioning. Also, the hands-first position allows the diver to more easily execute a forward or backward somersault (or swim out) on entry—these moves are critical to creating a good save for a nonvertical dive. Finally, the hands-first position provides a cleaner entry (ie, one with less of a splash) than a feet-first entry. For these reasons, Olympic and other elite divers always choose a hands-first entry over feet-first.[4]

The position of the diver's hands at the time of impact with the water has a direct effect on how much of a splash is created. Two principal types of hand positions have been used over the years. The older thumb-in-fist technique involved positioning the hands into side-by-side fists, with the radial sides of the hands together, and the thumb of the dominant hand held in the nondominant fist (**Fig. 1**).[3]

The newer technique involves creating a larger, flatter surface with which to contact the water. This has been referred to as the flat-hand grab.[5] With arms over the head and elbows in full extension, the wrists are both completely extended and the fingers then turned toward each other, so that the thumbs interlock, with the dominant hand placed palmar to the nondominant hand (**Fig. 2**A). The nondominant hand then grasps the dominant hand to further secure the position, pulling the dominant hand into an even more extended position (**Fig. 2**B). Finally, the shoulders are shrugged, pressing the arms against the diver's ears, eliminating as much potential space between the arms as possible. It was with this newer technique that ripping a dive became more predictable and less sporadic, as evidenced by the strong performance of the Soviet dive team in the 1972 Olympic Games.

Contact with the water accounts for a large proportion of diving injuries: 32.0% of men's injuries and 16.2% of women's injuries according to one report.[6] In hands-first entry techniques, the hands and wrists break the surface of the water first, taking the brunt of the initial impact on the upper extremity. The flat-hand grab position presents more than twice the contact surface area at the time of water penetration compared with the thumb-in-palm (closed fist) hand position (175 cm^2 vs 83 cm^2).[3] This larger surface area leads to a more pronounced braking effect using the flat-hand grab technique. At the moment of entry, the diver's speed slows abruptly from 31.5 mph to 20.5 mph, and the hands absorb the energy of this deceleration.

EPIDEMIOLOGY

A standard diving practice regimen involves approximately 200 dives per week.[7] Given the

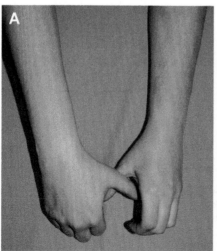
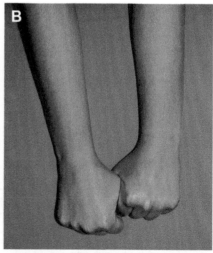

Fig. 1. Demonstration of the thumb-in-palm position. (*A*) The thumb of the dominant hand is placed within the palm of the nondominant hand. (*B*) In the final position, the nondominant fist grasps the dominant thumb.

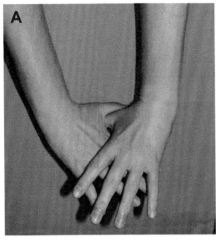
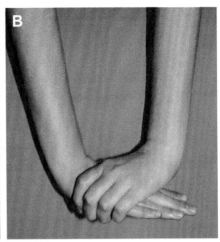

Fig. 2. Demonstration of the flat-hand grab position. (*A*) With both wrists completely extended, the thumbs are interlocked. The dominant hand is palmar to the nondominant hand. (*B*) In the final position, the nondominant hand grasps the dominant hand with the wrists in extension, pronation, and radial deviation.

laws of physics and the popularity of hands-first water entry, it is not surprising that many divers sustain upper extremity injuries. Calculation of exact injury rates is difficult, because most injury reports are case series rather than prospective studies, and the definition of injury varies between reports. In one rare prospective study, a researcher in the Netherlands followed athletes for 3 months and documented an injury rate of 8.8 injuries per 1000 training hours among competitive divers. Injuries were defined as any inability to train or compete, which may overestimate the incidence of clinically significant injuries. Apropos of this, the report noted that only 25% of injuries detected by the researcher were reported by the divers' coaches.[8]

Data collected through the USA Diving Injury Surveillance Program and reported in 1992 put the rate of injury at approximately 6.5 injuries per 100 participants per year. Given that these data are based on the filing of insurance claims, it is not surprising that the reported incidence is much less than expected, because minor injuries not requiring any insurance payment were not included in this database.[8]

Kerr and colleagues[6] reported on the incidence of swimming and diving injuries in a sample of National Collegiate Athletic Association (NCAA) varsity sport teams, using data collected from athletic trainer reports. A reportable injury was defined as any injury that required attention from an athletic trainer or physician. Incidence was reported as injuries per 1000 athlete-exposures; 1 athlete-exposure was defined as 1 practice or competition during which the athlete was at risk. The risk of diving injury for men was found to be

1.94 injuries per 1000 athlete-exposures; for women the risk was higher: 2.49 injuries per 1000 athlete-exposures. Approximately 89% of diving injuries occurred during practice; the remainder occurred during competition.

Injuries do not seem to decline in frequency with time in the sport. Some reports suggest injuries increase in number with increasing years of training and competition.[8] In 1984, one Olympic coach estimated that more than 50% of divers are sidelined for some period of time for injuries related specifically to rip entry techniques, and 20% are out for periods longer than 7 to 10 days.[9] A study of 21 Olympic-level divers in 1991 found that 18 had at least occasional wrist pain, and 9 had injuries to the upper extremity that required medical care.[3]

Although the hands and wrists enter the water first, the more proximal aspects of the upper extremity are also susceptible to injury when diving. Rubin and Anderson[8] reported 80% of national diving team members have had shoulder injuries. Kerr reported that 32.0% of men's diving injuries were shoulder injuries, whereas hand and wrist accounted for 8.0% of injuries. In women, the shoulder accounted for just 5.4% of injuries, whereas 16.2% of injuries involved the hand and wrist. The upper arm and elbow are less likely injured, accounting for only 4.0% of men's and 2.7% of women's diving injuries.[6]

SPECIFIC INJURIES: HAND AND WRIST

The older thumb-in-fist technique of hands-first entry has been mostly abandoned. Only one case could be found in the literature with an injury specific to this technique (**Table 1**). The diver developed

Table 1
Specific diving injuries to the hand and wrist reported in the literature

Author, Year	Diving Activities	Hand Position	Injury/Findings	Treatment
Berkoff & Boggess,[11] 2011	Platform and springboard	Flat-hand grab	Multiple bony contusions (lunate, capitate, hamate, distal radius) and peripheral TFCC tear	Nonoperative (custom wrist brace, NSAIDs)
Dawson,[12] 1992	Springboard	Unspecified	EPL rupture	EIP to EPL transfer
Hosey et al,[13] 2006	Platform and springboard	Flat-hand grab	Scaphoid stress fracture	Open reduction internal fixation
le Viet et al,[3] 1993	Platform	Thumb-in-fist	Synovitis of EPL and EPB, rupture of radial collateral ligament of trapeziometacarpal joint	Synovectomy and ligament repair
le Viet et al,[3] 1993	Platform	Flat-hand grab	Intra-articular loose body, microfracture of radial styloid, TFC perforation	Excision of loose body
le Viet et al,[3] 1993	Platform	Flat-hand grab	Pseudoarthrosis of hook of hamate with tendinitis of ring and small finger flexor tendons	Excision of hook of hamate
Mohamed Haflah et al,[14] 2014	Platform	Flat-hand grab	Bilateral scaphoid stress fractures	Open reduction internal fixation (bilateral)

Abbreviations: EIP, extensor indicis proprius; NSAIDs, nonsteroidal anti-inflammatory drugs; TFC, triangular fibrocartilage.

painful swelling and instability of the right (dominant) hand trapeziometacarpal joint. Presumably this injury resulted from the repetitive strain (hyperextension and traction) on the right thumb, which was systematically held within the left fist at the time of water entry. At surgery, synovitis of the thumb extensors and rupture of the radial collateral ligament of the trapeziometacarpal joint were identified. Débridement of synovitis and repair of the ligament were performed, and the diver returned to training and was pain-free for at least a year.[3]

The flat-hand grab technique has been linked to a broad range of injuries. Many minor injuries respond to conservative treatment alone. Doyle and colleagues[10] report on a 17-year-old competitive female platform diver who sustained a partial tear of the ulnar collateral ligament (UCL) of the thumb metacarpophalangeal joint. They point out that the diver's UCL is vulnerable in 2 specific situations. First, if the diver does not completely grab the dominant hand prior to water entry, the thumbs are less protected from the impact force of the

water. Second, after water entry, at the instant the diver separates the clasped hands and moves into a forceful underwater swim out, the UCL of the dominant hand is subjected to ulnar deviation stress as the hands disengage quickly and move rapidly apart from each other. This diver was treated with splinting for 4 weeks but required a custom splint to return to practice, due to ongoing discomfort and fear of reinjury.

Berkoff and Boggess[11] reported on a 15-year-old Olympic-level diver who presented with 3 months of persistent dorsal wrist pain of the dominant right wrist. His preferred water entry technique was a flat-hand grab, with the dominant right hand positioned to contact the water first. He reported pain with any weight bearing, such as pushing up out of the pool and with turning door knobs and opening jars. Conservative treatment with taping was only temporarily helpful. Pain was localized to the dorsal ulnar wrist, including the region of the; triangular fibrocartilage complex (TFCC). The Watson scaphoid shift test was negative, although some generalized ligamentous laxity was noted. MRI was obtained showing contiguous contusions of the lunate, capitate, hamate, and distal radius in addition to a peripheral tear of the ulnar attachment of the TFCC. The patient was advised to try a custom-molded rigid wrist extension brace for diving activities to offer some protection and permit healing of these structures. He used the brace for 2 weeks but then returned to taping his wrist instead, because he found the brace to be too limiting. Nevertheless, over another 2 to 3 weeks, his symptoms improved enough that he was able to return to competitive diving without difficulty.[11]

More complex injuries, such as fractures or tendon injury, often require operative treatment. Dawson[12] reported a case of a 17-year-old male right-handed diver with sudden onset of the inability to extend his right thumb. He had recently increased his diving practice regimen in preparation for an upcoming competition. Physical examination confirmed apparent rupture of the right extensor pollicis longus (EPL) tendon. Radiographs were interpreted as normal. Thumb extension was restored with an extensor indicis proprius tendon transfer to EPL, and the patient was able to return to all activities 9 weeks after surgery.[12] Although the location of tendon rupture was not reported in the article, it can be speculated that this occurred in the watershed area at Lister tubercle where EPL ruptures are common. The fact that he had only mild, intermittent wrist discomfort in the weeks before the tendon rupture argues against a missed distal radius fracture, and some sort of tendinitis or overuse seems more likely.

Case reports of unilateral and bilateral scaphoid stress fractures in divers have been published. Hosey and colleagues[13] reported on a 13-year-old female high school diver with 2 months of right wrist pain exacerbated by using handstand technique for platform diving as well as hands-first water entry. She did not recall a specific inciting injury. Diagnosis of a scaphoid waist stress fracture was made on radiographs, and MRI confirmed this was an isolated injury with good perfusion of the proximal pole. The patient was treated with open reduction and internal fixation; no follow-up data were presented in the case report.[13]

A case of bilateral scaphoid fracture in a platform diver was reported by Mohamed Haflah and colleagues[14] in 2014. A 16-year-old right-handed male diver on a national team presented with 18 months of left wrist pain without any recollection of specific injury. On radiographs, he was found to have a right scaphoid waist fracture with bone resorption and cystic changes

suggestive of a long-standing nonunion. He declined surgical intervention for over a year but ultimately agreed to surgery when symptoms did not relent. During routine preoperative evaluation, he was found to have an asymptomatic left scaphoid stress fracture as well. Open reduction internal fixation with iliac crest bone graft was performed for both scaphoid fractures. At 4 months, the patient reportedly had full range of motion, no pain, and bony union on radiographs.

In their report on injuries observed in a group of championship platform divers, le Viet and colleagues[3] reported that 9 of 21 divers sustained injuries that required medical care. Two patients required surgery for their injuries. One such operative case was a 20-year-old man with mild chronic wrist pain who noted a sudden sharp wrist pain on water entry. Radiographs revealed an intra-articular loose body, presumed to be an avulsion fragment from the radial styloid. Surgical excision of this fragment led to a full recovery. One year later, he developed similar symptoms on the contralateral wrist and was found to have an identical lesion, which was also treated with excision. Although follow-up radiographs showed progressive destruction of the scaphotrapeziotrapezoidal joint, this was treated conservatively and the diver was able to return to Olympic-level competition.

The other operative patient in le Viet and colleagues' article[3] was discussed previously in the context of injury resulting from routine use of the thumb-in-palm hand position. Approximately 1 year after treatment of her right-sided hand injury, this diver switched to a flat-hand type grip and sustained a new left hand injury. She was found to have a pseudoarthrosis of the hook of the hamate, with associated tendinitis of the ring and small finger flexor tendons. Resecting the hook of the hamate relieved all her pain, and she was able to return to training, although she abandoned platform diving in favor of springboard diving, for fear of additional injuries.[3]

The author had the opportunity to treat a collegiate platform diver with bilateral wrist pain several years ago. The patient complained of ulnar-sided wrist pain that was exacerbated by hands-first water entry as well as the handstand position sometimes used at takeoff. Pain was localized to the pisotriquetral joint. Standard radiographs did not reveal any arthritis at this articulation, but bone scan and MRI confirmed localized hyperemia/hyperperfusion and bone marrow edema, respectively. Pisiform excision proved curative when conservative treatment with corticosteroid injection and splinting failed. The patient was able to return to competitive diving without limitations.

This collection of case reports and case series are not high-level evidence but do allow making some generalizations about hand and wrist diving injuries. First, injury is more common to the dominant hand, because both of the described hand positions (see **Figs. 1** and **2**) place the dominant hand at higher risk. Second, most of the injuries are localized to the carpal bones and distal radius; no reports of finger fractures or finger dislocations were found in the literature. In addition to the carpal fractures, contusions, and other maladies discussed previously, subtle forms of carpal instability have also been alluded to in the literature.[2] Unfortunately, the type and severity of these instability cases have not been specified in the literature at this time.

The frequency of carpal injuries, especially scaphoid fractures, should not be surprising, given what is known about the proposed mechanisms of scaphoid fractures. The 2 mechanisms proposed for scaphoid waist fractures are (1) palmar-directed force applied to the radial palm with the wrist extended/hyper-extended[15] and (2) axial force applied to a closed fist with the wrist in near-neutral position.[16] These 2 mechanisms closely resemble the 2 described hand positions in competitive diving.

ROLE OF PROTECTIVE DEVICES

Beginning divers, as well as divers with weak wrists, are encouraged to use various methods to reduce the impact of the repetitive wrist extension stress encountered with hands-first water entry techniques. Many divers use taping or wrapping of the wrist for support, though the adhesion of tape can be problematic when exposed to the wet environment of a diving pool.[11,17]

Orthoses designed to stabilize the thumb and/or wrist are used by many divers. Such braces can be used to treat acute problems, or may be used prophylactically to help avoid injury. Unfortunately, many of the commercial devices are not suitable for the competitive diver. Splints containing a metal stay are often too rigid and can create new injury on water entry. Other products that are comfortable and fit well may not be compatible with chlorine and tend to disintegrate after extended exposure to pool water. One viable alternative reported in the literature is a custom silicone orthosis for thumb protection. Silicone is compatible with chlorinated water, is firm enough to provide support without creating new injury, and holds its shape even in hot tub temperatures. Doyle and colleagues[10] provide a step-by-step guide to construction of this orthosis in their article.

SPECIFIC INJURIES: ELBOW AND SHOULDER

There are few case reports in the literature regarding elbow, shoulder, and clavicle injuries, despite that these injuries outnumbered hand and wrist injuries in NCAA male divers (**Table 2**).[6]

Shinozaki and colleagues[18] reported on a 14-year-old boy with 2 weeks of dull aching pain in his dominant right elbow. He had been tower diving at the 7-m level since age 7. No instability, swelling, or crepitus of the elbow was present; he had full range of motion. Radiographs suggested an olecranon stress fracture, which was later confirmed on MRI. Because displacement was minimal, the patient was simply advised to cease sports activities to allow this fracture to heal. Two months later, healing was confirmed on radiograph, and the patient was allowed to gradually return to diving.[18]

A case report by Waninger[7] describes a 19-year-old right-handed male collegiate athlete who developed left anterior shoulder pain 3 months after starting a diving training regimen; he had formerly been a swimmer and was new to the sport of diving. Pain was exacerbated on water entry, and point tenderness was present at the mid-clavicle. Radiographs showed a mild periosteal reaction at this location. A bone scan demonstrated focal intense activity in the left midclavicle also, confirming the diagnosis of stress fracture. The diver switched to a cross-training program

Table 2
Specific diving injuries to the elbow, arm, and shoulder reported in the literature

Author, Year	Diving Activities	Hand Position	Injury/Findings	Treatment
Shinozaki et al,[18] 2006	Platform (7 m)	Flat-hand grab	Olecranon stress fracture	Nonoperative (activity modification)
Waninger,[7] 1997	Platform	Flat-hand grab	Clavicle stress fracture	Nonoperative (activity modification)

and avoided diving for 8 weeks, which allowed the fracture to heal. He was then able to return to a full pain-free diving program.

Shoulder instability is mentioned in the literature as a consequence of diving, but detailed case reports have not been published. Altchek and colleagues[19] published a report on a modification of the Bankart procedure for treatment of shoulder instability in 42 athletes, at least 1 of whom was a diver. Individual case descriptions and outcomes were not reported in the article, but most patients did have a successful outcome.

The flat-hand grab water entry technique has been linked to chronic tendinitis of the shoulder and rotator cuff injuries. Inflamed cuff musculature leads to a decrease in the subacromial space and impingement of the deltoid tendons on the coracoacromial ligament. Tendon rupture has been reported, but details of these cases is not discoverable in the literature.[17]

Despite epidemiologic reports that show large numbers of shoulder injuries, no additional case reports could be found in the existing literature. A majority of these injuries, although significant enough to interrupt training, are assumed to not require surgical treatment in most cases. This is consistent with the epidemiologic data that the most common diving injury—in both men's and women's diving—is strain, followed by entrapment/impingement and tendonitis.[6] The stress fractures identified in the proximal upper extremity did not require operative intervention, in contrast to the scaphoid fractures discussed previously. It is impossible to estimate the incidence of chronic shoulder instability, but it seems to be low, based on scant case reports available.

SUMMARY

Due to the repetitive trauma of water entry, competitive divers are at risk for upper extremity injuries. Impact forces in the range of 2.0 to 2.4 times the force of gravity are transmitted to the upper extremity with each dive, and divers typically perform approximately 200 dives per week during training. The dominant hand is affected most often, although many conditions are bilateral. Shoulder injury is more common in epidemiologic studies, but injuries to the hand and wrist more commonly require surgical intervention. Upper extremity surgeons and specialists should be aware of the broad spectrum of possible injuries and have a high degree of suspicion for those that may require surgical treatment for a successful outcome.

ACKNOWLEDGMENTS

The author wishes to thank and acknowledge Madeleine M. Haase for her assistance with the creation of the figures in this article.

REFERENCES

1. Diving - summer olympic sport. Available at: https://www.olympic.org/diving. Accessed August 12, 2016.
2. Rubin BD. The basics of competitive diving and its injuries. Clin Sports Med 1999;18(2):293–303.
3. le Viet DT, Lantieri LA, Loy SM. Wrist and hand injuries in platform diving. J Hand Surg Am 1993; 18(5):876–80.
4. The Benefits of headfirst entries in diving. August 12, 2016. Available at: http://diving.isport.com/diving-guides/the-benefits-of-headfirst-entries-in-diving. Accessed August 12, 2016.
5. How to perfect the rip entry in diving. August 12, 2016. Available at: http://diving.isport.com/diving-guides/how-to-perfect-the-rip-entry-in-diving. Accessed August 12, 2016.
6. Kerr ZY, Baugh CM, Hibberd EE, et al. Epidemiology of national collegiate athletic association men's and women's swimming and diving injuries from 2009/2010 to 2013/2014. Br J Sports Med 2015;49(7): 465–71.
7. Waninger KN. Stress fracture of the clavicle in a collegiate diver. Clin J Sport Med 1997;7(1):66–8.
8. Rubin BD, Anderson SJ. Chapter 11: diving, in epidemiology of sports injuries. In: Caine DJ, Caine C, Lindner KJ, editors. Epidemiology of sports injuries. Champaign (IL): Human Kinetics Publishers, Inc; 1996. p. 176–85.
9. Mifflin, L. A 'rip' dive brings points–and pain. in The New York Times. Available at: http://www.nytimes.com/1984/07/25/sports/a-rip-dive-brings-points-and-pain.html. Accessed August 12, 2016.
10. Doyle C, Lastayo P, Damore E. A silicone splint to prevent diving injuries of the thumb. J Hand Ther 2006;19(4):425–9.
11. Berkoff D, Boggess B. Carpal contusions in an elite platform diver. BMJ Case Rep 2011;2011: 1–5.
12. Dawson WJ. Sports-induced spontaneous rupture of the extensor pollicis longus tendon. J Hand Surg Am 1992;17(3):457–8.
13. Hosey RG, Hauk JM, Boland MR. Scaphoid stress fracture: an unusual cause of wrist pain in a competitive diver. Orthopedics 2006;29(6):503–5.
14. Mohamed Haflah NH, Mat Nor NF, Abdullah S, et al. Bilateral scaphoid stress fracture in a platform diver presenting with unilateral symptoms. Singapore Med J 2014;55(10):e159–61.

15. Weber ER, Chao EY. An experimental approach to the mechanism of scaphoid waist fractures. J Hand Surg Am 1978;3(2):142–8.
16. Horii E, Nakamura R, Watanabe K, et al. Scaphoid fracture as a "puncher's fracture". J Orthop Trauma 1994;8(2):107–10.
17. Carter RL. Prevention of springboard and platform diving injuries. Clin Sports Med 1986;5(1):185–94.
18. Shinozaki T, Kondo T, Takagishi K. Olecranon stress fracture in a young tower-diving swimmer. Orthopedics 2006;29(8):693–4.
19. Altchek DW, Warren RF, Skyhar MJ, et al. T-plasty modification of the Bankart procedure for multidirectional instability of the anterior and inferior types. J Bone Joint Surg Am 1991; 73(1):105–12.

Hand and Wrist Injuries in Golfers and Their Treatment

Sang-Hyun Woo, MD, PhD[a], Young-Keun Lee, MD, PhD[b],*,
Jong-Min Kim, MD[a], Ho-Jun Cheon, MD[a],
William H.J. Chung[c]

KEYWORDS

- Golf injury • Swing mechanism • Trigger finger • De Quervain disease • Tendinopathy
- Pisiform ligament complex syndrome • Hook of hamate fracture

KEY POINTS

- Golf injuries of the hand and wrist are common and most of these injuries are related to overuse.
- To diagnose and to provide appropriate management for golf injuries of the hand and wrist, the kinematics of the golf swing should be understood.
- Initial treatment starts with cessation of golfing to rest the wrist and includes a splint or orthotic brace, nonsteroidal antiinflammatory drug medication with corticosteroid injection, and swing modification.
- Pisiform excision is the best treatment of the most severe chronic cases of pisiform ligament complex syndrome, especially if the patient's symptoms are intolerable and nonoperative treatment measures have failed.
- Delayed diagnosis of hook of hamate fracture may lead to complications, including flexor tendon rupture of the little or ring fingers and sensory or motor deficits of the ulnar nerve. Prompt surgical resection is recommended to hasten return to sport and to prevent further complications.

INTRODUCTION

Golf has become an increasingly popular sport, attracting new players from all ages and socioeconomic groups. Irrespective of physical condition or underlying diseases, most people can enjoy the sport and the health-related benefits of walking up to 7 or 8 km per 18 holes and relaxing in a pleasant natural environment. There are an estimated 60 million golfers worldwide, playing on 32,000 golf courses. With the rapid expansion and globalization of the sport, the International Olympic Committee has included it as an Olympic sport for 2016.

The potential causes of golf injuries usually involve overuse by too much practice, poor swing mechanism, inappropriate equipment, or striking the ground or an object other than the ball, such as a tree root. McCarroll and colleagues[1] reported that, in professional golfers, wrist injuries were most common, followed by injuries to the back, left hand, left shoulder, left knee, and left thumb in reference to a right-handed golfer. In amateur golfers, the back is the most common site of injury,

Disclosure Statement: The authors have nothing to disclose.
[a] W Institute for Hand and Reconstructive Microsurgery, W Hospital, 1632 Dalgubeol-daero, Dalseo-Gu, Daegu 42642, Korea; [b] Department of Orthopaedic Surgery, Chonbuk National University Hospital, 93, Changpo-gil, Deokjin-gu, Jeonju, Jeollabuk-do 54896, Korea; [c] Comprehensive Hand Center, University of Michigan, North Campus Research Complex, 2800 Plymouth Road, Building 14 G200, Ann Arbor, MI 48109, USA
* Corresponding author.
E-mail address: trueyklee@naver.com

followed by the elbow, hand, wrist, and shoulder. Compared with other sports, golf is a noncontact sport, is considered a low-risk activity, and does not require much physical skill or athletic ability to participate. However, with incorrect techniques, unexpected serious injuries can happen. In most sports in which a club, bat, or racket is held, the hand and wrist directly absorb all transmitted power from the impact.

A study of injuries and overuse syndromes in amateur golfers showed that almost 40% of players had injuries in more than 2 different sites.[2] On a driving range, amateur golfers tend to practice the same swing with the same clubs over and over again. In pursuit of perfection, they believe that the constant repetition of the swing is a good way to develop a reliable golf swing. Severity of reported injuries were minor in 52% of cases, moderate in 27%, and major in 22%.[2] Overuse proved to be the most important factor resulting in golf injuries. Even though professional and low-handicap golfers have a much better swing mechanism, they tend to experience more wrist and hand problems than amateurs do, because they have spent more time hitting balls, and their impact power is much greater than with amateurs. More experienced golfers intentionally aim to hit through the ball, taking a divot of turf with the club after ball contact, producing spin on the golf ball and thereby controlling its landing. This technique results in an increased contact force when the club hits the ball and ground, and this force is transmitted to the wrist and hand. A recent study of professional golfers showed that 30% had reported various wrist problems.[3] Most injuries (67%) occurred in the leading wrist (left side of a right-handed golfer) at the most common location, the ulnar side of the wrist (35%).

This article reviews the kinematics of the golf swing and provides a diagnosis and management recommendations for golf injuries of the hand and wrist. Traumatic thrombosis of the distal ulnar

artery and distal ulnar nerve neuropathy are presented in the article on nerve entrapment syndrome in cyclists.

BIOMECHANICS OF THE GOLF SWING

The ideal golf swing hits the ball a specific distance and direction following the trajectory the player wants. Therefore, the golf swing is a highly coordinated, multisegment, rotational, closed-chain activity that requires strength, explosive power, flexibility, speed, and balance.[4] Golf swing speeds can reach more than 50 m/s, producing high levels of stress in the joints. In simpler terms, the golf swing is divided into 5 stages: setup (address), backswing, downswing, impact, and follow-through.

Regarding the setup, a correct grip is the foundation of a good golf swing. An overlapping grip is currently by far the most popular. This grip enables golfers with large or strong hands to perform powerful shots. However, those with small or weak hands may find it more difficult to control the club. For right-handed golfers, the interlocking grip takes the small finger of the right hand and interlocks it with the index finger of the left hand, a grip often recommended for players with small hands, like women or children. In addition to the grip patterns, choosing the proper size of grip helps prevent tendinitis. Using a grip that is too small can cost the player some power, but, if it is too big, the player needs much greater flexion power to hit long or straight shots. Correct grip size permits the fingers in a golfers' top hand to barely touch the palm. People with hand arthritis usually benefit from using a bigger golf grip. The club should be gripped as lightly as possible in order to minimize tension in the swing.

During setup, the leading, nondominant wrist begins the golf swing in a position of ulnar deviation when addressing the ball (**Fig. 1**A). During the backswing, the club is lifted away from the

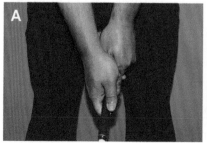
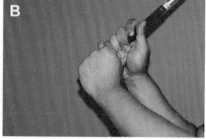

Fig. 1. (*A*) In the setup, the leading, nondominant left wrist begins the golf swing in a position of ulnar deviation when addressing the ball. (*B*) During the backswing, as the club is lifted away to the rear, the wrist moves into radial deviation until it sits maximally radially deviated at the top of the swing. The right wrist is in maximal extension at the top of the backswing.

player's core and the wrist moves into radial deviation until it sits maximally radially deviated at the top of the backswing (**Fig. 1**B). At this point, the club changes direction to begin the downswing and the leading, nondominant wrist returns to ulnar deviation until impact. An understanding of the opposing motion paths of ulnar to radial deviation for the leading, nondominant wrist and flexion/extension for the dominant wrist enables the mechanism of wrist and hand injuries in golf to be understood, especially when right-handed golfers use a driver. The right wrist is required to move in the planes of extension and flexion by 103° as well as radial and ulnar deviation by 45°.[5] In the left wrist, the arc is relatively small in flexion, with an extension of about 71° but slightly more radial and ulnar deviation of about 47°.[6] Through the downswing, most traumatic injuries occur at impact.

When the club hits the ball, it should strike the ball then the turf, taking a divot. However, hitting the ground before the ball can injure amateur golfers; this is known as a fat shot. By hitting fat shots, players can strike unseen tree roots, rocks, and other objects lying near the ball. The follow-through is the final phase of the swing, and it finishes in extension and radial deviation of both the leading and trailing wrists. Throughout the swing cycle, wrist motion is complex and serves as a potential source for injuries.

TYPES OF GOLF INJURIES

Golf injuries are the result of preexisting physical weaknesses that become manifest when following a specific activity. Moreover, because of overpractice, poor swing mechanism, or hitting the ground or an object, golf injuries can injure tendons, ligaments and joints, bones, vessels, and even nerves. Golf injuries are divided by timing as acute striking injury and repetitive strain injury. In the category of acute injury, there are triangular fibrocartilage complex (TFCC) injuries and carpal bone fractures, including scaphoid or hook of hamate fractures. Acute collateral ligament rupture of the digit may occur as a result of a loose grip. In amateur golfers, repetitive strain injury, such as of the trigger finger, is more common. Depending on the force transmission of the golf swing, repeated overpractice may result in tenosynovitis, like de Quervain disease, tendinitis of the flexor carpi ulnaris (FCU), extensor carpi ulnaris (ECU) dislocation, or even flexor tendon ruptures combined with hook of hamate fractures. Furthermore, peripheral nerve compression causes carpal tunnel syndrome and ulnar nerve compression at the Guyon canal.[7]

Anatomic location of the pathologic lesions can be divided into ulnar, radial, and dorsal wrist pain. The causes of ulnar wrist pain are ECU subluxation or tenosynovitis, or TFCC problems. In cases of radial wrist pain, there are de Quervain disease and intersection syndrome. Ganglia or extensor synovitis are the main causes of dorsal wrist pain from golf.

TRIGGER FINGER

With the pursuit of perfection through constant repetition of the swing, most beginner golfers feel stiffness and swelling of the digits the morning following an extended practice at a driving range. It commonly happens in golfers with a strong grip in the left hand. By practicing with the same clubs over and over again, the flexor tendons are impinged. With proximal interphalangeal (PIP) joint flexion, flexor tendons pass through a narrow A1 pulley. Particularly with a power grip, high angular loads are developed at the distal edge of the A1 pulley. It is like the effect of pulling a multifilament strand through the eye of a needle; bunching of the interwoven tendon fibers occurs,[8] resulting in reactive intratendinous swelling of the flexor tendon.[9] Moreover, the pulley shows gross hypertrophy that is whitish, cicatricial collarlike thickening. On ultrasonography, thickening and hypervascularization of the A1 pulley are the hallmarks of trigger fingers (**Fig. 2**A, B).

Symptoms vary greatly depending on the severity and the golfer. It usually starts as a vague pain on the palm and stiffness of the involved digits. Golfers feel catching of the digits and cannot actively extend the digit, requiring passive extension. In addition, the digits show catching with a fixed flexion contracture of the PIP joint, sometimes accompanied by pain on the dorsal aspect of PIP joint.

Trigger digit in golfers is usually spontaneously resolved in the early stage. First, the grip habit should be changed. A player's grip should not be tight, but it should be gentle. Because a worn grip causes the golfer to grasp the club tighter, clubs should be regripped regularly. The traction that a fresh grip provides lets golfers hold the club lightly. Most trigger digits can be treated with steroid injection, nonsteroidal antiinflammatory drugs (NSAIDs), and/or splinting. Corticosteroid injection has a high satisfaction rate, particularly in nondiabetic patients with involvement of a single digit, a discrete palpable nodule, and a short duration of symptoms. All patients with trigger digits should be offered 2 or 3 trials of corticosteroid injections. Two corticosteroid injections followed by surgery was the least costly

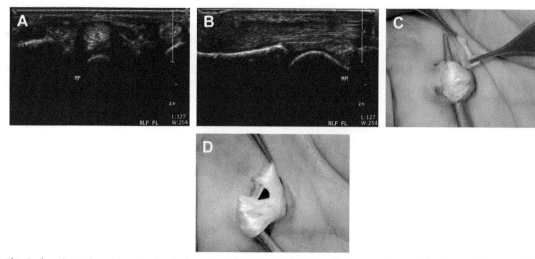

Fig. 2. (*A, B*) Axial and longitudinal ultrasonography images show mild hypoechoic thickening of the A1 pulley with minimal peritendinous fluid along the flexor tendon. (*C, D*) Beginner golfer: a 45-year-old man practiced 7 days a week at a driving range for 3 months. He hit more than 200 balls every day. On the A1 pulley release of the right long finger, the flexor tendon ruptured longitudinally and tenosynovium was hypertrophied.

algorithm and was less expensive than immediate surgical release.[10] Patients with trigger digits caused by rheumatoid arthritis or diabetes are recommended to have a second injection. When the open surgical release is scheduled, a corticosteroid injection should be avoided in the first 6 weeks before the operation. Under local anesthesia, the A1 pulley is released through a transverse, oblique, or vertical incision (**Fig. 2**C, D). After operation, immediate motion of the digits is advised. The incidence of postoperative complications is neither high nor serious. Pain in the incision site, fluid collection, and mild flexion contraction or stiffness of the digits resolve spontaneously. Rarely are there serious complications, including nerve transection, infection, or contracture of the PIP joint requiring secondary surgery.

DE QUERVAIN DISEASE

The first extensor compartment of the wrist, which is over the styloid process of the radius, contains the abductor pollicis longus (APL) and extensor pollicis brevis (EPB) tendons. These tendons pass through the fibro-osseous tunnel, about 2 to 2.5 cm in length, which is covered by tough, overlying transverse fibers of the dorsal ligament. De Quervain disease is friction at the rigid retinacular sheath, with subsequent swelling or narrowing of the tunnel. It is caused by chronic inflammation of the APL and EPB, or aberrant slips of APL tendons, or presence of ganglion.

De Quervain happens more often in female golfers when they are between their 30s and 60s.

Most cases are caused by poor swing mechanism. An excessive radial deviation of the left wrist in the backswing of right-handed golfers is a causal factor of de Quervain disease. Repeated thumb extension at the top of the backswing and a sudden deceleration at impact can produce or exacerbate symptoms. Beginner golfers or higher-handicapped golfers tend to release the hand early instead of retaining it in the cocked position. Early release of hand results in an off-plane swing following an outside to inside path, causing a slice of the golf ball and a significant loss of distance. In right-handed golfers, this motion allows an abrupt ulnar deviation of the left wrist, whereas the left thumb is more or less trapped in a fixed position between the right hand and the golf club.

Diagnosis is easily made by localized pain on the radial side of the wrist and is aggravated by the movement of the thumb. The Finkelstein test is the classic diagnostic test for de Quervain disease.[11] To perform the test, the examiner grasps the thumb and ulnar deviates the hand. However, it often leads to misdiagnosis. Eichhoff[12] modified the test by asking patients to flex the thumb and to clench the fist over the thumb before ulnar deviation. This process of ulnar deviation is performed by the practitioner (**Fig. 3**A).[12] Repetition of the patient's symptoms confirms a positive result, but it is essential to compare this with the normal contralateral side. Wrist hyperflexion and abduction of the thumb is a dynamic test that isolates the tendons within the first extensor compartment.[13] With the wrist maximally flexed, the patient is asked to abduct the thumb against

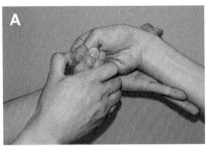
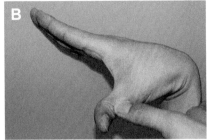

Fig. 3. (A) Eichhoff modification of the Finkelstein test. (B) The wrist hyperflexion and abduction of the thumb test is a dynamic test that isolates the tendons within the first extensor compartment.

resistance by the examiner (**Fig. 3**B). A positive test reproduces the patient's symptoms. With a sensitivity of 0.99 and specificity of 0.29, this test may allow clinician to more accurately diagnose de Quervain disease rather than using the Eichhoff test alone with a sensitivity of 0.89 and specificity of 0.14.[13]

Sonography is useful to diagnose de Quervain disease and to identify the presence of intracompartmental septum or ganglion as well as the number of aberrant slips of APL tendons in the first extensor compartment[14] (**Fig. 4**A, B).

Swing modification is the first treatment of de Quervain disease in golfers.[15] Initial treatment starts with the cessation of playing golf to rest the wrist. A thumb spica splint or orthotic brace is recommended with the wrist gently extended and the thumb abducted. NSAIDs are also helpful. The most effective conservative treatment is corticosteroid and lidocaine injection for relief of persistent symptoms. A satisfactory response to a diagnostic injection should precede the decision for surgery. Corticosteroid injection is successful in 50% to 80% of patients after 1 to 2 injections,

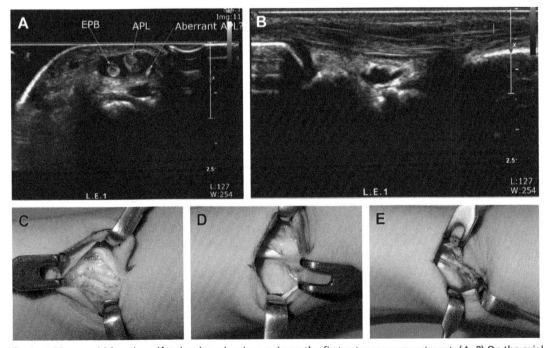

Fig. 4. A 28-year-old female golfer developed serious pain on the first extensor compartment. (A, B) On the axial and longitudinal ultrasonography views, aberrant APL tendon with fluid collection was found within the first extensor compartment. (C) Through the zigzag skin incision, the most dorsal part of the first extensor compartment opened revealing fluid collection and longitudinal rupture of the tendons. (D) Inside the first compartment, there was a septum with an aberrant tendon. (E) Intracompartmental septum was completely released.

and is particularly effective in acute cases.[16] Because of local complications of insoluble steroid, including localized atrophy of the subcutaneous tissues, fat necrosis, and discoloration, water-soluble dexamethasone or betamethasone mixed with 1% lidocaine is preferred.

A zigzag skin incision is made over the first dorsal compartment about 1 cm proximal to the tip of the radial styloid process. During incision of skin and dissection of the extensor retinaculum and tendons, care is taken to avoid iatrogenic injury to even small branches of the superficial sensory nerves. The hypertrophied annular ligament of the first compartment is sharply incised on its most dorsal margin to prevent tendon subluxation volarly. On traction of all exposed tendons, a thorough exploration for hidden aberrant tendons inside intracompartmental septum is necessary. Failure to identify and release a separate compartment is the main cause of recurrence of pain (**Fig. 4**C–E).

Wound massage is recommended after the stitches are removed. Short iron practice or approach shot with wedge clubs can commence about 4 to 6 weeks postoperatively.

INTERSECTION SYNDROME

Intersection syndrome is a localized inflammation of the peritendinous tissue at the intersection of the APL, the EPB, and the radial wrist extensors just proximal to the wrist's dorsal retinaculum.[17] In this condition the APL and EPB are irritated at the point where they cross over the second dorsal compartment of extensor carpi radialis longus and brevis. It should be differentiated from de Quervain disease. The tenderness point and significant soft tissue swelling with marked crepitus is about 6 to 8 cm more proximal to the Lister tubercle than de Quervain disease. These overuse-type injuries should be treated similarly to de Quervain disease. Conservative treatment includes rest, splinting, stretching and strengthening exercises, and NSAIDs. If this therapy is not effective, corticosteroid injection or surgical decompression may be required. It is frequently seen in golf swings that require repetitive wrist flexion and extension against resistance. Nonoperative treatment is usually successful. Initial measures include NSAIDs, avoidance of aggravating activities, and splint immobilization. When this fails, steroid injection is advocated into the area of the APL bursa. Following injection, immobilization should be continued for 1 to 2 weeks. In recalcitrant cases, surgical exploration and debridement of inflamed tenosynovium may be necessary. Postoperative immobilization should be limited following surgery to start gentle range-of-motion exercises. When the patient has regained range of motion and strength, golf participation can be resumed.

FLEXOR CARPI RADIALIS TENDINITIS

Flexor carpi radialis (FCR) tendinitis is usually found in the right hand of right-handed golfers. Repetitive wrist flexion against resistance causes FCR tendinitis in the right hand during the swing. The pain and tenderness are most prominent at the palmar wrist crease over the scaphoid tubercle where it is enveloped by its fibro-osseous sheath. In addition, localized swelling or ganglion may be present at that site. Resisted wrist flexion and radial deviation increase pain and are pathognomonic signs in FCR tendinitis.[18]

FCR tendon deviates about an average of 45° relative to the longitudinal axis of the forearm in the tunnel before inserting at the base of the index and long finger metacarpals.[19] This characteristic anatomic feature makes this tendon vulnerable to repetitive flexion and extension of the wrist.

Successful relief of pain after infiltration of the tendon sheath with 1 mL of 1% lidocaine can confirm the diagnosis. However, the multiplicity of other diagnoses, including basal joint degenerative disease, scaphotrapezium-trapezoid degenerative osteoarthritis, ganglion cyst, scaphoid fractures and nonunion, and de Quervain disease, may lead to misdiagnosis. Therefore, MRI can be used to differentiate between these conditions and confirm the diagnosis.[18,20]

Nonoperative treatment is recommended initially, with a period of splint, ice, NSAIDs, wrist extensions, stretching exercises, and the avoidance of golf for 4 to 6 weeks. Corticosteroid injection into the FCR tendon sheath can be used.[15,18] In cases in which nonoperative treatment is ineffective, decompression of the FCR fibro-osseous tunnel may be required.[21,22]

FLEXOR CARPI ULNARIS TENDINOPATHY

The FCU tendon of the wrist may be injured because of microtrauma from forces produced by the golf swing just before impact. When the club hits the ground before the ball and takes a divot (a fat shot), there is a sudden overload on the flexor tendon, leading to injury.[15] FCU tendinopathy is more common in the right hand of right-handed golfers because of the range of flexion and extension during the golf swing. The most common presentation is calcified tendinitis of the FCU.

The FCU is a large muscle and the most powerful wrist motor, but it does not have a synovial sheath. It inserts into the proximal and anterior aspect of the pisiform, a sesamoid bone located within the FCU, which articulates with the volar surface of the triquetrum. Because there is no inherent stability of the pisotriquetral joint, stability depends on the pisohamate and pisometacarpal ligaments.[23] The ulnar neurovascular bundle lies on the radial side of the FCU tendon just proximal to the wrist joint. It passes just radial to the pisiform at the Guyon canal, which may cause associated ulnar nerve symptoms.

Usually, carpal tunnel view and tangential radiographs of the volar and ulnar aspects of the wrist reveal calcium deposits distal to the ulna (**Fig. 5**). MRI reveals the signs of tendinopathy with increased signal on T1-weighted and T2-weighted images and can also show the calcification deposition of calcified tendinitis.

The first treatment of tendinopathy of the FCU is decreased practice intensity, or grip or swing alteration. It is most commonly treated with nonoperative options, including rest, immobilization, NSAIDs, and occasionally corticosteroid injection. At least 6 months of conservative management is recommended before adopting surgical treatment. FCU tendinitis that does not respond to nonoperative treatment may be relieved by 5-mm Z-plasty lengthening of the tendon proximal to its insertion on the pisiform.[24] Because FCU tendinopathy is degenerative tendinosis of extrasynovial tendons, surgical debridement of the pathologic tendinosis tissue is also an effective treatment of patients who fail nonsurgical management. Minor tendon slips branching from the main tendon to the adjacent soft tissue should be released. In a scraping fashion, excision of the degenerative tissue should proceed until only healthy tissue remains.[23] Excision of calcific deposits, lysis of peritendinous adhesions, and repair of the FCU tendon are necessary.[25] If the pathologic process primarily involves the pisiform, excision of the pisiform is the most commonly used surgical procedure.

PISOTRIQUETRAL ARTHRITIS

Pisotriquetral (PT) arthritis or PT instability is another potential cause of ulnar-sided wrist pain in golfers. PT arthritis is associated with local pain and tenderness that are aggravated by the grinding of the pisiform dorsally against the triquetrum. Instability may be subtle and more difficult to diagnose. A diagnostic injection of local anesthetic in combination with appropriate radiographic imaging can confirm both diagnoses.

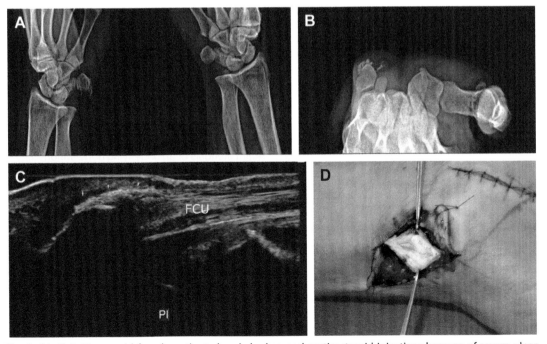

Fig. 5. (*A–C*) A 56-year-old female patient already had several corticosteroid injections because of severe ulnar-side pain. On pisiform bone view and carpal tunnel view, ultrasonography showed marked calcific deposits around the FCU and pisiform (PI). (*D*) Intraoperative view of calcification.

Pisiform ligament complex (PLC) syndrome is defined as ulnar palmar wrist pain in the vicinity of the pisiform and is caused by injury to the components of the PLC leading to PT joint instability with subsequent arthrosis. Primary osteoarthritis of the PT joint is uncommon and many arthritic disorders of this joint are posttraumatic, preceded by chronic PT joint instability. FCU tendinopathy is often associated with PT instability and PT arthritis. Narrowing of PT joint space while the wrist is in a neutral position is common in patients who have chronic instability of the PT joint and moderate arthrosis. The patient's radiograph shows marked widening of PT joint space during wrist flexion (**Fig. 6**).

Paley and colleagues[26] analyzed pathologic conditions of the pisiform from 216 cases identified from the literature and classified them into 4 pathologic groups: primary osteoarthritis (2.3%), secondary osteoarthritis (48.4%), other arthritides (4.7%), and FCU enthesopathy (44.6%). The most common causes were acute and chronic trauma and instability. Pisiform excision is the best treatment of the most severe chronic cases of PLC syndrome, especially if the patient's symptoms are intolerable and if nonoperative treatment measures have failed. Indications for pisiformectomy are painful nonunion of the pisiform, PTA, and FCU tendinitis.[27] A recent study on wrist function after pisiform excision showed that there is no significant difference in patients' grip and pinch strength, flexion and extension forces, ulnar and radial deviation, and flexion between the operated and nonsurgical wrists. However, wrist extension was significantly reduced in operated wrists compared with patients' nonsurgical wrists.[28]

EXTENSOR CARPI ULNARIS DISORDERS

During the golf swing, when the wrist supinates, the ulnar deviates and flexes during impact, and a painful snapping or clicking sensation can occur over the dorso-ulnar side of the wrist as the tendon shifts in and out of the shallow sulcus. In higher-handicapped golfers, a casting maneuver at the start of the golf swing risks development of this condition. Casting maneuver is an early release of the hand instead of leaving it in the retained cocked position, which allows wrist release at impact. A similar condition can be caused by the sudden ulnar load to the wrist from the club striking the ground with a fat shot or striking a stone instead of the golf ball.

Anatomically, the ECU muscle's actions vary depending on the forearm position. During supination, the ECU tendon moves dorsally closer to the extensor digiti minimi. In full supination, it is subjected to maximal traction and exits the sixth compartment at an angle of 30°, resulting in a greater contribution to true wrist extension. During pronation, the ECU tendon lies more in the palmar and ulnar positions of the ulnar head, far from the extensor digiti minimi, and exits the sixth compartment in a straight direction, resulting in a diminishing of its contribution to wrist extension. Therefore, tension on the ECU subsheath and retinaculum is increased in forearm supination with the wrist in flexion and ulnar deviation.[29]

The hallmark of the physical examination pointing to localized ECU disorder includes pain and tenderness directly over the ECU tendon and the sixth dorsal compartment where the pain is exacerbated by resisted wrist active extension with ulnar deviation. Swelling along the course of the ECU tendon is evident. In the case of ECU tendon instability, active supination, flexion, and ulnar deviation often produce visible subluxation of the tendon. In diagnosis, plain radiographs occasionally show calcification within the ECU tendon. However, in most cases, it is difficult to diagnose ECU tendinopathy and instability with only plain radiographs and clinical presentation. Therefore, ultrasonography and/or MRI are the imaging modalities of choice in the diagnosis of ECU tendinopathy and instability.[30,31] ECU tendon disorder can be broken down anatomically into 3 components that sometimes create multifactorial problems. The first is inflammation or tenosynovitis surrounding the ECU tendon; the second is tendinopathy caused by intrinsic damage or tendinosis; the third is mechanical failure resulting from bowstringing and subluxation/dislocation of the ECU tendon.

EXTENSOR CARPI ULNARIS TENOSYNOVITIS

Acute ECU tenosynovitis is defined by inflammation of the tenosynovium of the ECU without significant stenosis or an underlying bony abnormality of the sixth dorsal compartment. Ultrasonography shows compressible anechoic fluid surrounding the tendon with minimal or no vascularity on Doppler (**Fig. 7**). The treatment of acute ECU tenosynovitis includes the cessation of golf until symptoms subside, short-arm splinting of the wrist in a position of 30° to 40° of extension for 2 weeks, and oral NSAIDs.[15,30] If symptoms persist, a corticosteroid injection into the sixth dorsal compartment is recommended.

EXTENSOR CARPI ULNARIS TENDINOPATHY

ECU tendinopathy develops gradually. In general, it is possible to continue to play golf despite the

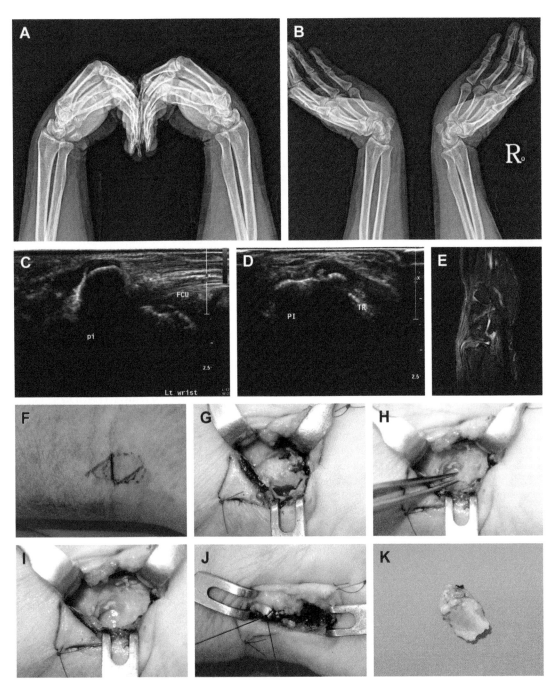

Fig. 6. (A, B) A 55-year-old female patient with severe pain in the left wrist. On semisupination oblique view of the wrist (pisiform bone view), the pisotriquetral joint of the left wrist showed marked joint space widening and sclerotic change. (C, D). Axial and longitudinal images of ultrasonography show mild FCU tendon thickening and some fluid collection around the pisiform. (E) Fat-suppression T2-weighted sagittal image showed FCU thickening with increased signal intensity and osteophytes and cartilage loss of the pisotriquetral joint. (F, G) Through the Z-shaped incision on the volar crease of the ulnar wrist, pisiform was subperiosteally dissected through the midline splitting of the FCU tendon. (H) Incidental osteophyte in the pisotriquetral joint was removed. (I) Cartilage of the triquetrum was denuded. (J) After excision of the pisiform, the flexor carpi ulnar tendon was repaired with 4-0 PDS suture in a continuous figure-of-eight method. (K) Excised pisiform showed almost totally denuded cartilage of the pisiform. TR, triquetrum; PI, pisiform.

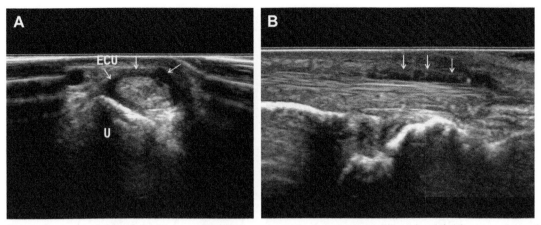

Fig. 7. Ultrasonography of the right wrist ECU tenosynovitis. Longitudinal (*A*) and axial (*B*) views showed anechoic fluid in the tendon sheath (*white arrows*). U, ulna.

pain or failure of a patient with tenosynovitis to respond to appropriate treatment. As the disease progresses, tendon thickening becomes more pronounced, resulting in stenosing tenosynovitis. The tendon can become unstable and dislocated from attenuation or tearing of its subsheath.[30,32] The ECU tendon can be ruptured partially by gliding over the ulnar ridge of the groove or a bony spur. MRI shows moderate increased signal intensity at the area of tendinopathy and tendon thickening. In the case of partial tendon tears, MRI reveals clefts or splits within the tendon substance (**Fig. 8**). Initial treatment should be conservative. If symptoms are not relieved by conservative measures, it can also be treated by corticosteroid injection into the sheath. In patients

with recalcitrant symptoms, sixth dorsal compartment release should be considered.[33] After the division of retinaculum and subsheath, the tendon should be inspected for tearing of the sheath; spur and prominent ridges should be repaired or trimmed.

EXTENSOR CARPI ULNARIS TENDON INSTABILITY

The ECU tendon is stabilized by a unique fibro-osseous sheath (subsheath) deep to the extensor retinaculum. This deep subsheath maintains the tendon's normal position.[30,34] Therefore, instability of the ECU can result following disruption of the subsheath even if the extensor retinaculum was

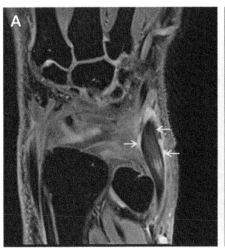
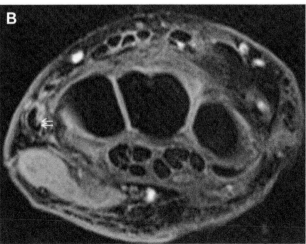

Fig. 8. (*A*) Coronal section of fat-saturated T2-weighted magnetic resonance images of ECU tendinopathy show moderately increased signal intensity at the area of tendinopathy and tendon thickening (*white arrows*). (*B*) Axial section shows a linear area of high signal intensity within the ECU tendon (*white arrows*) representing a partial tear.

intact. The exact mechanism is not clear, but generally this condition is seen with forceful supination with wrist flexion and ulnar deviation.[33,35] During impact, a painful snapping sensation can occur over the ulnar aspect of the wrist. Confirmed diagnosis can be made with dynamic ultrasonography and MRI. Treatment of the acute ECU tendon instability consists of 4 to 6 weeks of long-arm splinting or casting with the wrist in extension, radial deviation, and forearm in pronation followed by an additional 4 weeks of removable splint.[36] In chronic ECU tendon instability, surgical reconstruction of the ECU subsheath may be indicated.[37]

HOOK OF HAMATE FRACTURE

Most patients do not realize that a hamate fracture can happen from a golf swing error. Hook of hamate fractures occur almost exclusively in the leading hand. Anatomically, the prominent hook of hamate is easily broken when the golfer strikes the ground abruptly. After repetitive practice of golf swing or a sudden painful event such as hitting the ground or stone, players may feel a vague pain and focal tenderness on the hypothenar eminence. Tenderness to palpation is felt over the hamate hook approximately 2 cm distal and radial to the pisiform. Patients complain of pain aggravated by active grasping. Sometimes, patients complain of numbness of the ring and small fingers. However, standard radiographs of the hand and wrist fail to show a definite fracture line. Even hand surgeons tend to misdiagnose this as a repetitive strain injury or nerve-related problem. Over time, finger flexion of the small and/or ring fingers becomes affected, resulting in complete rupture of the flexor tendons.

The mechanism of fracture is the force directly transmitted through the butt of the golf club to the hook of hamate. Prevention of this injury is by selecting golf clubs of appropriate length. Correct fitting and a proper club grip should allow the butt of the club to extend beyond the hypothenar border of the hand. If the clubs are short, the club end is directly against the hamate.

Diagnosis of a hook of hamate fracture mainly depends on the history of overpractice or painful memories of club strike and physical examination. On the radiograph, the carpal tunnel view is the best tool to check the profile of the hook of hamate (**Fig. 9**). Computed tomography scan can show definite fracture line with high sensitivity and accuracy.[38] In suspicious cases of combined flexor tendon ruptures, ultrasonography provides real-time dynamic images of a moving flexor tendon, unlike static images. Ultrasonography may be a viable diagnostic tool in preoperative identification of the proximal tendon stump. High-resolution 3-T MRI can diagnose complete or partial tendon tears, helps determine the location of the tears and the degree of tendon retraction, and excludes any associated fractures. On T2-weighted fat-suppressed and proton density–weighted fat-suppressed sequences, flexor tendon tears are seen as fluid signal at the site of the tear. Electromyography and nerve conduction study are required in cases of paresthesia or numbness of the ring and small fingers to confirm the ulnar nerve neuropathy.

Delayed diagnosis of this injury may lead to complications, including flexor tendon rupture of the little or ring fingers and sensory or motor deficits of the ulnar nerve. Thus, prompt surgical treatment is recommended to hasten the return to sport and to prevent further complications. Successful cast immobilization within 7 days of injury is required. The average period of immobilization is 11 weeks.[39] The hook of hamate has a tenuous blood supply. Pull of the pisohamate ligament along with the origins of the flexor digiti minimi brevis and opponens digiti minimi displaces the fracture fragment, causing nonunion. Failure rates after conservative management ranged from 80% to 100% in previous studies because of nonunion and associated complications.[40–42] Excision remains the operation of choice for most surgeons.[43] In high-level amateur athletes especially, excision of hook of hamate fractures is an effective procedure.

Incision for decompression of the Guyon canal provides a good approach for excision of ununited hook of hamate fractures.[44] Some of the complications reported, such as injury to the motor branch of the ulnar nerve, superficial palmar arch injury, or median nerve paresthesia secondary to retraction, are complications of surgical exposure rather than of the excision itself. The open carpal tunnel approach is another option. Its familiarity, ease of performance, excellent visualization, and low morbidity make it a successful technique for open excision of symptomatic ununited hook of hamate fractures. A slightly curved linear incision is taken just ulnar to the midline in line with the ring finger and over the carpal tunnel with a slight proximal extension above the transverse wrist crease. After the release of the transverse carpal ligament in carpal tunnel syndrome, the ulnar wall of the carpal tunnel is exposed to be palpated in the nonunion area. Dissection starting from the radial aspect of the ulnar wall of the carpal tunnel proceeds in careful subperiosteal excision. A rectangular floor-based periosteal flap can be used to cover the raw bony surface of the hamate. Almost

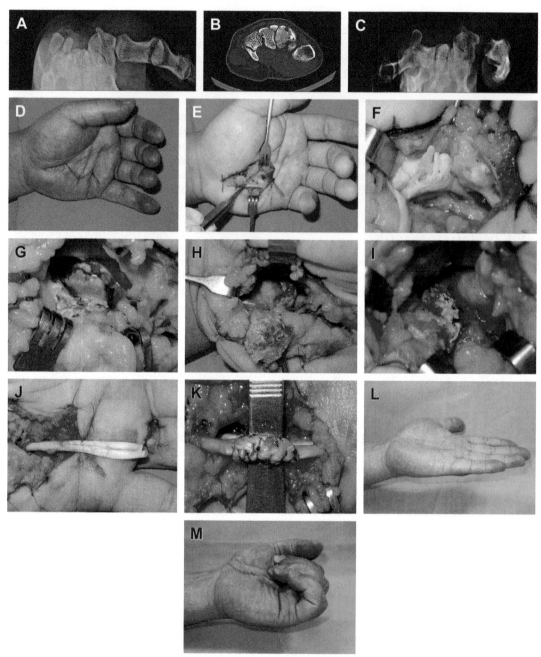

Fig. 9. Beginner golfer: a 56-year-old male patient had chronic pain on the left palm and limitation of flexion on the ring and small fingers after intensive golf practice for 3 months. (*A*, *B*) On the radiograph of the carpal tunnel view and computed tomography, the base portion of the hook of hamate was fractured. (*C*) Postoperative carpal tunnel view after resection of the fracture segment. (*D*) The preoperative view showed destroyed cascade of the ring and small finger and preoperative design for resection of the fractured segment of the hook of hamate, and fourth flexor digitorum superficialis (FDS) tendon transfer for the reconstruction of the fifth flexor digitorum profundus (FDP) together. (*E*) Complete ruptured fifth FDP at zone III. (*F*) The fourth FDP was also longitudinally torn. (*G*) Fractured hook of hamate was identified and periosteal flap based from the ulnar wall of carpal tunnel was designed with gentian violet. (*H, I*) The fracture segment was excised and then the raw surface was resurfaced with periosteal flap. (*J, K*) The fourth FDS was harvested from the small transverse incision on the metacarpophalangeal volar crease. Pulvertaft interweaving suture was performed between the proximal end of the fifth FDP and distal end of the fourth FDS. (*L, M*) 36 months postoperation.

all cases show longitudinal tearing of the fourth or fifth flexor tendons. Debridement or sometimes tendon repair is necessary.

In case of associated flexor tendon ruptures, incision should be extended to identify and expose the proximal and distal end of ruptured tendons. The preferred treatment of these ruptures is interposition tendon grafting. A tendon gap at the palm or wrist level can be reconstructed by the transfer of an adjacent intact flexor digitorum superficialis tendon passed deep to the neurovascular bundle or median nerve and sewn to the distal segment of the injured tendon. Flexor digitorum superficialis tendon transfer from the ring to the little finger has proved to be another good option, but has been considered less favorable because it may compromise ring finger function and overall grip strength.[45] Because adjusting tension of the transfer has always been difficult, tendon transfer is best performed using wide-awake surgery. With the patient being awake, the digits and the hand can move actively to determine correct tension of the transfer.[46,47] Intraoperatively, unsedated patients can observe active motion of their digits in a pain-free state. Patients also develop a much stronger desire for rehabilitation.

TRIANGULAR FIBROCARTILAGE COMPLEX SPRAIN/TEARS

TFCC is the term most commonly used to describe the interconnected soft tissues that span and support the distal radioulnar joint (DRUJ) and ulnocarpal articulations. The role of the TFCC is to stabilize the bones in the wrist. It acts as a shock absorber and enables smooth movement. However, cartilages and ligaments of the complex are prone to degeneration and wear-and-tear injuries, which can lead to ulnar-side pain, weakness of grip strength, and instability of the DRUJ. During the golf swing, rotational injuries may occur when hitting the ball out of deep rough. When the club head gets trapped and twisted in long grass, it produces a sudden strain on the structures that stabilize wrist rotation, thus resulting in acute tears of the TFCC. The wrists are locked when a golfer holds a club, but, once the club swings, the wrist movement may cause pain in the TFCC region. A poor golf shot on the little-finger side of the wrist may also sprain or tear the TFCC.

Magnetic resonance arthrography of the wrist is a valuable tool in diagnostic evaluation to detect full-thickness tears of the TFCC. Arthroscopy is sensitive in identifying traumatic TFCC tears or degeneration of the central portion of the disk, chondromalacia, and ulnocarpal ligament injuries.

Arthroscopy is more sensitive and more accurate than noninvasive imaging modalities.[48]

Most acute, isolated TFCC tears do not require prompt aggressive treatment. The treatment modality usually depends on the presence of persistent joint pain from mechanical irritation or synovitis caused by the tear or DRUJ instability. Conservative treatment consists of rest, immobilizing the wrist with a splint, ice application, and taking NSAIDs. Most golf-induced wrist injuries are caused by overuse and are successfully treated without surgery, although the golfer may need to give up the game for an extended period of time. If initial treatments fail, cortisone injections may provide relief. If a sudden injury causes a wrist sprain or a tear of the TFCC, the wrist should be immobilized for 3 to 4 weeks. After that, depending on the injury, the golfer can slowly return to play. If a golfer experiences persistent pain and instability, wearing a wrist brace may help. For the treatment of degenerative TFCC lesions, debridement of the joint, reduction of load across the ulnocarpal joint, DRUJ stability, DRUJ articular congruity, and presence of developmental or acquired skeletal deformities should all be considered. In severe cases, surgery is usually necessary to reconstruct the TFCC. Symptomatic and complete tears with grossly unstable or even chronic injury can be repaired by arthroscopic-assisted techniques, including transosseous or direct capsular suture repair.

Following TFCC reconstruction, the wrist and forearm should be immobilized for 4 to 6 weeks. By 6 weeks, the golfer is usually able to initiate up and down palm motions and wrist flexion and extension. The main goals of physical therapy are to achieve full range of motion in the forearm and the wrist, and for the patient to be able to return to playing pain-free golf.

CARPAL TUNNEL SYNDROME

Although playing golf is not a direct cause of carpal tunnel syndrome, the repetitive swing or strong grip can contribute. Playing a few rounds of golf every month is not a major factor in the development of carpal tunnel syndrome, but serious amateurs, beginners, or professional golfers spend countless hours in practice and play. In this case, inflammation and swelling of flexor tendons and tenosynovium causes crowding and increased pressure on the median nerve (**Fig. 10**). The increased pressure on the nerve causes it to malfunction, resulting in the symptoms of carpal tunnel syndrome. Flexor tenosynovitis and carpal tunnel syndrome result from repetitive grasping and wrist motions. Repetitive digital flexion in individuals

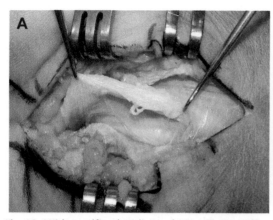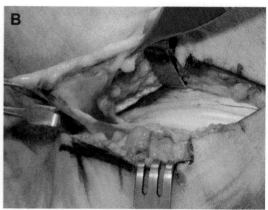

Fig. 10. With a golfing handicap of 10, a 45-year-old male patient developed numbness of the right thumb and index, long, and ring fingers after aggressive practice and 3 to 4 rounds of golf a week. (*A, B*) After confirmed diagnosis of carpal tunnel syndrome with the nerve conduction test, open carpal tunnel release was performed with long incision. Severe synovial hypertrophy was found around all flexor tendons and there was longitudinal tearing of the fourth and fifth FDS tendon in the carpal tunnel.

unaccustomed to such activity can induce significant tenosynovitis of the digital flexors.[49]

Rest, wrist splinting at night, NSAIDs, and steroid injections are frequently used as initial treatments for carpal tunnel syndrome. For beginner golfers, easing up on grip pressure during the address phase of the swing and the replacement of worn golf grips may reduce stress on the wrists and hands. Wearing a glove on each hand should also provide extra cushioning. Decreasing the frequency of rounds of golf played and the number of balls hit at the range each week may help injured nerves to recover.

Surgery is the treatment of choice when nonsurgical treatments fail or when abductor pollicis brevis and/or sensory denervation are problematic. Release of the transverse carpal ligament may be performed using an open or endoscopic technique. Open carpal tunnel release is the most common method of decompression and can be performed under local anesthesia or through wide-awake anesthesia. Practicing approach shots with wedge clubs or short iron clubs may resume as little as 4 weeks after operation. At 10 to 12 weeks after surgery, the use of all clubs, including a long iron and driver, is possible without restriction.

SUMMARY

Golf injuries of the hand and wrist are preventable through proper understanding of swing mechanics, avoidance of repetitive and excessive golf practice and play, and ensuring that the hands are appropriately placed on the club to minimize impact injuries. A thorough understanding of the swing phases and mechanisms of injury in golf facilitates accurate diagnosis, treatment, and future prevention of injuries. Initial treatment starts with the cessation of practice to rest the wrist, a splint or orthotic brace, and NSAIDs with corticosteroid injection. Swing modification is recommended for trigger finger, de Quervain disease, and tendinopathy. Pisiform excision is the best treatment of the most severe chronic cases of PLC syndrome, especially if the patient's symptoms are intolerable and nonoperative treatment measures have failed. Delayed diagnosis of hook of hamate fracture may lead to complications, including flexor tendon rupture of the little or ring fingers and sensory or motor deficits of the ulnar nerve. Prompt surgical resection is recommended to hasten return to sport and to prevent further complications.

REFERENCES

1. McCarroll JR, Retting AC, Shelbourne KD. Injuries in the amateur golfer. Phys Sports Med 1990;18:122–6.
2. Gosheger G, Liem D, Ludwig K, et al. Injuries and overuse syndromes in golf. Am J Sports Med 2003;31(3):438–43.
3. Hawkes R, O'Connor P, Campbell D. The prevalence, variety and impact of wrist problems in elite professional golfers on the European Tour. Br J Sports Med 2013;47(17):1075–9.
4. Gordon BS, Moir GL, Davis SE, et al. An investigation into the relationship of flexibility, power, and strength to club head speed in male golfers. J Strength Cond Res 2009;23(5):1606–10.
5. Chao EY, Cooney WP 3rd, Cahalan TD, et al. Biomechanics of golf swing and a comparison of club handle design. Biomed Sci Instrum 1987;23:23–7.

6. Cahalan TD, Cooney WP 3rd, Tamai K, et al. Biomechanics of the golf swing in players with pathologic conditions of the forearm, wrist, and hand. Am J Sports Med 1991;19(3):288–93.

7. Hsu WC, Chen WH, Oware A. Distal ulnar neuropathy in a golf player. Clin J Sport Med 2005;15(3):189–90.

8. Hueston JT, Wilson WF. The aetiology of trigger finger explained on the basis of intratendinous architecture. Hand 1972;4(3):257–60.

9. Fahey JJ, Bollinger JA. Trigger-finger in adults and children. J Bone Joint Surg Am 1954;36(6):1200–18.

10. Kerrigan CL, Stanwix MG. Using evidence to minimize the cost of trigger finger care. J Hand Surg Am 2009;34(6):997–1005.

11. Finkelstein H. Stenosing tendovaginitis at the radial styloid process. J Bone Joint Surg Am 1930;1(2):509–40.

12. Eichhoff E. Zur pathogenese der tenovaginitis stenosans. Bruns Beitr Klin Chir 1927;139:746–55.

13. Goubau JF, Goubau L, Van Tongel A, et al. The wrist hyperflexion and abduction of the thumb (WHAT) test: a more specific and sensitive test to diagnose de Quervain tenosynovitis than the Eichhoff's test. J Hand Surg Eur 2014;39(3):28692.

14. Kwon BC, Choi SJ, Koh SH, et al. Sonographic identification of the intracompartmental septum in de Quervain's disease. Clin Orthop Relat Res 2010;468(8):2129–34.

15. Murray PM, Cooney WP. Golf-induced injuries of the wrist. Clin Sports Med 1996;15(1):85–109.

16. Weiss AP, Akelman E, Tabatabai M. Treatment of de Quervain's disease. J Hand Surg Am 1994;19(4):595–8.

17. Mastey RD, Weiss APC, Akelman E. Primary care of hand and wrist athletic injuries. Clin Sports Med 1997;16(4):705–24.

18. Wolfe SW. Tendinopathy. In: Wolfe SW, Hotchkiss RN, Kozin SH, et al, editors. Green's operative hand surgery. 7th edition. Philadelphia: Elsevier; 2017. p. 1904–25.

19. Bishop AT, Gabel G, Carmichael SW. Flexor carpi radialis tendinitis. Part I: operative anatomy. J Bone Joint Surg Am 1994;76(7):1009–14.

20. Parellada AJ, Morrison WB, Reiter SB, et al. Flexor carpi radialis tendinopathy: spectrum of imaging findings and association with triscaphe arthritis. Skeletal Radiol 2006;35(8):572–8.

21. Gabel G, Bishop AT, Wood MB. Flexor carpi radialis tendinitis. Part II: results of operative treatment. J Bone Joint Surg Am 1994;76(7):1015–8.

22. Brink PR, Franssen BB, Disseldrop DJ. A simple blind tenolysis for flexor carpi radialis tendinopathy. Hand (N Y) 2015;10(2):323–7.

23. Budoff JE, Kraushaar BS, Ayala G. Flexor carpi ulnaris tendinopathy. J Hand Surg Am 2005;30(1):125–9.

24. Palmieri TJ. Pisiform area pain treatment by pisiform excision. J Hand Surg Am 1982;7(5):477–80.

25. Wood MB, Dobyns JH. Sports-related extraarticular wrist syndromes. Clin Orthop Relat Res 1986;202:93–102.

26. Paley D, McMurtry RY, Cruickshank B. Pathologic conditions of the pisiform and pisotriquetral joint. J Hand Surg Am 1987;12(1):110–9.

27. Rayan GM. Pisiform ligament complex syndrome and pisotriquetral arthrosis. Hand Clin 2005;21(4):507–17.

28. van Eijzeren J, Karthaus RP. The effect of pisiform excision on wrist function. J Hand Surg Am 2014;39(7):1258–63.

29. Ghatan AC, Puri SG, Morse KW, et al. Relative contribution of the subsheath to extensor carpi ulnaris tendon stability: implications for surgical reconstruction and rehabilitation. J Hand Surg Am 2016;41(2):225–32.

30. Campbell D, Campbell R, O'Connor P, et al. Sport-related extensor carpi ulnaris pathology: a review of functional anatomy, sports injury and management. Br J Sports Med 2013;47(17):1105–11.

31. O'Connor PJ, Hawkes R. Imaging the elite golfer. Skeletal Radiol 2013;42(5):607–9.

32. Montalvan B, Parier J, Brasseur JL, et al. Extensor carpi ulnaris injuries in tennis players: a study of 28 cases. Br J Sports Med 2006;40(5):424–9.

33. Hajj AA, Wood MB. Stenosing tenosynovitis of the extensor carpi ulnaris. J Hand Surg Am 1986;11(4):519–20.

34. Graham TJ. Pathologies of the extensor carpi ulnaris (ECU) tendon and its investment in the athlete. Hand Clin 2012;28(3):345–56.

35. Inoue G, Tamura Y. Surgical treatment for recurrent dislocation of the extensor carpi ulnaris tendon. J Hand Surg Br 2001;26(6):556–9.

36. Ek ET, Suh N, Weiland AJ. Hand and wrist injuries in golf. J Hand Surg Am 2013;38(10):2029–33.

37. MacLennan AJ, Nemechek NM, Waitayawinyu T, et al. Diagnosis and anatomic reconstruction of extensor carpi ulnaris subluxation. J Hand Surg Am 2008;33(1):59–64.

38. Andresen R, Radmer S, Sparmann M, et al. Imaging of hamate bone fractures in conventional X-rays and high-resolution computed tomography: an in vitro study. Invest Radiol 1999;34(1):46–50.

39. Walsh JJ 4th, Bishop AT. Diagnosis and management of hamate hook fractures. Hand Clin 2000;16(3):397–403.

40. David TS, Zemel NP, Mathews PV. Symptomatic, partial union of the hook of the hamate fracture in athletes. Am J Sports Med 2003;31(1):106–11.

41. Stark HH, Chao EK, Zemel NP, et al. Fracture of the hook of the hamate. J Bone Joint Surg Am 1989;71(8):1202–7.

42. Carroll RE, Lakin JF. Fracture of the hook of the hamate: acute treatment. J Trauma 1993;34(6):803–5.

43. Devers BN, Douglas KC, Naik RD, et al. Outcomes of hook of hamate fracture excision in high-level amateur athletes. J Hand Surg Am 2013;38(1):72–6.

44. Tolat AR, Humphrey JA, McGovern PD, et al. Surgical excision of ununited hook of hamate fractures via the carpal tunnel approach. Injury 2014;45(10): 1554–6.
45. Yamazaki H, Kato H, Nakatsuchi Y, et al. Closed rupture of the flexor tendons of the little finger secondary to non-union or fractures of the hook of the hamate. J Hand Surg Br 2006;31(3):337–41.
46. Lalonde DH. Wide-awake flexor tendon repair. Plast Reconstr Surg 2009;123(2):623–5.
47. Tang JB. Wide-awake primary flexor tendon repair, tenolysis, and tendon transfer. Clin Orthop Surg 2015;7(3):275–81.
48. Cooney WP. Evaluation of chronic wrist pain by arthrography, arthroscopy, and arthrotomy. J Hand Surg Am 1993;18(5):816–22.
49. Fulcher SM, Kiefhaber TR, Stern PJ. Hand and wrist injuries: upper-extremity tendinitis and overuse syndromes in the athlete. Clin Sports Med 1998;17(3): 433–48.

Hand and Wrist Injuries in Boxing and the Martial Arts

Benjamin Todd Drury, MD[a], Thomas P. Lehman, MD[b],
Ghazi Rayan, MD[c],*

KEYWORDS

- Hand • Injury • Boxing • Judo • Taekwondo • Karate • Prevention

KEY POINTS

- Hand and wrist injuries in martial arts are a reflection of the combat nature of this discipline.
- There is clear evidence to support that hand protection reduces the risk of hand injury in martial arts.
- A key component of injury prevention in martial arts is the use of proper techniques for both striking and grappling.

INTRODUCTION

A wide variety of hand injuries are encountered in combat sports. These are often specific to the combat and contact techniques that are unique to each sport. With the introduction of mixed martial arts in the 1990s, the blending of disciplines has introduced an increasing number of hand and wrist injuries that reflect the violent nature of modern combat sports.

A 2012 survey of martial arts participants demonstrated that 53% of upper extremity martial arts injuries occur in the hand and wrist, followed by the shoulder and elbow at 27% and 19%, respectively.[1]

Overall injury rates in martial arts are less frequent than those reported in soccer, volleyball, and gymnastics but perhaps are substantially underreported.[2,3] Most studies investigating injury statistics in martial arts report primarily tournament competition and do not accurately include training injuries. Therefore surveys performed among martial arts participants at all levels may offer further insight into the prevalence of related injuries.

The Olympic combat sports include boxing, judo, taekwondo, and wrestling (Greco-Roman and freestyle). For purposes of discussion, wrestling is not included in this narrative, as much of this sport has been introduced into mixed martial arts competition and carries a similar injury profile to judo. Combat sports can be classified into 3 main categories: striking sports, grappling sports, and hybrids of these 2 sports. The hand and wrist injuries associated with these categories are unique to these methods of combat.

Striking sports include boxing, kickboxing, karate, and taekwondo. Grappling sports include Brazilian jiu-jitsu and judo. Hybrids of striking and grappling are generally referred to as mixed martial arts, and these include combinations of striking, kicking, and grappling to achieve submission of the opponent.

Most combat sports have evolved to include the use of some type of protective gear on the hands,

Disclosure: None of the authors have any commercial or financial conflict of interest to disclose.
[a] Texas Orthopedic Specialists, 2425 Highway 121, Bedford, TX 76021, USA; [b] OUHSC Department of Orthopedic Surgery, College of Medicine Building, 800 Stanton L. Young Boulevard Suite 3400, Oklahoma City, OK 73104, USA; [c] University of Oklahoma Health Sciences Center, 3366 Northwest Expressway # 700, Oklahoma City, OK 73112, USA
* Corresponding author.
E-mail address: ouhsgmr@aol.com

Hand Clin 33 (2017) 97–106
http://dx.doi.org/10.1016/j.hcl.2016.08.004
0749-0712/17/© 2016 Elsevier Inc. All rights reserved.

to potentially reduce the risk of injuries to the extremity when performing a strike, and reduce the risk of injury to the head or other organs. Boxing requires padded gloves of specific weight depending on the level of competition. Taekwondo participants often wear forearm pads, as they use this portion of the extremity frequently to inflict strikes and defend them (**Fig. 1**).

Diesselhorst and colleagues,[1] in a survey among martial arts participants, found that the use of hand protection significantly reduced the likelihood of injury to the hand during participation, and recommended the use of hand protection during training and competition. However, they did note a slight increase in injuries to the arm and shoulder, which was attributed to possible force dissipation more proximal in the limb with the use of hand protection. Other investigators have noted an actual potential increase in injuries with the use of hand protection in striking sports. Johannsen and Noerregaard[4] noted in their study that the use of knuckle pads in karate competition did not change the overall rate of injury, but head injuries were slightly increased with the use of knuckle pads, noting that the pattern differed significantly, with more contusions and fewer nasal fractures and lacerations reported. However, they noted that hand injuries were reduced dramatically with the use of knuckle pads, with only 1 hand injury reported in 2 tournaments in which knuckle padding was used, compared with 17 injuries in the 2 tournaments conducted previously in which no hand protection was used.

Diesselhorst and colleagues[1] also noted in their survey of 758 martial arts participants that the most common injury patterns to the hand in competition and practice were sprains/strains (47%) and bruises/abrasions (26%). Thirty-nine percent of their respondents reported sustaining fractures of the upper extremity during

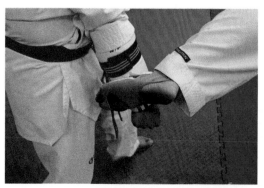

Fig. 1. Taekwondo athlete demonstrating the use of forearm padding to protect the ulna when blocking a kick.

participation, and 47% reported upper extremity dislocations. More injuries were noted during defensive positions than offensive maneuvers, and these more commonly occurred from strikes (56%) than from grappling submissions (33%). Zetaruk and colleagues[5] compared 5 different martial art disciplines and noted that the overall risk of injury in martial arts participation increased with years of participation, doubling once engaged in the sport for more than 3 years. These findings were supported in other studies that showed as the level of training and competition increases, so does the inherent risk of injury to the upper extremity requiring surgery, as well as the risk of cumulative and chronic injuries to the hand and wrist.[1,6] However, Stricevic and colleagues[7] noted that in karate competitions, acute injury rates decreased as the skill level of the participant increased.

Gender differences exist for both the rates and type of upper extremity injuries sustained during combat sport competition. Diesselhorst and colleagues[1] noted that male participants were more likely to injure their hand and fingers, whereas female participants were more likely to injure their shoulder or elbow, and that male participants had a significantly higher rate of upper extremity injuries requiring surgery. Similar findings were also observed by Birrer.[6]

The term Iron Palm training is unique to striking martial arts, particularly those with Chinese origins. It refers to the practice of conditioning the palm of the hand through repetitive striking of progressively harder objects, followed by application of herbal liniments that are often of a closely guarded mixture of specific substances. This training is concurrent with striking technique that concentrates force and maximizes strength.[8]

Mixed martial arts is a modern combat sport that represents combat using a variety of martial art disciplines that combine striking and grappling techniques. Bledsoe and colleagues[9] reported an overall injury rate of 28.6 injuries per 100 fights in mixed martial arts, with 13% of those reported being hand injuries. Lystad and colleagues[10] found similar overall rates and patterns of hand injuries related to mixed martial arts. The specific injuries of mixed martial arts are not different from those described herein for the various specific grappling and striking martial arts, and thus are not discussed under separate headings.

Boxing

History and epidemiology

Boxing was introduced as an Olympic sport in 688 BC, and remained a popular sport in ancient Roman times for nearly 300 years before it waned.

It historically reappeared in the seventeenth century and evolved into organized amateur competitions in the late 1800s, making its reappearance in the Olympics in 1904.[11] Olympic boxing matches consist of 4 rounds of 2 or 3 minutes each and require the use of 10-ounce (284 g) padded gloves. Boxing is unique among the combat sports in that it involves striking only with the gloved part of the hand; therefore, hand injuries in boxing are generally limited to those that occur in an offensive striking maneuver.

Estwanik and colleagues[12] reported that upper extremity injuries in boxing represented 44% of the overall boxing injuries recorded in their study, with more than 90% of those occurring in the hand and fingers. Noble[13] reported that hand injuries in boxing occurred most commonly to the thumb, followed closely by injuries to the base of metacarpals 2 to 5, which he related to forced wrist flexion during impact.

Prevention

Prevention of hand injury in boxing centers around 4 main concepts: hand and wrist wraps/taping, modifications of glove padding and design, proper striking technique, and proper conditioning.

Hand and wrist wraps are traditionally used to brace and cushion the hand. The various methods of wrapping the hand are steeped in boxing tradition and have had very little investigative attention as to their effectiveness. The goals of taping are first to prevent forced abduction of the border metacarpals during impact, second to pad the metacarpophalangeal (MP) joints and prevent their injury by providing a firmer area beneath the glove to lessen impact, and third to protect the wrist during impact. The wraps are usually a combination of tape and cushioned wrap to achieve these goals. Rules and restrictions regarding taping in amateur boxing may limit the wrap to one yard, but most require only that the taped hand fit into the legal glove.

Boxing glove design has made significant improvements in the past 20 years with the introduction of improved impact-absorbing and force-dissipating materials. The separation of the thumb component from the remainder of the glove is a step to reduce the risk of injuries to the thumb, which comprises more than a third of all hand injuries in boxing. Generally there are 3 types of gloves used: bag gloves (for use on a punching bag), sparring gloves with extra padding, and competition gloves.

Emphasis on proper striking technique seeks to direct the force to the middle finger metacarpal head. The teaching of correct alignment of the elbow and wrist at impact creates a direct line of force to the middle finger metacarpal with secondary dissipation to the index metacarpal head, which both are the fixed unit of the hand. Off-angle or poorly coached striking technique can result in impact to the ring and small finger metacarpals that may result in their fracture.

Common hand injuries

Sagittal band/metacarpophalangeal joint capsule (Boxer's knuckle) The MP joints are continually impacted during training and competitions, resulting in potential injury to the MP joint and to the overlying extensor hood.[14] The term "Boxer's knuckle" is often used interchangeably to describe an injury to either the sagittal band resulting in pain or instability of the extensor tendon as it traverses the MP joint, or to the dorsal MP joint capsule.[14,15] On occasions with severe impact, both the sagittal band and MP joint dorsal capsule may be injured. In the senior author's (GR) experience, sagittal band injuries from boxing are more common than isolated dorsal capsule tears. The condition most often affects the middle finger metacarpal, as this is the intended impact point and the most prominent of the metacarpal heads (**Fig. 2**).

The injury to sagittal bands usually involves the radial side of the long finger. This can result in pain with or without extensor tendon instability. Rayan and Murray[16] reported 3 types of sagittal band injuries:

- Type I is injury without extensor digitorum communis (EDC) tendon instability
- Type II is injury with EDC tendon subluxation
- Type III is frank dislocation of the EDC tendon

These injuries when mild (type I with stable EDC tendon), whether acute or chronic, can often be treated with rest and immobilization, but when severe with EDC tendon dislocation (type III) may require surgical reconstruction via a variety of methods.[16]

Injury to the dorsal MP joint capsule may be difficult to differentiate clinically from type I sagittal band injury. Posner and Ambrose[14] described 4 cases in boxers, all recalling a specific traumatic event that resulted in a swollen MP joint and subsequent pain that gradually resolved, then recurred as a chronic swelling and pain and aggravated by sparring sessions. Each of these patients had symptoms more than 2 years before seeking surgical treatment. The most typical finding in these patients was a palpable defect over the dorsal capsule of the MP joint that corresponded to the maximum area of tenderness.

Carpometacarpal joint dislocation Chronic or acute instability of the carpometacarpal joints,

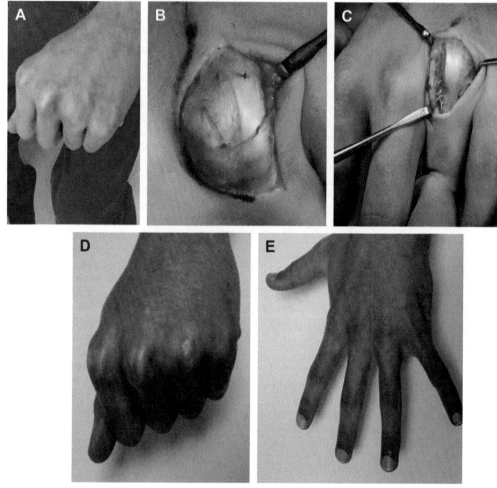

Fig. 2. (*A*) Preoperative photo of taekwondo athlete with ring finger type III sagittal band injury. (*B*) Intraoperative picture demonstrating type III radial sagittal band injury in a boxer intraoperatively and (*C*) status post reconstruction of the sagittal band to achieve centralization of the tendon. (*D, E*) Eight weeks postoperative demonstrating full motion with stable centralization of the tendon.

particularly the index and middle, is a common problem among amateur and professional boxers. Nazarian and colleagues[17] described a series of 13 elite boxers with this injury who were unable to continue competing due to pain and instability. These investigators advocated open reduction and Kirschner wire fixation for acute injuries, and arthrodesis of the carpometacarpal (CMC) joints if the instability and pain are chronic in nature. All boxers in their series were able to return to elite-level competition after surgical treatment.

Fractures Fractures in boxing are often related to poor striking technique and are more likely to occur during competition than in sparring or training.[18] Noble[14] noted that up to 39% of all hand injuries in boxing involve the thumb, with fractures of the remaining hand bones (excluding fractures of the metacarpal base) making up

approximately 29% of all injuries. The fracture pattern varies greatly depending on the force vector direction, which is influenced by the angle of attack and the surface struck. The term "Boxer's fracture" is often used to describe those of the metacarpal neck, particularly of the fourth and fifth metacarpals, and is not often seen in competitive elite boxing. This injury is more commonly the result of nongloved altercations among amateurs and is the product of a poorly thrown punch that shifts the impact point to the ulnar digits, rather than to the radial-central fixed axis of the hand.

Taekwondo

History and epidemiology
Taekwondo has its ancient roots in Korea and China but its modern form began in Korea in the 1950s and has gained widespread popularity

throughout the world, becoming an Olympic sport in 2000. The style of taekwondo is based with emphasis on speed, and the predominance of striking originating from the lower extremities in a variety of spinning and jumping kicks delivered at head or chest height. Koh and Watkinson[19] noted that point-scoring striking in taekwondo is approximately 90% delivered by the lower extremity, and 10% by the upper extremity. Traditional taekwondo training involves nonconflict-based drills or "forms" and scripted noncontact or semicontact sparring. Full contact is primarily reserved for competition, although sparring may involve limited striking.

Kazemi and colleagues[20] noted that although the lower extremity is the most commonly injured in taekwondo, the upper extremity represents up to 18% of overall injuries. Zetaruk and colleagues[5] found that up to 40% of taekwondo injuries involve the upper extremity. Pieter[21] described upper extremity injuries in detail, noting that a slight increase in distal upper extremity injuries among female competitors (12% male vs 15% female). Of these injuries, 5% occurred in the hand, 3% in the fingers, and 2% in the wrists. Koh and colleagues[22] found a much higher incidence of upper extremity injuries in female competitors (26% for males and 46% for females), noting that female competitors have equal distributions of hand, finger, and wrist injuries with a tendency to more proximal upper extremity injuries. Male competitors showed similar distributions of injuries to Pieter's study,[21] with the exception of an increase in the number of finger injuries.

Zetaruk and colleagues[5] reviewed taekwondo training injuries that resulted in fewer than 7 days of missed participation, and observed that belt rank did not predict time loss.

The use of the hands in taekwondo as an offensive weapon is very limited, particularly in the variety used for Olympic competition, which outlaws the use of the hand to strike the head or face. Therefore, most upper extremity injuries sustained in taekwondo occur in a defensive position, where the upper extremities are used to protect the trunk from kicks. However, there are multiple hand strikes taught in taekwondo that can result in acute or chronic injuries to the hand.

Prevention

Prevention of taekwondo injuries is centered primarily on the following: maintenance of strength and flexibility, relaxation techniques to absorb impact forces and reduce tissue damage, teaching proper striking techniques, and the use of limited padding in training. Padding of the upper extremity

typically consists of forearm pads that protect this area from kicks, particularly the ulna, in addition to the head and trunk. Hand protection is typically used in sparring and only recently in competition, consisting of a lightweight glove to absorb impact inflicted on the MP joints and proximal phalanx during striking.

Common hand injuries

There is a dearth of literature relative to specific hand injuries in taekwondo. Publications reporting hand injuries in taekwondo invariably describe regions of injury (wrist, hand, fingers) and/or type of injury (sprain, fracture) without specifics. A review of common hand strikes in taekwondo and their potential for injury are listed in **Box 1**.

Defensively in taekwondo, the forearm takes the most forceful blows to the upper extremity, with a high risk of nightstick injury to the ulna. Padding of the forearm may reduce the risk of this injury, although there are no known studies documenting its true efficacy (see **Fig. 1**).

Pecht and Raschka[23] reported a single case of a taekwondo athlete who deformed his fist with fibrous tissue between the heads of the metacarpals by striking progressively harder materials (eg, sand, dried peas, small stones) over a 25-year period. This led to development of a flatter knuckle profile. *The fighter believed this* reduced his risk of injury to the metacarpal head by reducing its prominence (**Fig. 3**).

Judo

History and epidemiology

Founded in Japan in 1882 by Jigoro Kano, judo is primarily a grappling martial art that has roots in jujitsu. It consists of grappling techniques done from both a standing and ground position and includes 4 basic movement categories: the throw, the hold down, choke, and arm lock. Each of these has potential for serious injury. Judo became an Olympic demonstration sport in 1964 and an official sport for men in 1972. It became an Olympic sport for women in 1992.

Pocecco and colleagues[24] conducted a systematic review of the literature regarding judo injuries. In their 2013 study, they identified an overall risk of injury during Olympic competition of approximately 12%. They noted that other studies showed risks that were double that and attributed this potentially to a wider range of skill levels in those studies. Their meta-analysis showed a trend toward sprain injuries in higher-level competitors, and upper body fractures in less-experienced competitors. Up to 30% of the injuries affected the hand and fingers, with some studies showing the fingers to be the most common site of injury,

---

Box 1
Common strikes used in taekwondo and their risks of injuries

Jab

A quick, straight punch from shoulder level with the most forward arm, with the fist clenched.

Risks of injury are to the finger extensor mechanism, particularly the radial sagittal band of the long finger, metacarpal neck or base fracture, carpometacarpal joint dislocation.

Reverse Punch

A straight powerful punch using the rear arm and a pivot of the body to develop more force.

Risks are the same as for the jab.

Back Fist

Uses the dorsum of the hand and metacarpophalangeal (MP) joints to strike the opponent as the arm moves from the opposite shoulder across the chest. Impact occurs on the dorsal aspect of the metacarpal head.

Risk is for metacarpal fracture.

Hammer Fist

Uses the hypothenar eminence and fifth metacarpal in a clenched fist position to strike the opponent.

Risks are fifth metacarpal fracture, carpal fracture, ulnar-sided wrist injury (triangular fibro cartilage complex) with forced radial deviation.

Spear Hand Strike

Hand open, fingers clenched together, strike occurs in a jabbing motion with the tips of the index, middle, and ring fingers.

Risks are mallet finger injury and phalangeal fracture (see **Fig. 4**).

Knife Hand Strike

Uses the ulnar side of the open hand to strike the opponent,

Risks are fracture of the fifth metacarpal and/or phalanges.

Ridge Hand Strike

Uses the radial side of the hand to strike, with the thumb tucked to prevent injury to the MP joint ulnar collateral ligament.

Risk is injury to the index metacarpal and phalanges.

---

primarily due to grappling during standing position of judo combat.[25] Other studies have shown that although finger injuries are most common during standing combat, shoulder injuries are more prevalent when being thrown by or throwing an opponent.[26]

Overall, 85% of judo injuries are sustained in the standing position and are related to the gripping

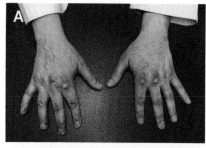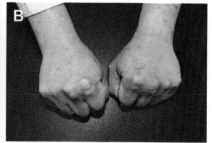

Fig. 3. (*A, B*) Note the formation of fibrous knuckle pads over the second and third metacarpophalangeal joints in this 50-year-old taekwondo participant. These were developed with repetitive daily striking of various firm objects to condition the hands and theoretically reduce the risk of injury.

that occurs when engaging the opponent before an attack, or engagement with grip when throwing or being thrown. Pierantozzi and colleagues[27] found the hand and fingers to be the most common site of injury in judo, noting that they represented nearly 30% of all injuries. Other investigators have found consistent rates of injury varying between 11% and 17% involving the hand and fingers.[26,28,29]

Prevention
Prevention of injury in judo primarily revolves around proper technique for hand positioning when being thrown or "break-fall training." In general, most throws begin with gripping of the opponent's judogi (judo clothing) and use tremendous leverage through the grip to facilitate the throw. The opponent is taught to strike the mat with the palm or dorsum of hand during the fall to minimize the risk of injury to the upper extremity and to reduce the impact of the fall. As there is very little striking in judo, it is not common to wear protective hand gear. Taping is used occasionally in training, but no literature exists as to its effectiveness in preventing injury in judo training or competition. Barsottini and colleagues[28] noted that more than 70% of judo injuries occur during training, and particular attention must be paid to injury prevention during training to reduce time loss from competition.

Common hand injuries
There is paucity of literature relative to hand injuries in judo. Clearly the injury patterns in this grappling sport are much different from those seen in the striking martial arts. Virtually all published studies on judo injury classify sprains as the most common injuries, although no study identifies or classifies specific hand injuries.

Jersey finger Jersey finger is likely a common injury in judo due to the gripping nature of standing combat. Often judo athletes refer to "Jersey finger" as the soreness that occurs during training from repetitive forced gripping, but the true Jersey finger is the disruption of the flexor digitorum profundus tendon from its distal attachment, either with or without a bony fragment. Typically the ring finger is the most frequently affected.

Sprains/dislocations of finger interphalangeal joints The force required for executing a throw in judo is often initiated via grip on the judogi, resulting in potential for interphalangeal and metacarpophalangeal joint ligament injury. Although no specific case reports exist in the literature, Barsottini and colleagues[28] conducted a survey of judo athletes and noted that they reported that finger sprains accounted for 10% of injuries. They also found no relationship between any particular judo techniques or "strokes" and hand or finger injuries. To our knowledge, no study has clearly documented the potential association of finger injury and judo, such as joint ligament injuries, or tendon injuries, such as mallet finger (**Fig. 4**), or central tendon disruption with resultant Boutonniere deformity.

Chronic injuries Both Strasser and colleagues[30] and Frey and Müller[31,32] found that degenerative changes of the proximal interphalangeal and distal interphalangeal joints were very common in long-term judo athletes. Frey and Müller[31] noted the presence of Heberden nodes over the distal interphalangeal joints of nearly 30% of the members of the Swiss national team, noting that examined members of the other Olympic martial arts disciplines lacked this finding.

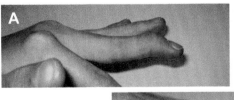
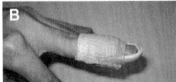
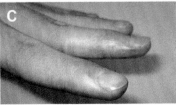

Fig. 4. (*A*) Mallet finger injury sustained by taekwondo athlete blocking a kick. (*B*) Injury was treated in a splint maintaining extension at the distal interphalangeal joint. He continued to train and compete with the splint taped and padded. (*C*) Full correction of the deformity 6 weeks later. He continued to wear the splint for 6 additional weeks during taekwondo activities only.

Karate

History and epidemiology

Karate began as an ancient Japanese striking martial art that has its origins in the Ryukyu Islands, and its name means "empty hands." It evolved into its more modern form in the late 1800s and was brought to the United States and Europe in the late 1940s. It became very popular with pop culture martial art movies of the 1970s, and the World Karate Federation estimates that the sport has up to 100 million participants worldwide. There are efforts to establish karate as an Olympic sport but it has not yet reached the voting threshold to be included as an Olympic sport.

Despite some similarities in hand and foot strikes to taekwondo, Zetaruk and colleagues[5] found that the overall injury rate in karate to be half of that noted in taekwondo. There are quite a few similarities in the 2 disciplines, although karate may emphasize hand strikes more, and in particular open palm or strikes with the base of the thenar and hypothenar eminences while the wrist is extended (palm heel strike).

Injury rates in karate are inconsistently reported, primarily due to wide discrepancies in the level of contact allowed in various tournaments. Overall injury rates are reported to be 0.25 to 0.30 injuries per bout in multiple studies done with and without the use of hand padding.[4,7,33] McLatchie and colleagues,[34,35] in a large series spanning a decade, noted a fivefold reduction in overall injury rate with the addition of hand padding in bouts, but other studies noted previously show no reduction in overall rates.[4,7,33] However, Johannsen and Noerregaard[4] in a Danish study of karate championships noted that although overall injury rates did not decrease with the use of gloves, the rate of hand injuries decreased from 0.045 per match to 0.010. They did note that all but one of the reported hand injuries in their series occurred without gloves, and were caused by punching into a block or from poor technique of striking of an opponent's bony prominence.

There are 3 basic components of most karate training: the "kihon" are basic movements practiced alone, the "kata" are a continuation of more sophisticated movements also done alone, and "kumite," which encompasses all combat with an opponent. Modern karate tournaments are divided into 5 levels with increasing amounts of contact allowed, with "full contact" being the least restrictive and involving full force of hand and foot strikes.[36] Specific hand strikes in karate are virtually identical to those previously listed (see **Box 1**) for taekwondo, with the addition of the "palm heel strike," which, although used in taekwondo, is emphasized more in karate training.

Prevention

Prevention of injury in karate seems more centered on control of strikes and the level of contact in competition. Various investigators have noted the strict enforcement of striking rules and controlled striking as the most important contributor to the reduction of injuries in karate.[4,36] In particular, reduction of hand injuries by avoidance of poor technique and inaccurate target selection is emphasized in traditional teaching (**Fig. 5**). Hand padding, as noted previously, has been shown to reduce hand injuries and is now mandatory for all bouts that involve full contact. Macan and colleagues[37] noted that rule changes implemented by the World Karate Federation in 2000, which standardized glove wear and restricted the use of open palm and palm heel strikes, have reduced the rate of injury, particularly among young competitors.

Common injuries

Injuries in karate follow the same logic as other striking martial arts, with the position of the hand and the object struck determining patterns of fracture, sprain, or contusion. Of particular

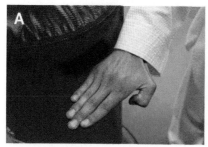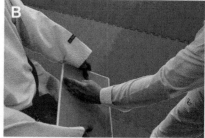

Fig. 5. (*A*) Karate athlete demonstrating the knife hand strike with proper technique that dissipates force along the length of the metacarpal and phalanges, and protects the thumb. (*B*) Off camber knife hand strike demonstrating the deforming forces that occur at the fifth metacarpophalangeal joint with less than perfect technique.

interest, the palm heel strike can lead to the formation of an ulnar artery aneurysm (hypothenar hammer syndrome), even from a single traumatic event.[38] Vidal and colleagues[39] reported a case of a triple dislocation involving the MP, proximal interphalangeal, and distal interphalangeal joints of the small finger in a karate participant who was struck on the tip of the finger, most likely in a defensive maneuver.

Chronic injuries in karate were also reported in the literature. Gardner[40] described an incident of hypertrophic infiltrative tendinitis of the long finger extensor tendon secondary to the "abused karate hand," describing this as an entrapment of the tendon at the MP joint requiring surgical release similar to a trigger finger. Rao and Culver[41] noted in their series of 10 patients with midcarpal instability in 1 patient who sustained this injury from karate, but more from a twisting mechanism than a strike. They treated this successfully with triquetrohamate arthrodesis. Crosby[42] reviewed hand radiographs of 22 karate instructors with a minimum of 5 years of experience. Although he noted the presence of 10 healed fractures, there were no considerable degenerative changes or other signs of chronic trauma noted in his cohort. Chiu[43] reported a case of a 12-year-old karate athlete with segmental perineural and interfascicular fibrosis of the dorsal cutaneous branch of the ulnar nerve in the small finger that developed from repeated karate strikes against various hard objects. This was treated with microsurgical internal neurolysis with satisfactory results. Nieman and Swann[44] reported a similar case involving temporary paralysis of the deep branch of the ulnar nerve that resolved with cessation of knife hand strikes on hard surfaces as part of karate training.

SUMMARY

Hand and wrist injuries in martial arts are typically a reflection of the primary combat nature of this discipline. In striking sports, the axial load mechanism of injury is common and causes fractures and dislocations, whereas in grappling sports sprain injuries and degenerative changes predominate. Although there is some debate as to the effectiveness of hand protection in reducing overall rates of injury in martial arts, there is clear evidence that it does reduce specifically the risk of injury to the hand. Traditional training in martial arts on proper technique and target selection in striking sports reduces the risk of hand injury, and is an important component of hand and wrist injury prevention.

REFERENCES

1. Diesselhorst M, Rayan G, Pasque C, et al. Survey of upper extremity injuries among martial arts participants. Hand Surg 2013;18:151–7.
2. Tenvergert EM, Duis HJ, Klasen HJ. Trends in sports injuries 1982-1988: an in depth study on four types of sport. J Sports Med Phys Fitness 1992;32(2):214–20.
3. Birrer RB, Birrer CD. Unreported injuries in the martial arts. Br J Sports Med 1983;17(2):131–4.
4. Johannsen HV, Noerregaard FO. Prevention of injury in karate. Br J Sports Med 1988;22(3):113–5.
5. Zetaruk MN, Violan MA, Zurakowski D, et al. Injuries in martial arts: a comparison of five styles. Br J Sports Med 2005;39:29–33.
6. Birrer R. Trauma epidemiology in the martial arts: the results of an eighteen-year international survey. Am J Sports Med 1996;24(6):S72–9.
7. Stricevic MV, Patel MR, Okazaki T, et al. Karate: historical perspective and injuries sustained in national and international tournament competitions. Am J Sports Med 1983;11(5):320–4.
8. Anta J. Shaolin physical conditioning: what's old is new again. J Asian Martial Arts 2009;18(1):72–80.
9. Bledsoe GH, Hsu EB, Grabowski JG, et al. Incidence of injury in professional mixed martial arts competitions. J Sports Med Sci 2006;5:136–42.
10. Lystad RP, Gregory K, Wilson J. The epidemiology of injuries in mixed martial arts a systematic review and meta-analysis. Orthop J Sports Med 2014;2(1). 2325967113518492.
11. Zazryn T, McCrory P. Boxing. In: Caine DJ, Harmer PA, Schiff MA, editors. Epidemiology of injury in Olympic sports. Hoboken (NJ): Blackwell; 2010. p. 92–106.
12. Estwanik JJ, Boitano M, Ari N. Amateur boxing injuries at the 1981 and 1982 USA/ABF national championships. Phys Sportsmed 1984;12(10):123–8.
13. Noble C. Hand injuries in boxing. Am J Sports Med 1987;15(4):342–6.
14. Posner MA, Ambrose L. Boxer's knuckle—dorsal capsular rupture of the metacarpophalangeal joint of a finger. J Hand Surg 1989;14(2):229–36.
15. Hame SL, Melone CP. Boxer's knuckle in the professional athlete. Am J Sports Med 2000;28(6):879–82.
16. Rayan GM, Murray D. Classification and treatment of closed sagittal band injuries. J Hand Surg 1994; 19(4):590–4.
17. Nazarian N, Page RS, Hoy GA, et al. Combined joint fusion for index and middle carpometacarpal instability in elite boxers. J Hand Surg Eur Vol 2014; 39(3):242–8.
18. Porter M, O'Brien M. Incidence and severity of injuries resulting from amateur boxing in Ireland. Clin J Sport Med 1996;6(2):97–101.
19. Koh JO, Watkinson EJ. Video analysis of blows to the head and face at the 1999 World Taekwondo

Championships. J Sports Med Phys Fitness 2002; 42(3):348–54.

20. Kazemi M, Shearer H, Choung YS. Pre-competition habits and injuries in Taekwondo athletes. BMC Musculoskelet Disord 2005;6(1):26.

21. Pieter W. Taekwondo. In: Caine DJ, Harmer PA, Schiff MA, editors. Epidemiology of injury in Olympic sports. Hoboken (NJ): Blackwell; 2010. p. 249–59.

22. Koh JO, de Freitas T, Watkinson EJ. Injuries at the 14th world taekwondo championships in 1999. Int J App Sports Sci 2001;13(1):33–48.

23. Pecht VS, Raschka C. Deformation of the fist due to Taekwondo training. MMW Fortschr Med 2005; 147(42):48–9 [in German].

24. Pocecco E, Ruedl G, Stankovic N, et al. Injuries in judo: a systematic literature review including suggestions for prevention. Br J Sports Med 2013; 47(18):1139–43.

25. Green CM, Petrou MJ, Fogarty-Hover ML, et al. Injuries among judokas during competition. Scand J Med Sci Sports 2007;17(3):205–10.

26. Souza M, Monteiro H, Del Vecchio F, et al. Referring to judo's sports injuries in São Paulo State Championship. Sci Sports 2006;21(5):280–4.

27. Pierantozzi E, Muroni R. Judo high level competition injuries. Medit J Musc Surv 2009;17:26–9.

28. Barsottini D, Guimarães AE, Morais PR. Relationship between techniques and injuries among judo practitioners. Revista Brasileira de Medicina do Esporte 2006;12(1):56–60.

29. Yard EE, Knox CL, Smith GA, et al. Pediatric martial arts injuries presenting to emergency departments, United States 1990–2003. J Sci Med Sport 2007; 10(4):219–26.

30. Strasser P, Hauser M, Häuselmann HJ, et al. Traumatic finger polyarthrosis in judo athletes: a follow-up study. Z Rheumatol 1997;56(6):342–50 [in German].

31. Frey A, Müller W. Heberden arthroses in judo athletes. Schweiz Med Wochenschr 1984;114(2):40–7.

32. Harmer P. Judo. In: Caine DJ, Harmer PA, Schiff MA, editors. Epidemiology of injury in Olympic sports. Hoboken (NJ): Blackwell; 2010. p. 161–75.

33. Tuominen R. Injuries in national karate competitions in Finland. Scand J Med Sci Sports 1995;5(1):44–8.

34. McLatchie GR, Morris EW. Prevention of karate injuries–a progress report. Br J Sports Med 1977; 11(2):78–82.

35. McLatchie GR, Commandre FA, Zakarian H, et al. Injuries in the martial arts. Clin Pract Sports Inj Care 1994;5:609–23.

36. Critchley GR, Mannion S, Meredith C. Injury rates in Shotokan karate. Br J Sports Med 1999;33(3):174–7.

37. Macan J, Bundalo-Vrbanac D, Romić G. Effects of the new karate rules on the incidence and distribution of injuries. Br J Sports Med 2006;40(4): 326–30.

38. Marie I, Hervé F, Primard E, et al. Long-term follow-up of hypothenar hammer syndrome: a series of 47 patients. Medicine 2007;86(6):334–43.

39. Vidal N, Barrera-Ochoa S, Lluch A, et al. Simultaneous triple dislocation of the small finger. J Hand Surg 2013;38(1):206.

40. Gardner RC. Hypertrophic infiltrative tendinitis (HIT syndrome) of the long extensor: the abused karate hand. JAMA 1970;211(6):1009–10.

41. Rao SB, Culver JE. Triquetrohamate arthrodesis for midcarpal instability. J Hand Surg 1995;20(4):583–9.

42. Crosby AC. The hands of karate experts. Clinical and radiological findings. Br J Sports Med 1985; 19(1):41–2.

43. Chiu DT. "Karate kid" finger. Plast Reconstr Surg 1993;91(2):362–4.

44. Nieman EA, Swann PG. Karate injuries. Br Med J 1971;1(5742):233.

Wrist Arthroscopy for Athletic Injuries

Rick Tosti, MD[a],*, Eon Shin, MD[b]

KEYWORDS

- Wrist arthroscopy • Wrist injuries • Sports • Athletes

KEY POINTS

- Management of wrist pain in athletes must take into consideration the timing and achievement of sport-specific goals.
- Wrist arthroscopy is the standard for diagnosing intracarpal derangements.
- A variety of wrist procedures can be safely and effectively performed through the arthroscope.

INTRODUCTION

Hand and wrist injuries are common in athletes, accounting for approximately 3% to 9% of all sports-related injuries.[1] Specific sports, such as football, gymnastics, and combat sports may have a higher incidence. Trauma to the hand and wrist is the second most common injury in mixed martial artists and boxers.[2–4] Hand and wrist injuries may affect up to 46% to 87% of gymnasts.[1] Management strategies for athletes are often tailored to their sport-specific goals, which can involve a combination of operative repair, early rehabilitation, and/or minimally invasive techniques.

The goal is to provide reliable healing with expeditious return to sport. Wrist arthroscopy is a useful tool in the surgeon's armamentarium; it is widely considered the most sensitive and specific method of evaluating carpal derangements,[5,6] and in appropriate cases, may provide a minimally invasive solution. This article reviews the relevant anatomy of the carpus, clinical evaluation of the patient with wrist pain, and sports-related injuries that are commonly treated using arthroscopy.

ANATOMY

The carpus is composed of 8 bones arranged in 2 rows. The proximal row articulates with the radius to form the radiocarpal joint and with the distal row to form the midcarpal joint. The distal row articulates with the 5 metacarpals to form the carpometacarpal joints. The intrinsic ligaments directly connect the bones within a row. In the proximal row, the scapholunate interosseous ligament (SLIL) provides static volar and dorsal stability to the scaphoid and lunate. The lunotriquetral interosseous ligament (LTIL) similarly connects the lunate and triquetrum.

The distal row consists of multiple intercarpal connections similarly named according to their intercarpal origins and insertions. The volar extrinsic ligaments confer stability across the radiocarpal joint and are arranged in a "double V" orientation (**Fig. 1**). The dorsal extrinsic ligaments include the dorsal intercarpal ligament and the radiotriquetral ligament. The triangular fibrocartilage complex (TFCC) separates the wrist from the distal radioulnar joint. It consists of the articular disk, meniscus homologue, volar and dorsal radioulnar ligaments, extensor carpi ulnaris

Disclosure: The authors have nothing to disclose.
a Department of Orthopaedic Surgery, Massachusetts General Hospital, Harvard Medical School, 55 Fruit Street, Boston, MA 02114, USA; b The Philadelphia Hand Center, Sidney Kimmel Medical College, Thomas Jefferson University, 834 Chestnut Street, Philadelphia, PA 19107, USA
* Corresponding author.
E-mail address: rjtosti@gmail.com

hand.theclinics.com

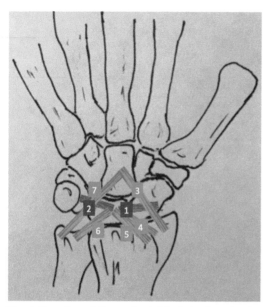

Fig. 1. Drawing of the major intrinsic (*red*) and volar extrinsic (*blue*) ligaments: (1) Scapholunate, (2) luno-triquetral, (3) radioscaphocapitate, (4) long radiolunate, (5) short radiolunate, (6) ulnolunate, and (7) ulnotriquetral capitate complex.

(ECU) subsheath, and the ulnolunate and ulnar triquetral ligaments. In an ulnar neutral wrist, it absorbs 18% of the load across the carpus.[7] The radioulnar ligaments of the TFCC also impart stability to the distal radioulnar joint (DRUJ).

Motion of the wrist is passively transmitted through the crossing tendons and guided by the bony geometry and ligamentous architecture. As a result of the helicoid geometry of the midcarpal joint, motion at the wrist is often "paired"

for most sports-related movements. The "dart-throwers motion" nicely illustrates the combinations of radial deviation/extension and ulnar deviation/flexion, which guide smooth and synchronous movement.

EVALUATION OF WRIST PAIN

A thorough history provides useful information in making the diagnosis. The character and onset of pain, mechanism of injury, location of pain, and associated, relieving, and exacerbating symptoms help focus the examination. We find it helpful to ask patients to point with 1 finger to the 1 area of the most intensity. As many structures comprise and cross the carpus, the differential diagnosis includes many possibilities, which can be organized by location (**Table 1**). The treating physician should ask additional questions regarding hand dominance, sport-specific season and goals, sport-specific difficulties, and level of competitiveness.

Physical examination should begin with inspection for skin lesions, wounds, swelling, and deformity. Palpation along the carpus begins away from the side of pain (eg, if the patient has radial wrist pain, then start by palpating ulnar structures). When palpating the wrist, the examiner should systematically palpate each osseous, tendinous, and ligamentous structure in that region. Range of motion, grip strength measurements, and neurovascular testing are included in the examination. Special provocative maneuvers are performed last and may provide injury-specific information (**Table 2**). Radiographs, arthrography, computed tomography, and MRI are useful diagnostic

Table 1		
Differential diagnosis for wrist pain		
Radial Wrist Pain	**Dorsal Wrist Pain**	**Ulnar Wrist Pain**
Thumb basal joint arthritis	Intersection syndrome	TFCC tear
STT arthritis	Extensor tendon synovitis	DRUJ instability
Radioscaphoid arthritis	Keinbock disease	Ulnocarpal abutment
deQuervain tenosynovitis	SLIL tear	ECU tendinitis
Radial artery aneurysm	Occult ganglion	FCU tendinitis
Scaphoid fracture	Radiocarpal arthritis	Pisotriquetral arthritis
FCR tendinitis	DRUJ arthritis	Lunotriquetral ligament tear
Preiser disease	Distal radius fracture	Hook of Hamate fracture
SLIL tear	Inflammatory arthritis	Ulnar styloid fracture
Radial styloid fracture	Septic arthritis	Hypothenar hammer syndrome
Radial sensory neuritis	Perilunate dislocation	Ulnar sensory neuritis

Abbreviations: DRUJ, distal radioulnar joint; ECU, extensor carpi ulnaris; FCR, flexor carpi radialis; FCU, flexor carpi ulnaris; SLIL, scapholunate interosseus ligament; STT, scaphotrapeziotrapezoid; TFCC, triangular fibrocartilage complex.

Table 2
Provocative tests for wrist pain

Test	Pathology	Maneuver	Positive Result
Watson	SL ligament tear	Examiner places dorsal directed pressure on the scaphoid tubercle. Wrist is moved into radial deviation.	Clunk and pain as the proximal scaphoid subluxes dorsally.
Ballottement for LT	LT ligament tear	Examiner ballots to lunate and triquetrum in a dorsal and volar direction.	Pain and laxity as the bones glide against each other.
Catch Up Clunk	Midcarpal instability	Axial load on the wrist as it is moved from radial to ulnar deviation.	Clunk and pain as the proximal row snaps from flexion to extension.
Ballottement for DRUJ	DRUJ instability	Examiner stabilizes the radius and ulna in neutral rotation and ballots the radius. Perform also in pronation and supination.	Clunk and pain as the radius subluxes out of the DRUJ.
Compression Rotation	DRUJ instability	Examiner compresses the radius and ulna at the DRUJ and rotates through supination and pronation.	Clunk and pain as the radius subluxes out of the DRUJ.
ECU snap test	ECU subluxation	Examiner palpates the ECU at the wrist while supinating the DRUJ.	ECU subluxes volarly with supination.
Allen	Arterial occlusion	Radial and ulnar arteries are occluded. The hand opens and closes to remove venous blood. One artery is released.	The hand should return to pink color with a patent artery. Pallor signals an occlusion.
Finkelstein	deQuervain tenosynovitis	Patient holds own thumb as wrist moves into ulnar deviation.	Pain over the first dorsal compartment.
CMC grind	Thumb basal joint arthritis	Circumduction of the thumb metacarpal with axial load.	Pain at the base of the metacarpal.
Tinel	Neuritis	Tapping on peripheral nerve.	Electrical shock along nerve distribution.

Abbreviations: DRUJ, distal radioulnar joint; ECU, extensor carpi ulnaris; LT, lunotriquetral; SL, scapholunate.

adjuncts and are discussed in subsequent sections.

BASIC WRIST ARTHROSCOPY

The patient is positioned supine on a hand table. The index and middle fingers are placed into finger traps. The wrist is distracted 10 to 15 lb across the wrist articulations by an overhead boom or traction tower. The arthroscopic portals are named by their position relative to the dorsal extensor compartments (**Fig. 2**). The 3 to 4 and 6-R portals are the most common working portals. The 3 to 4 portal is located approximately 1 cm distal to Lister tubercle in the "soft spot" between the scaphoid and lunate. The joint is insufflated with 5 to 7 mL saline through this interval, aiming the needle

10° volarly to accommodate the volar tilt. An 11 blade is used to nick the skin followed by a curved hemostat, which spreads the soft tissue and punctures the capsule. The blunt trochar and cannula are inserted into the portal, followed by the arthroscope, which is usually a short barrel scope approximately 2 to 3 mm in diameter.

Although a variety of inflow systems are available, we prefer a manual hand pump. The 6-R portal is placed under direct visualization. The surgeon pierces the capsule with an 18-g needle just radial to the ECU tendon, which is followed by a hemostat and a blunt probe. Diagnostic arthroscopy begins with a systematic evaluation of structures from radial to ulnar. The radioscaphocapitate ligament is the most radial structure seen on the volar side, and the short and long

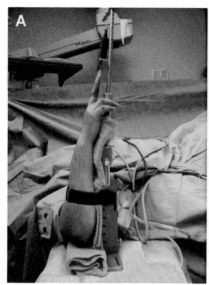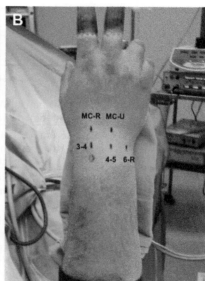

Fig. 2. (A) Traction tower setup for wrist arthroscopy. All bony prominences should be appropriately padded. (B) Wrist portals for arthroscopy. MC, midcarpal; R, radial; U, ulnar.

radiolunate ligaments are just ulnar. The surgeon should note and probe the condition of the cartilage on the radius and carpal bones. The SLIL and LTIL are also probed for structural integrity. The arthroscope is advanced ulnarly where one can evaluate the TFCC. Particular attention should be paid to the most common areas of TFCC injury, which include centrally, ulnar fovea, ulnocarpal attachment, and radioulnar origins.

Accessory proximal portals are less commonly used. The 1 to 2 portal is entered just distal to the radial styloid between the extensor carpi radialis longus and the extensor pollicis brevis; the superficial radial nerve and dorsal radial artery are at risk. The 4 to 5 portal is placed between the extensor digitorum communis and extensor digiti minimi. The 6-U portal is placed just ulnar to the ECU. It may be used as an outflow portal but risks injuring the dorsal sensory branch of the ulnar nerve.

The midcarpal joint should be routinely viewed. The 2 most common working portals are the midcarpal-radial (MC-R) and midcarpal-ulnar (MC-U) portals, which are located 1 cm distal to the 3 to 4 and 4 to 5 portals, respectively. The midcarpal joint also can be entered through a torn SLIL. Through the midcarpal portals, the distal SLIL, LTIL, and scaphotrapeziotrapezoid (STT) joints are visualized. Less commonly, an STT portal can be used to visualize the distal pole of the scaphoid, or the triquetrohamate portal can be used as an outflow. The STT portal is placed just ulnar to the extensor pollicis longus;

it is helpful to view its placement through the MC-R portal.

Volar portals may be occasionally needed. A volar-radial portal can be made by making an incision over the flexor carpi radialis at the wrist crease, retracting it ulnarly, and dissecting to the wrist capsule with tenotomy scissors. The joint can be localized with a 22-gauge needle. Alternatively, a switching stick can be driven through the 3 to 4 portal just radial to the radioscaphocapitate ligament. The switching stick is pushed through the volar capsule and found through dissection on the volar side. The volar-ulnar portal is made similarly by incising the skin over the wrist crease along the ulnar edge of the finger flexors.

Portals for the DRUJ are occasionally needed as well. The dorsal portal is made in line with the 6-R portal approximately 1 to 2 cm proximally. The volar portal can be made through the volar-ulnar skin incision by angling the trochar proximally.

Before completing the diagnostic arthroscopy, we also remove synovitis and/or loose bodies with a 2-mm shaver or grasping tools. A final lavage of the joint is performed before closure.

SPORTS-RELATED INJURIES TREATED WITH ARTHROSCOPY

A variety of injuries can occur in athletes. Serious injuries such as perilunate instability, radiocarpal instability, and most carpal bone fractures are traditionally treated with open procedures and are not discussed in this article. Additionally, the presence of an infectious or oncogenic diagnosis should never be underestimated. The following athletic injuries may be treated by arthroscopy or with arthroscopic assistance.

Scapholunate Ligament Rupture

SLIL tears usually occur from an extension and ulnar deviation force with an intercarpal supination moment. A fall onto an outstretched pronated hand is a common mechanism in sports. Patients present with dorsal wrist pain in the scapholunate interval. They may complain of clicking in the wrist. The scaphoid shift test may be positive. Radiographs may be normal in partial tears, but dynamic instability becomes evident with an ulnar deviated and clenched fist view. However, a clenched fist view always should be compared with the uninjured side, as generalized laxity may produce a false-positive result. Signs of instability include a gap greater than 3 mm between the scaphoid and lunate (Terry Thomas sign) and a flexed scaphoid posture (signet ring sign). The lateral view may demonstrate dorsal intercalary segmental instability (DISI) deformity, seen when the scapholunate angle measures greater than 60°.

MRI may be useful in identifying an SL ligament tear, especially in the presence of normal radiographs; however, the degree of tearing and the condition of the cartilage is best determined by arthroscopy. Dissociative carpal instability is classified by the severity of injury, malalignment, and degenerative disease (**Table 3**).[8] Acute partial and complete tears are amenable to arthroscopic treatment. Irreparable tears that require reconstruction (chronic or severe tears), reduction (malaligned carpus), or arthrodesis (degenerated carpus) should undergo an open procedure.

After performing a diagnostic arthroscopy, the surgeon examines and grades the severity of the SLIL tear. A grading system is used in the decision-making process (**Table 4**).[9] In Geissler grade 1, the ligament loses tension but is still intact. In Geissler grades 2 and 3, partial tearing is seen. No gross instability or malalignment is seen in grades 1 to 3. Geissler grade 4 (complete) tears are identified arthroscopically with a positive drive-through sign from the midcarpal articulation into the radiocarpal joint space through the SL interval. Pain is thought to be from increased motion, shearing, and synovitis.

For Geissler grades 1 and 2, the surgeon may decide to

Table 3
Stages of SL ligament dissociation

Stage	Pathology	Treatment Options
Partial tear	Partial ligament tear.	1. Proprioceptive education 2. Debridement ± thermal shrinkage 3. SL pinning
Complete tear Repairable	Acute or subacute complete tear.	1. Reduction SL interval, repair of ligament, protection with intercarpal wires or screw ± capsulodesis
Complete tear Not repairable No malalignment	Chronic complete tear. Secondary stabilizers intact.	1. Dorsal capsulodesis 2. Bone ligament bone grafts 3. RASL
Complete tear Not repairable Malalignment Reducible	Chronic complete tear. Loss of secondary stabilizers.	1. Ligament reconstruction with tendon autograft 2. RASL
Complete tear Not repairable Malalignment Irreducible	Chronic tear. Loss of secondary stabilizers. Fibrosis preventing reduction.	1. Partial (selective) arthrodesis
Complete tear Arthritis (SLAC)	Chronic tear. Degenerative changes in cartilage.	1. Radial styloidectomy 2. Wrist denervation 3. Proximal row carpectomy 4. 4 corner fusion 5. Total wrist arthrodesis 6. Total wrist arthroplasty

Abbreviations: RASL, reduction and association of scaphoid and lunate; SL, scapholunate; SLAC, scapholunate advanced collapse.

Table 4
Geissler arthroscopic classification or tear of the intracarpal ligaments

I	Attenuation or hemorrhage of the interosseous ligament as seen from the radiocarpal space. No incongruency of carpal alignment in midcarpal space.
II	Attenuation or hemorrhage of the interosseous ligament as seen from the radiocarpal space. Incongruency or step off of the carpal space. There may be a slight gap (less than width of probe) between carpal bones.
III	Incongruency or step off of carpal alignment as seen from both radiocarpal and midcarpal space. Probe may be passed through gap between carpal bones.
IV	Incongruency or step off of carpal alignment as seen from both radiocarpal and midcarpal space. There is gross instability with manipulation. A 2.7-mm arthroscope may be passed through gap between carpal bones.

Data from Geissler WB, Freeland AE, Savoie FH, et al. Intra-carpal soft-tissue lesions associated with an intra-articular fracture of the distal end of the radius. J Bone Joint Surg Am 1996;78(3):357–65.

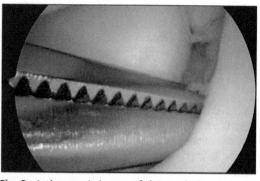

Fig. 3. Arthroscopic image of the scapholunate interval from the midcarpal portal. Note the straight snap is passed in the interval, which classifies the tear as a Geissler grade 3. (*Courtesy of* B. Ting, MD, Boston, MA.)

1. Choose nonoperative strengthening of the flexor carpi radialis and extensor carpi radialis brevis to act as dynamic stabilizers
2. Debride the tear and perform thermal capsule shrinkage, or
3. Perform arthroscopic-assisted pinning of the scapholunate interval.

At present, no one technique has been proven superior. For athletes, our opinion is that pinning would be the least desirable option, owing to 8 to 10 weeks of immobilization following surgery.

Direct repair is best indicated for Geissler grade 3 or 4 cases that are acute and have minimal or no malalignment (**Fig. 3**). In such cases, the secondary stabilizers of the STT joint and dorsal intercarpal ligaments are intact, and usually only dynamic instability is noted preoperatively. Otherwise, direct repair in the presence of static instability with attenuated secondary stabilizers is less likely to be successful.[10] At the time of arthroscopy, the surgeon may decide to convert to an open repair, or alternatively perform the repair arthroscopically. Arthroscopic ligamentoplasty also has been described, but we have no direct experience with this technique.[11]

We prefer to make a 3-cm incision over the SL interval. Slight DISI deformity can be corrected with dorsally placed Kirschner wires to act as "joy-sticks" rotating the scaphoid and lunate out of flexion and extension, respectively. The scaphoid and lunate are then immobilized in the reduced position with either two 0.062-inch Kirschner wires or a 2.4-mm headless compression screw. Midsubstance ruptures of the SLIL can be repaired with nonabsorbable suture. Avulsion injuries usually originate from the scaphoid and can be repaired using 1 to 2 suture anchors or transosseous tunnels securing the ligament with horizontal mattress stitches. In athletes, our preference for Geissler grade 3 or 4 tears would be repair of the ligament and placement of a headless screw for protection. Range of motion can be started in 2 weeks with this technique, as opposed to Kirschner wire fixation, which would require 2 months.[12] The disadvantage of screw fixation is that a second surgery is performed to remove the screw at 5 to 6 months.

Outcomes data for SLIL injury are difficult to interpret due to heterogeneity. Darlis and colleagues[13] studied 16 patients with Geissler grade 1 to 2 SLIL tears treated with debridement and thermal shrinkage. They found 14 had significant relief, grip strength returned to 78% of the contra-lateral side, and none had evidence of radiographic arthritis at 19 months. Similar results showing pain improvement and prevention of arthritis with thermal shrinkage for Geissler 1 and 2 injuries were reported by Lee and colleagues.[14]

Pomerance[15] reported on 17 wrists with dynamic instability treated with direct ligament repair, Kirschner wire fixation, and dorsal capsulodesis at an average of 22 weeks from injury. He found improvement in radiographic parameters postoperatively; however, he noted that the average Disabilities of the Arm, Shoulder, and Hand (DASH) score was 31, 8 of 17 had moderate or severe pain, and 3 had degenerative changes at 66 months.[15]

Wyrick and colleagues[10] reported on 24 wrists with static instability treated within 3 months of injury with repair and capsulodesis. They noted overall poor improvement in radiographic findings at final follow-up. Although the optimal method of surgical management for SLIL injury remains unproven, a few studies have noted better results if the severity of the injury is less, reduction and fixation are performed before 3 months, and the patient has a lower-demand occupation.[15,16]

Lunotriquetral Ligament Rupture

LTIL rupture occurs in a manner opposite of SLIL rupture; the wrist is hyperextended with radial deviation and intercarpal pronation. In sports, this can be seen with a fall backward on an outstretched hand. Patients complain of ulnar wrist pain. A ballottement test may be positive (**Table 2**). Radiographs are usually normal, although volar intercalary segmental instability deformity is possible. MRI may show various degrees of tearing, but arthroscopy remains the most reliable method of diagnosis. LTIL tears associated with perilunate instability or chronic tears with carpal collapse should be treated with open procedures. Acute or chronic tears without deformity may be treated with arthroscopic methods.

Arthroscopic debridement of partial LTIL tears was studied by Ruch and Poehling,[17] who noted pain relief in 13 of 14 patients with no evidence of carpal collapse at 34 months. Osterman and Seidman[18] reported results of 20 wrists treated with debridement and arthroscopic-assisted pinning of the LT interval (**Fig. 4**). They noted pain relief in 80% of patients, albeit with a mild decrease in grip strength and range of motion.[18]

Triangular Fibrocartilage Complex Tear

Isolated TFCC tears result from hyperextension of the wrist with radial deviation. These may be acute or chronic/degenerative (**Table 5**).[19] More commonly, distal radius fractures also may cause TFCC injury from excessive displacement. Up to 43% of distal radius fractures may have a concurrent TFCC tear.[9] By definition, Galeazzi fractures of the radius have avulsed radioulnar ligaments. TFCC tears associated with DRUJ instability after distal radius fractures are often stable with anatomic fixation of the radius. Occasionally, the DRUJ must be immobilized, pinned, or secured with TFCC repair via open or arthroscopic-assisted methods. This section focuses on isolated traumatic TFCC tears.

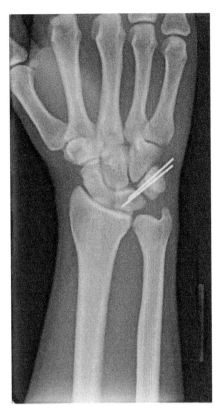

Fig. 4. Radiograph of a wrist showing LT interval pinning after arthroscopic diagnosis.

Table 5	
Palmer classification of acute triangular fibrocartilage complex (TFCC) tears	
Traumatic	
1A	Central perforation
1B	Ulnar avulsion (+/− styloid fracture)
1C	Distal avulsion (ulnocarpal ligaments)
1D	Radial avulsion (+/− sigmoid notch fracture)
Degenerative	
2A	TFCC wear
2B	TFCC wear + lunate or ulna chondromalacia
2C	TFCC perforation + lunate or ulna chondromalacia
2D	TFCC perforation + lunate or ulna chondromalacia + lunotriquetral interosseous ligament perforation
2E	Ulnocarpal arthritis

Adapted from Palmer AK. Triangular fibrocartilage complex lesions: A classification. J Hand Surg Am 1989;14(4):596; with permission.

Depending on the location and severity of the tear, patient complaints may range from vague ulnar-sided wrist pain to instability of the DRUJ. On physical examination, tenderness may be palpated in the fovea and painful crepitus may be elicited from extension/supination maneuvers. Grip strength is also consistently diminished. One also should examine the DRUJ and ECU for signs of instability (see **Table 2**).

Radiographs are often unrevealing, but positive ulnar variance may raise suspicion for a central tear or abutment syndrome. Triple injection arthrography is most useful for diagnosing radial or LTIL tears, but less accurate for peripheral tears; it is performed less commonly, as an undesirable rate of false-positive and false-negative results have been reported.[20] MRI has approximately 64% to 97% accuracy for diagnosing TFCC tears using arthroscopy as a reference standard.[21,22]

Nonoperative treatment includes rest, immobilization in a long-arm cast or splint, steroid injection, and therapy. Early operative intervention can be considered in athletes depending on their timing requirements for return to play.

Palmer type 1A tears are usually treated with debridement of the central tear. As the central articular disk is relatively avascular, repair is often not successful. When using a probe to bounce on the articular disk, a brisk bounce-back (ie, "trampoline effect") is lost. We remove unstable tissue flaps with a 2-mm shaver, biters, and a thermal wand (**Fig. 5**). Up to 80% of the central TFCC can be removed without creating instability.[23] Removing the tear and restoring the peripheral rim tension may reduce pain in 81% to 88% of cases.[20,24] The patient is splinted for 1 to 2 weeks and may usually return to sport by 4 weeks. In the ulnar-positive patient, a surgeon may consider shortening the ulna via wafer resection or a shortening osteotomy; however, these are more substantial procedures that would significantly sideline the athlete for a longer period of time. Our preference is to attempt a debridement first and then later consider ulnar shortening osteotomy to unload the ulnar-positive variance and tighten the extrinsic ligaments.

Palmer type 2A lesions are the most amenable to arthroscopic repair. Acute isolated injuries with DRUJ instability are the best indication, but repair can be considered for pain as well. During arthroscopy, the radioulnar ligaments are found avulsed from the ulnar fovea with a probe. The fovea and the flap edges are debrided with a shaver. The tear can be repaired with a variety of techniques including inside-out, outside-in, or all-inside. Open repair can also be considered.

In athletes, we prefer the inside-out technique described by de Araujo and colleagues.[25] A Tuohy needle is inserted into the 1 to 2 or 3 to 4 portal and directed ulnarly toward the tear. The TFCC edge is pierced with the needle and advanced out of the skin. A skin incision is made to protect the ulnar sensory nerve and to retrieve one free end of the 2 to 0 PDS suture. The needle is retracted back into the radiocarpal joint enough to create some slack in the suture. The needle is then advanced again 2 mm dorsal or volar to the previous puncture site and advanced through the TFCC and capsule again. The beveled needle prevents the suture from being cut. The suture is retrieved outside the capsule, and a knot is tied over it. The patient is placed into a 45° supination splint or cast preventing forearm rotation for 6 weeks followed by 6 weeks of motion and strengthening. Return to sports usually occurs approximately 12 weeks after surgery. Using an inside-out technique, Trumble and colleagues[26] reported pain relief in 10 of 11 ulnar-sided TFCC repairs, and 7 of 11 returned to original work or sport.

Palmer 1C tears are rare and are often found as a ligamentous fraying on the volar-ulnar rim. A partial tear with fraying and synovitis can be debrided

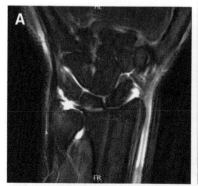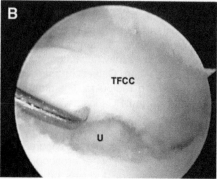

Fig. 5. (A) MRI showing a TFCC tear and (B) post debridement viewed from the 3 to 4 portal.

with a shaver. A larger tear with associated instability should undergo open repair.

Palmer 1D tears are radial-sided tears often associated with distal radius fractures. Small tears not extending significantly into the radioulnar ligaments and without instability can be debrided. Larger tears, especially those with instability of the DRUJ, are indicated for repair. We perform the repair as described by Sagerman and Short.[27] The tear is debrided with a shaver exposing the sigmoid notch, which is prepared with a bur to create a healing surface. A 0.045 Kirschner wire is introduced though the 6-R portal and aimed radially and proximally starting at the sigmoid notch and emerging on the radial side of the radius. A second drill hole is prepared adjacent to the first one. A cannula is introduced into the 6-R portal, and 2.0 meniscal suture needles are introduced through the cannula. The needles are connected by the suture. The first needle pierces the articular disk and then is shuttled into the drill hole to tent the skin. An incision is made here to protect the radial sensory nerve. The second meniscus repair needle is passed through the articular disk and through the second drill tunnel. The sutures create a horizontal mattress that is tied over a bone bridge on the radial side.

Palmer type 2 repairs are treated in a similar fashion to 1A tears. Central degenerative tears are debrided and an ulnar shortening osteotomy is considered for ulnar impaction syndrome, which is evidenced by chondromalacia on arthroscopy. Cases with advanced arthritis are usually not candidates for arthroscopic procedures and are often considered for selective fusions or other salvage procedures.

Hamatolunate Impingement

A type II lunate morphology is one in which an additional facet on the lunate articulates with the hamate. Impingement between the lunate and hamate occurs in some patients causing vague ulnar-sided wrist pain. Radiographs show a medial lunate facet for the hamate. MRI may reveal bone edema with the hamate head. Arthroscopy confirms the diagnosis; chondromalacia is viewable through the MC-U portal. Although not much is known about this entity, small case series have reported encouraging results with arthroscopic resection of the hamate head using a small-caliber bur (**Fig. 6**).[28,29]

Arthroscopic-Assisted Reduction of Fractures

An exhaustive review of indications and surgical reduction techniques is out of scope for this article. However, a few investigators have noted arthroscopy as a useful adjunct for reduction of intracarpal fractures. Surgical fixation may be desired in an athlete wishing to quickly return to play. Arthroscopic-assisted fixation of scaphoid fractures has been suggested to identify displacement before and after fixation and also to assist in achieving an accurate starting point for a dorsal percutaneous screw.[30,31] The fracture reduction is viewed through the midcarpal portals, whereas the start point is visualized through the 3 to 4 portal.

More recently, investigators have suggested nonunion surgery for scaphoid fractures is technically possible through arthroscopic methods; however, the long-term efficacy of this method remains unproven.[32] Reduction of acute distal radius fractures also can be assessed via arthroscopy. We find the most useful indication for arthroscopic assistance to be for intra-articular malunions. Corrective osteotomy can be performed under direct visualization through the 6-R portal. Volar and dorsal portals can be used to guide the osteotomy and manipulate the fracture fragments (**Fig. 7**). The fracture is then fixed using standard techniques.

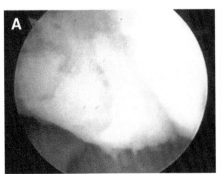
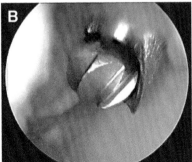

Fig. 6. Hamate chondromalacia. (*A*) Arthroscopic view demonstrating proximal pole hamate arthritis from the radial midcarpal portal. (*B*) A 2.9-mm burr is used to resect the proximal pole of the hamate. (*From* Yao J, Osterman AL. Arthroscopic techniques for wrist arthritis (radial styloidectomy and proximal pole hamate excisions). Hand Clin 2005;21(4):524; with permission.)

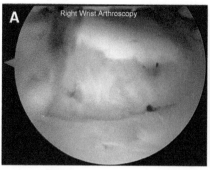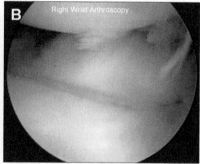

Fig. 7. Arthroscopic-assisted osteotomy of a distal radius showing (*A*) a malunited lunate facet through a 3 to 4 portal. The osteotomy was performed under direct visualization, facilitating (*B*) accurate articular reduction. (*Courtesy of* N. Chen, MD, Boston, MA.)

SUMMARY

Wrist injuries are common in athletes. An understanding of the variety of conditions that cause wrist pain is critical in achieving the most optimal outcome. Wrist arthroscopy is an effective adjunctive tool in the diagnosis of wrist derangements. In special situations, minimally invasive procedures can be performed through the arthroscope.

REFERENCES

1. Rettig AC. Athletic injuries of the wrist and hand. Part 1. Traumatic injuries of the wrist. Am J Sports Med 2003;31:1038–48.
2. Lystad RP, Gregory K, Wilson J. The epidemiology of injuries in mixed martial arts: a systematic review and meta-analysis. Orthop J Sports Med 2014; 2(1). 2325967113518492.
3. Zazryn T, Finch C, McCrory P. A 16-year study of injuries to professional boxers in the state of Victoria, Australia. Br J Sports Med 2003;37:321–4.
4. Zazryn T, Cameron P, McCrory P. A prospective cohort study of injury in amateur and professional boxing. Br J Sports Med 2006;40:670–4.
5. Weiss APC, Akelman E, Lambiase R. Comparison of the findings of triple-injection cinearthrography of the wrist with those of arthroscopy. J Bone Joint Surg Am 1996;78:348–56.
6. Chung KC, Zimmerman NB, Travis MT. Wrist arthrography versus arthroscopy: a comparative study of 150 cases. J Hand Surg Am 1996;21:591–4.
7. Palmer AK, Werner FW. Biomechanics of the distal radioulnar joint. Clin Orthop 1984;187:26–35.
8. Garcia-Elias M, Lluch AL, Stanley JK. Three-ligament tenodesis for the treatment of scapholunate dissociation: indications and surgical technique. J Hand Surg Am 2006;31:125–34.
9. Geissler WB, Freeland AE, Savoie FH, et al. Intracarpal soft-tissue lesions associated with an intra-articular fracture of the distal end of the radius. J Bone Joint Surg Am 1996;78(3):357–65.
10. Wyrick JD, Youse BD, Kiefhaber TR. Scapholunate ligament repair and capsulodesis for the treatment of static scapholunate dissociation. J Hand Surg Br 1998;23B:776–80.
11. Corella F, Del Cerro M, Ocampos M, et al. Arthroscopic ligamentoplasty of the dorsal and volar portions of the scapholunate ligament. J Hand Surg Am 2013;38(12):2466–77.
12. Souer JS, Rutgers M, Andermahr J, et al. Perilunate fracture-dislocations of the wrist: comparison of temporary screw versus K-wire fixation. J Hand Surg Am 2007;32(3):318–25.
13. Darlis NA, Weisser RW, Sotereanos DG. Partial scapholunate ligament injuries treated with arthroscopic debridement and thermal shrinkage. J Hand Surg Am 2005;30(5):908–14.
14. Lee JL, Nha KW, Lee GY, et al. Long-term outcomes of arthroscopic debridement and thermal shrinkage for isolated partial intercarpal ligament tears. Orthopedics 2012;35(8):1204–9.
15. Pomerance J. Outcome after repair of the scapholunate interosseous ligament and dorsal capsulodesis for dynamic scapholunate instability due to trauma. J Hand Surg Am 2006;31(8):1380–6.
16. Whipple TL. The role of arthroscopy in the treatment of scapholunate instability. Hand Clin 1995;11(1): 37–40.
17. Ruch DS, Poehling GG. Arthroscopic management of partial scapholunate and lunotriquetral injuries of the wrist. J Hand Surg Am 1996;21:412–7.
18. Osterman AL, Seidman GD. The role of arthroscopy in the treatment of lunatotriquetral ligament injuries. Hand Clin 1995;11:41–50.
19. Palmer AK. Triangular fibrocartilage complex lesions: a classification. J Hand Surg Am 1989;14: 594–606.
20. Osterman AL. Arthroscopic debridement of triangular fibrocartilage complex tears. Arthroscopy 1990;6(2):120–4.

21. Haims AH, Schweitzer ME, Morrison WB, et al. Limitations of MR imaging in the diagnosis of peripheral tears of the triangular fibrocartilage of the wrist. AJR Am J Roentgenol 2002;178: 419–22.

22. Potter HG, Asnis-Ernberg L, Weiland AJ, et al. The utility of high-resolution magnetic resonance imaging in the evaluation of the triangular fibrocartilage complex of the wrist. J Bone Joint Surg Am 1997; 79:1675–84.

23. Adams BD, Holley KA. Strains in the articular disk of the triangular fibrocartilage complex: a biomechanical study. J Hand Surg Am 1993;18:919–25.

24. Minami A, Ishikawa J, Suenaga N, et al. Clinical results of treatment of triangular fibrocartilage complex tears by arthroscopic debridement. J Hand Surg Am 1996;21:406–11.

25. de Araujo W, Poehling GG, Kuzma GR. New Tuohy needle technique for triangular fibrocartilage complex repair: preliminary studies. Arthroscopy 1996; 12(6):699–703.

26. Trumble TE, Gilbert M, Vedder N. Isolated tears of the triangular fibrocartilage: management by early arthroscopic repair. J Hand Surg Am 1997;22(1): 57–65.

27. Sagerman SD, Short W. Arthroscopic repair of radial-sided triangular fibrocartilage complex tears. Arthroscopy 1996;12:339–42.

28. Thurston AJ, Stanley JK. Hamato-lunate impingement: an uncommon cause of ulnar-sided wrist pain. Arthroscopy 2000;16(5):540–4.

29. Yao J, Osterman AL. Arthroscopic techniques for wrist arthritis (radial styloidectomy and proximal pole hamate excisions). Hand Clin 2005;21:519–26.

30. Geissler WB. Carpal fractures in athletes. Clin Sports Med 2001;20:167–88.

31. del Pinal F, Cagigal L, Garcia-Bernal FJ, et al. Arthroscopically guided osteotomy for management of intra-articular distal radius malunions. J Hand Surg Am 2010;35A:392–7.

32. Slutsky DJ. Current innovations in wrist arthroscopy. J Hand Surg Am 2012;37(9):1932–41.

Finger Injuries in Ball Sports

David T. Netscher, MD[a],*, Dang T. Pham, MD[b], Kimberly Goldie Staines, ORT, CHT[c]

KEYWORDS

- Finger injuries • Ball sports • Athlete • Return to play • Orthoses

KEY POINTS

- Knowledge of bony and ligamentous anatomy of the digit is vital in treatment of finger injuries.
- Treatment of finger injuries in elite athletes remains a challenge for hand surgeons given the inherent demand for an expeditious return to play.
- Communication with the athlete and the coach is important to understand the particular sport and position of play, what orthosis may be allowable, and financial constraints.
- Occupational therapy and functional orthoses may greatly facilitate return to full activities.

INTRODUCTION

Ball sports are the leading cause of hand injuries in professional athletes.[1] The use of the hand for ball control and contact with the opponent leaves the fingers exposed to injury. Management of finger injuries in athletes often presents a challenge for hand surgeons. Multiple factors must be considered, such as appropriate timing of treatment, long-term functional outcome, and (often the most difficult issue) return to play. This article discusses the management of common finger injuries in ball sports and provides return-to-play recommendations for professional athletes.

MALLET FINGER

Mallet finger injuries are common in ball sports such as baseball, basketball, and football.[2] They are usually a result of forced hyperflexion of an extended finger on a ball or direct contact with another player (**Fig. 1**). The middle, ring, and small fingers are the most frequently involved digits.[3]

The athlete typically presents with a flexed posture at the distal interphalangeal (DIP) joint and impaired active extension (extension lag). Plain radiographs including posterior-anterior and lateral views of the affected finger are recommended to evaluate for fractures and joint subluxation. Mallet injuries can be categorized as soft tissue or bony mallet injuries.[2,3] Soft tissue mallet injuries are described as terminal extensor tendon avulsion from the insertion on the distal phalanx with no associated bone fragment. When there is a fragment of bone associated with the terminal extensor tendon avulsion from the distal phalanx, it is a bony mallet injury. A bone fragment involving greater than a third of the articular surface may result in loss of joint congruency and volar subluxation.

Closed mallet injuries that involve tendon only or that have a small avulsed bone fragment can be treated nonoperatively with DIP joint extension splinting. The splint should span the width of the finger and the length extend from fingertip to just distal to the proximal interphalangeal (PIP) joint

Disclosure Statement: The authors have nothing to disclose and have no conflicts of interest.
[a] Division of Plastic Surgery, Department of Orthopedic Surgery, Baylor College of Medicine, 6624 Fannin Street, Suite 2730, Houston, TX 77030, USA; [b] Department of Surgery, Houston Methodist Hospital, Weill Medical College of Cornell University, 6550 Fannin Street, Smith Tower 1661, Houston, TX 77030, USA; [c] Department of Physical Medicine and Rehabilitation, Michael E. DeBakey Veterans Affairs Medical Center, 2002 Holcombe Boulevard, RCL117, Houston, TX 77030, USA
* Corresponding author.
E-mail address: Netscher@bcm.edu

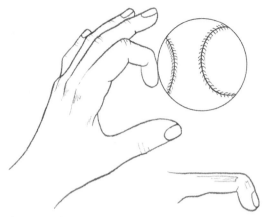

Fig. 1. Mechanism of injury of mallet finger. A flexion force on the tip of an extended finger by a ball can result in avulsion of the terminal extensor tendon on the dorsal lip of the distal phalanx base.

to allow for PIP joint motion.[2] Care should be taken to avoid skin ischemia, which can result from direct pressure on the skin by a tightly applied splint or by hyperextension of the DIP joint. With regard to splint type, a systematic review revealed that there are no substantial differences in treatment between prefabricated or custom-made orthoses (**Fig. 2**).[4] The key to treatment success is patient compliance with splinting. It is recommended to splint the DIP joint in full extension for 6 to 8 weeks followed by a similar period of nighttime splinting.[3] Patient compliance with wearing and properly positioning the splint is necessary for a good outcome.

Operative management is considered when there is volar subluxation of the distal phalanx with significant joint incongruity. Closed reduction and percutaneous internal fixation of the DIP joint using a Kirschner wire (K-wire) by extension block pinning is the preferred technique.[3] With the DIP

joint maximally flexed, a K-wire is introduced at a 45° angle into the head of the middle phalanx to create an extension block for the fragment and allow reduction of the volar fracture piece to the dorsal fragment (**Fig. 3**). Another K-wire is introduced axially from the distal to the middle phalanx to maintain the reduction. An alternative is to perform an open repair with pull-out button suture (**Fig. 4**). It can be used with either soft tissue mallet or bony mallet. Open reduction has the advantage of direct access to the extensor tendon but has significant risk of complications, including skin necrosis, infection, nail dystrophy, osteoarthritis, and stiffness.[5]

Wehbe and Schneider[6] advocated nonsurgical management of closed mallet fractures with large fracture fragments, even with volar subluxation of the distal phalanx. They found that subluxated mallet fractures heal and remodel the DIP joint articular surface with preservation of the joint space. In a study with 22 closed mallet finger fractures, it was shown that even nonoperative treatment of mallet injuries involving greater than one-third of the articular surface with or without subluxation resulted in satisfactory outcomes.[7] Based on the current literature, there is no clear indication for surgical treatment and insufficient evidence to support operative rather than nonoperative treatment of mallet fractures. Most clinicians consider operative intervention when there is volar subluxation and loss of DIP joint congruency. Close follow-up with lateral radiographic views is needed to guide treatment and ensure maintenance of DIP joint congruency.

Return to Play

Immobilization of the DIP joint in full extension may prevent optimal play for athletes and some may opt to delay treatment or to have no treatment.[8] Effective treatment of stable, closed mallet finger

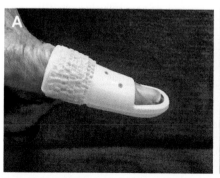
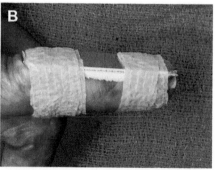

Fig. 2. (*A*) Stack splint. Prefabricated stack splint immobilizes the DIP joint in full extension. (*B*) Dorsal aluminum splint. Dorsal aluminum splint for mallet finger should be secured with 2 strips of tape to maintain the DIP joint in an extended position.

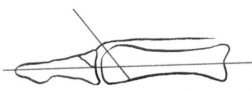

Fig. 3. Extension block pinning of mallet finger. A K-wire is inserted into the head of the middle phalanx at a 45° angle and proximal to the fractured fragment to create an extension block. The volar fracture is reduced and a second K-wire is passed retrograde across the DIP joint to maintain reduction.

injuries involves full-time splinting for at least 6 to 8 weeks followed by nighttime splinting of a similar duration. Athletes are expected to adhere strictly to the full treatment course and continue with immobilization during strenuous activity, including return to training.[9–11] Splinting during training and play runs the risk of maceration, loss of immobilization, and injury to other joints. During immobilization, consider including the adjacent joints in the splint, using a circumferential cast (QuickCast, Patterson Medical) and buddy taping to limit risk of injury to PIP and metacarpophalangeal (MCP) joints (**Fig. 5**). Also, the use of Dynamic Tape (Vanuatu) or Kinesio Tape (Kinesio Holding Corporation) in conjunction with the splint or cast can greatly decrease the risk of maceration.[12]

If players cannot tolerate the external splint because of the demands of their positions, some investigators have advocated internal splinting by percutaneous pins, also for at least 6 weeks.[8] However, there is a risk of another jamming injury breaking the pin in the joint of for pin migration.

As with all injuries, options need to be tailored to the urgency to return to play, the position and type of sport, and the specific injured finger.

Following discontinuation of immobilization, players are permitted to return to play and to resume ball handling as tolerated. Athletes must be aware that even with strict compliance with splinting, a residual 5° to 10° extensor lag and dorsal joint prominence may be present. Without treatment, permanent flexion deformity, swan neck deformity, and DIP joint osteoarthritis can develop.[5]

CHRONIC MALLET INJURIES AND SWAN NECK DEFORMITY

Chronic mallet deformities, categorized as more than 4 weeks from injury, may be successfully treated with extension splint even several weeks after the injury.[13] Swan neck deformity is characterized by hyperextension of the PIP joint and flexion of the DIP joint. It can result from failed treatment of mallet finger injuries and is most common in athletes with a hyperextensible PIP joint. A trial of splinting of the DIP in extension and the PIP in flexion for 4 to 6 weeks is initiated. Adjustments to the splint are made as the deformity begins to correct itself. The duration of splinting may be switched to part-time or nighttime splinting for maintenance. If there is a persistent deformity after nonoperative treatment of chronic mallet deformities, tendon rebalancing with a central slip tenotomy or spiral oblique retinacular ligament (SORL) reconstruction can be considered.[3,13] The athlete should be examined for the degree of

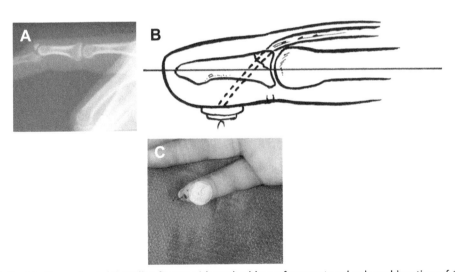

Fig. 4. Pullout button suture. (*A*) Mallet finger with avulsed bone fragment and volar subluxation of the distal phalanx. (*B*) A pullout button suture is used to secure the terminal tendon to bone. (*C*) An axial or oblique wire inserted through the DIP joint is necessary to maintain reduction.

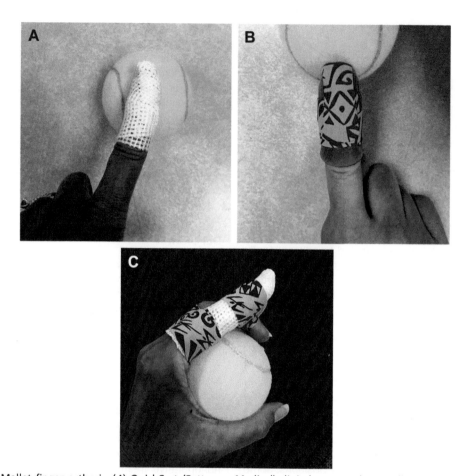

Fig. 5. Mallet finger orthosis. (*A*) QuickCast (Patterson Medical) digital cast can be rapidly applied and easily removed for the duration of the sporting activity. (*B*) Custom dorsal mallet orthosis can be sufficiently rigid to avoid repeated jamming injuries. (*C*) Full-finger digital cast with buddy taping provides even better support provided the positional play allows this. Full-finger immobilization, in contrast with only distal immobilization, avoids placing the PIP joint at risk for a new jamming injury. Splinting, where possible, should not only protect the injured joint but also avoid the risk of loading adjacent joints and sustaining a new injury.

extension lag at the DIP and PIP joint. An extension lag at the DIP joint less than 36° is best treated with Fowler central slip tenotomy.[14] SORL procedure is recommended when there is an extension lag at the DIP joint greater than 45°.[3]

The Fowler central slip tenotomy is designed to reduce the extensor tone at the PIP joint resulting from retraction of the extensor apparatus. It involves transecting the central slip proximal to its insertion into the middle phalanx base and allowing the extensor mechanism to slide proximally to correct the DIP extensor lag. Care is taken not to violate the triangular ligament so that development of extensor lag at the PIP joint and boutonnière deformity is avoided. The timing of the operation is delayed until at least 6 months after injury to allow for tendon maturation.[3] Fowler central slip tenotomy in several case series showed good results. In a series of 20 patients with chronic mallet finger treated with central slip tenotomy, an average extensor lag of 37° before the operation corrected to 9° after the operation.[15] Houpt and colleagues[16] found that, in 35 patients with mallet finger and an average extensor lag of 45°, 26 patients achieved full extension after treatment with Fowler central tendon tenotomy. The postoperative splinting protocol involves splinting the PIP joint at 25° of flexion and the DIP joint in full extension for 10 to 14 days, followed by a finger cast immobilizing the DIP joint only for 2 additional weeks. After the pin is removed at 4 weeks, full active range of motion of the DIP joint is begun. The PIP joint is started on full active and passive range of motion. By 6 months, maximal range of motion of both joints is obtained.

The SORL reconstruction is intended to restore the tenodesis of the oblique retinacular ligaments in promoting DIP joint extension with active PIP joint extension (**Fig. 6**).[3] A free tendon graft, typically the palmaris longus or toe extensor tendon, is harvested and secured distally to the dorsal base of the distal phalanx. The graft is then passed volar in a spiral fashion around the radial aspect of the middle phalanx and is secured proximally to the ulnar side of the flexor tendon sheath at the level of the proximal phalanx or directly to bone. Next, the DIP joint may be pinned in extension and the PIP joint in 10° to 15° of flexion with an oblique K-wire.[3] In a series of 12 patients who underwent the SORL reconstruction for chronic mallet finger caused by terminal tendon disruption, the mallet finger deformity was corrected in all cases.[17] One patient required flexor tenolysis for adhesions to obtain full range of motion and another patient required lengthening of the oblique retinacular ligament graft to obtain full PIP joint extension. An alternative to SORL reconstruction is flexor digitorum superficialis (FDS) tenodesis with combined flexor digitorum profundus joint fusion (**Fig. 7**).

Rehabilitation after SORL is challenging because the structures are so delicate. The goals of rehabilitation are to dynamically facilitate DIP extension with PIP flexion, allowing for functional grasp and prehension in a tenodesis manner.[18,19] Initial immobilization includes a dorsal gutter splint incorporating the PIP and DIP joints for 6 weeks followed by a figure-of-eight orthosis for an additional 4 weeks. Return to play should be discouraged for the initial 4 to 6 weeks for any team sports. Immobilization at the time of return to play should include the PIP in a flexed posture and DIP in an extended posture using a custom orthosis or digital cast. Again, maceration is a common complication, so consider using Dynamic Tape or Kinesio Tape under the cast or orthosis. Return to play with buddy taping can be entertained at 12 to 16 weeks as per tendon healing and strength assessment.

BOUTONNIÈRE DEFORMITY

A boutonnière deformity is characterized by flexion at the PIP joint and hyperextension at the DIP joint.[20] The precipitating injury leading to this chronic flexion deformity is disruption of the central slip, which causes continued flexion at the PIP joint and leads to attenuation of the triangular ligament followed by volar subluxation of the lateral bands (**Fig. 8**).[3] In athletes, disruption of the central slip can be caused by forced

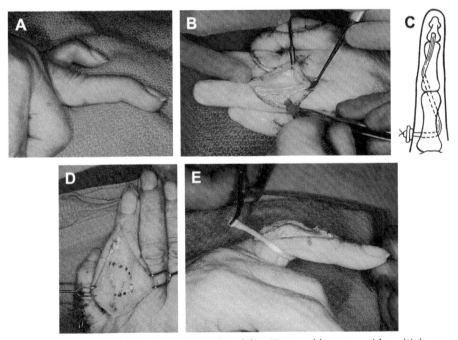

Fig. 6. Spiral oblique retinacular ligament reconstruction. (*A*) A 45-year-old woman with multiple swan neck deformities. (*B*) Dorsal capsulotomy of the PIP joint proximal to the central slip was performed. (*C*) The tendon graft is fixed to the distal phalanx, passed volar in a spiral fashion around the middle phalanx, tunneled through the shaft of the proximal phalanx, and secured with a bone anchor or suture button. The direction and course of the tendon graft is shown in the (*D*) dorsal and (*E*) lateral views.

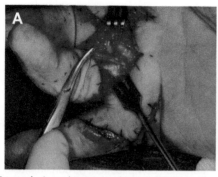
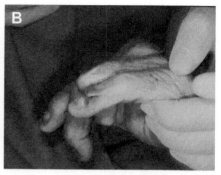

Fig. 7. FDS tenodesis and DIP joint fusion. (*A*) One slip of the FDS is transected proximal to the PIP joint, leaving the distal attachment intact. With the PIP joint flexed 20° to 30°, the detached FDS slip is passed under and wrapped around the A1 pulley. (*B*) FDS tenodesis can be combined with an arthrodesis of the DIP joint if the flexion lag of the DIP joint is severe.

hyperflexion at the PIP joint, such as when catching a ball with an outstretched hand. It can also result from an occasional open injury with laceration to the central slip or from crushing injury, or volar dislocation at the PIP joint.

Early recognition and intervention is key to preventing boutonnière deformity. If the athlete reports jamming the finger or having a finger put back into place after any injury, the clinician should be suspicious for central slip rupture.[20] Volar dislocation of the PIP joint reduced on the field can result in a boutonnière deformity if a central slip injury is unrecognized and left untreated.[21] The Elson test is a useful clinical assessment to determine whether the patient has a central slip tear before the deformity develops (**Fig. 9**).[22] It is performed by flexing the PIP joint to 90° and having the athlete extend the middle phalanx against resistance. The test is positive if the DIP joint is able to extend because of the recruitment of the lateral bands in the setting of a central slip deficient finger. A digital block may be necessary to accurately perform this test because pain may prevent performance of the test. Plain radiographs should be obtained to evaluate for dorsal fracture of the middle phalanx with or without volar subluxation or dislocation of the PIP joint.[20]

Early diagnosis of closed central slip injury can be treated nonoperatively with splinting of the PIP joint in extension for 6 weeks to promote healing of the central slip to the middle phalanx followed by 6 weeks of nighttime splinting. The DIP joint is left free to allow flexion, which promotes dorsal translation of the lateral bands. Athletes are encouraged to perform DIP joint active and passive flexion exercises hourly throughout the splinting course.[3]

Operative management is recommended for open injuries, large avulsion fractures, volar dislocation, or fracture-dislocation of the PIP joint.[20] Central slip injuries associated with small avulsion fractures that are nondisplaced can be managed nonoperatively. Larger, displaced fragments can be repaired with K-wire or screw fixation. Central slip laceration warrants open repair with reattachment of the tendon and placement of a transarticular K-wire to maintain the PIP joint in extension during healing.[3]

Return to Play

For closed central slip injury, athletes are generally allowed to return to play as long as it does not obviate use of the splint and buddy taping is recommended as an adjunct for game time protection.[23] Merritt[24] advocates relative motion splinting, which permits immediate full active motion of the injured extensor tendon if it is placed in

Fig. 8. Mechanism of injury of boutonnière deformity. A boutonnière deformity may develop in the acute setting from forced hyperflexion of the PIP joint, causing disruption of the central slip at the base of the middle phalanx.

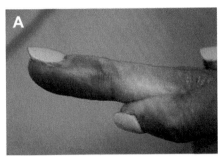
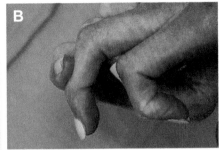

Fig. 9. Elson test. (*A*) With the PIP joint extended, the DIP joint can actively extend. (*B*) With the PIP joint flexed, the DIP joint cannot actively extend. In the presence of central slip injury, the DIP joint can be extended when the PIP joint is flexed because of the recruitment of the lateral bands.

15° to 20° less relative motion than adjacent tendons. The rationale for relative motion splinting is for the injured tendon to experience less force than adjacent tendons during motion. In boutonnière deformity, attenuation of the triangular ligament enables the lumbricals to act as flexors at the PIP joint and to extend the DIP joint without an opposing force. Placing the injured digit into 15° to 20° greater MCP flexion relative to adjacent digits allows the lumbricals to relax, which increases the tension on the extensor hood and promotes dorsal migration of the lateral bands.[24] Using the relative motion flexor splint when not playing enables extensor tendon rehabilitation but caution is needed when using this orthosis for return to play because of the high risk of injury to the adjacent fingers or unprotected hyperflexion injury of the affected finger (**Fig. 10**). Return-to-play protection should include Dynamic Tape

and/or circumferential digital casting with the PIP and DIP joints in full extension.

CHRONIC BOUTONNIÈRE DEFORMITY

Chronic boutonnière deformities can be categorized by the Burton classification. Stage I is a supple, passively correctable deformity; stage II consists of extensor mechanism contracture that is not passively correctable but does not involve the joint; stage III is a fixed contracture with involvement of the volar plate, collateral ligament, and intra-articular joint; and stage IV is stage III plus PIP joint arthritis.[3] Stages I and II can undergo a trial of dynamic splint or serial casting to regain passive extension of the PIP joint. If this is unsuccessful, an open joint contracture release can be performed. If an active extensor lag persists but full passive PIP joint was obtained, there are tendon rebalancing

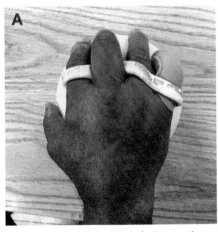
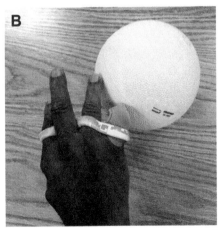

Fig. 10. Relative motion splint. (*A*) Relative motion splint allows for neuromuscular retraining of extension. (*B*) The PIP joint is left unprotected for repeated hyperflexion jamming injury. It also exposes the athlete to other injuries. For example, a forceful extension fall on an outstretched hand may lead to proximal phalangeal fracture. Rigid entrapment of adjacent fingers by the orthosis may lead to susceptibility to ligament injuries in these fingers.

procedures that can be considered. Before undergoing any surgical correction of a chronic boutonnière deformity, patients should be fully informed of the risks and expected outcomes of the procedure, particularly the possibility of jeopardizing flexor function in an attempt to gain extension.

Terminal tendon tenotomy (distal Fowler or Dolphin tenotomy) was designed to decrease the extensor tone at the DIP joint and to allow the extensor mechanism to retract and increase the extensor tension to the PIP joint.[25] It is most valuable in patients who report more difficulty with DIP joint hyperextension rather than the lack of PIP joint extension.[26]

Staged reconstruction of boutonnière deformity, described by Curtis and colleagues,[27] is performed with wide-awake anesthesia to allow assessment of active extension intraoperatively at each stage (Fig. 11). In stage I, an extensor tenolysis is performed. If active extension is not present, the surgeon proceeds to stage II, in which the transverse retinacular ligament is transected to allow dorsal translation of the lateral bands. In stage III, if full correction is not achieved and the PIP joint extensor lag is less than 20°, a Fowler tenotomy is performed. If PIP joint extensor lag is greater than 20°, the surgeon proceeds directly to stage IV, in which the central tendon is dissected free from its insertion and advanced to the middle phalanx base after 4 to 6 mm of scar tissue are removed from its terminal end.

A pseudoboutonnière deformity should be differentiated from a boutonnière deformity. Pseudoboutonnière deformities are usually caused by a hyperextension injury to the PIP joint resulting in volar plate and collateral ligament damage with no disruption of the central slip.[28] Scarring of the damaged structures leads to a PIP joint flexion contracture with a secondary mild DIP joint hyperextension deformity. Serial static or dynamic splinting and casting techniques are used to gradually restore extension of the PIP joint. For persistent PIP joint flexion contracture, surgical release may be necessary.[21]

Return-to-play guidelines are the same for conservative management of pseudoboutonnière and chronic boutonnière. Consider Dynamic Tape support to prevent further injury with or without orthosis. Most athletic trainers or athletes can be educated on independent application of this tape on the field of play for long-term management.[20]

PULLEY RUPTURE

Injuries to the finger flexor pulley system are common in rock climbers but have also been found in baseball pitchers.[29] The transfer of high forces to the A2, A3, and A4 pulleys during the crimp-grip position (MCP and DIP joints extended and resisted flexion at the PIP joint) is the likely injury mechanism for pulley rupture. Clinical findings include localized swelling at the level of the injured

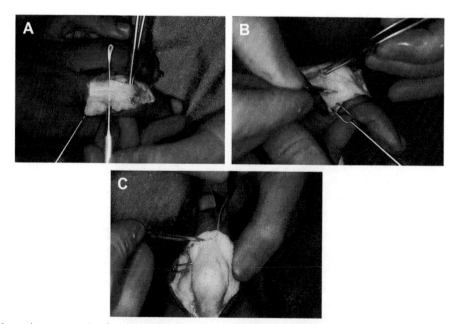

Fig. 11. Staged reconstruction for chronic boutonnière deformity. (*A*) Tenolysis of extensor tendon. (*B*) Release of the transverse retinacular ligament enables the lateral band to swing dorsally. (*C*) Fowler tenotomy can be performed if full extension is not obtained.

pulley and tendon bowstringing if the A2 and/or A4 pulleys are involved.[20] MRI can be useful in differentiating between a pulley strain and a partial or complete rupture (**Fig. 12**). The staging of pulley injuries and treatment protocol have been well described by Schoffl and colleagues[30] and this can be helpful in guiding treatment of professional athletes.

Return to Play

Grade I injuries are pulley strains that can be managed conservatively with nonsteroidal antiinflammatory medications. Easy sport activities can be started after 4 weeks and full sport activities after 6 weeks. Grade 2 injuries are complete A4 or partial A2/A3 ruptures that can be treated similarly to grade 1 injuries with the exception of a 10-day immobilization period. Complete A2/A3 ruptures are grade 3 injuries that can still be treated conservatively, but easy sport activities are restricted until 6 to 8 weeks and full sport activities until 3 months. Grade 4 injuries involve multiple pulley ruptures or single rupture combined with lumbrical muscle or ligament trauma. These injuries require pulley reconstruction, 14-day immobilization period after surgery, and 4 to 6 months of recovery before returning to sport activities. External pulley reinforcement can facilitate early return to play for athletes (**Fig. 13**).

PROXIMAL INTERPHALANGEAL JOINT DISLOCATION

Of the injuries in the hand, the PIP most commonly sustains ligamentous injuries.[31,32] The collateral ligaments and volar plate of the PIP joint create a three-dimensional ligament box that resists joint displacement until 2 sides of the box are disrupted (**Fig. 14**). These stabilizing structures of the PIP joint are vulnerable to the axial loading and extension force that is applied on an outstretched finger. Athletes who participate in ball sports are at risk for PIP joint injuries, either while catching a ball or falling. The spectrum of PIP joint injuries ranges from a minor volar plate strain to an irreducible dislocation of the joint. The joint should be inspected for an irreducible dislocation and any residual deformity or gross laxity.[33] Plain radiographs must be obtained to evaluate for avulsion fractures and the approximate percentage of the involved articular surface. The dorsal V sign may be a subtle indication of an incongruent or dorsally subluxated joint (**Fig. 15**).[31] PIP joint dislocations are classified by the direction of the middle phalanx in relation to the proximal phalanx, which can occur in one of 3 directions: dorsal, lateral, or volar.

Dorsal Dislocations

Dorsal dislocations are the most common type of PIP joint dislocations and usually occur secondary

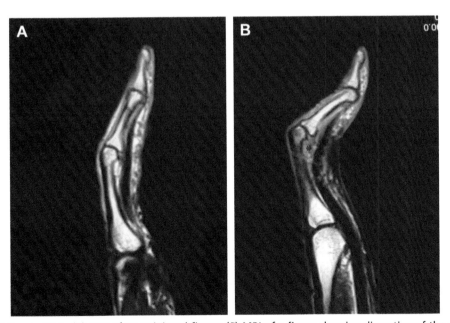

Fig. 12. Pulley rupture. (*A*) MRI of an uninjured finger. (*B*) MRI of a finger showing disruption of the A2 pulley with associated bowstringing deformity. The patient has also developed a fixed PIP joint flexion contracture with pseudoboutonnière hyperextension of the DIP joint. Asterisk shows scarring dorsal to the tendon and volar to the PIP joint.

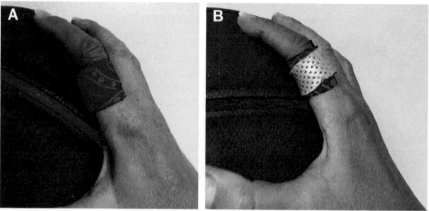

Fig. 13. Pulley ring. (*A*) Taped pulley reinforcement can allow early return to play in grade 1 and 2 pulley rupture injuries. (*B*) For grade 3 and 4 pulley ruptures, the use of a custom pulley ring with tape and padding is recommended during play for 4 to 6 months.

to hyperextension injury. Pure dorsal dislocations result in an avulsion of the volar plate at its distal attachment with the collateral ligaments remaining intact and joint congruity maintained.[31] With more longitudinal force, one of the collateral ligaments can be injured and result in a type I dorsal dislocation in which the joint surfaces are still touching or a type II dorsal dislocation in which there is a bayonet appearance (**Fig. 16**). Type I dorsal dislocation can be reduced with volar translation and flexion. Type II dorsal dislocation requires hyperextension of the middle phalanx followed by palmar force because the volar plate acts as a block to reduction with pure longitudinal traction.

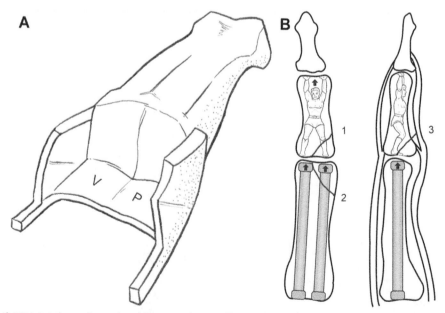

Fig. 14. (*A*) PIP joint three-dimensional ligament box. Collateral ligaments and volar plate of the PIP joint make up the ligament box. At least 2 sides of the box must be disrupted for joint displacement. (*B*) PIP joint bony stability. The 2 proximal phalangeal condyles provide 2 lateral columns for strength. The stability of the PIP joint is inherently provided by the congruency of the articular surface. Fracture lines 1, 2, and 3 result in lateral or volar to dorsal instability. (*Adapted from* [*A*] Merrell G, Slade JF. Dislocations and ligament injuries in the digits. In: Wolfe SW, Hotchkiss RN, Pederson WC, et al, editors. Green's operative hand surgery. 6th edition. Philadelphia: Elsevier Churchill-Livingstone; 2011. p. 292; with permission.)

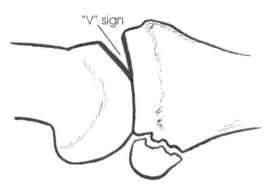

Fig. 15. Dorsal V sign. On a lateral radiograph of a joint, dorsal joint widening can be a sign of joint incongruity and subluxation. (*Adapted from* Merrell G, Slade JF. Dislocations and ligament injuries in the digits. In: Wolfe SW, Hotchkiss RN, Pederson WC, et al, editors. Green's operative hand surgery. 6th edition. Philadelphia: Elsevier Churchill-Livingstone; 2011. p. 292; with permission.)

Return to play

If the joint is stable and has full range of motion after reduction, the athlete is allowed to return to play immediately with buddy taping for protection. If the joint is unstable, the player is placed in an extension block orthosis for at least 4 weeks with weekly reassessment and splint adjustments (**Fig. 17**). For irreducible dislocations, open reduction with extraction of the volar plate from the joint is the best option. Postoperative return to play requires 12 to 16 weeks with an extension block orthosis during play.

Lateral Dislocations

Lateral dislocations of the PIP joint result from rupture of the collateral ligament on one side and partial avulsion of the volar plate on the side of injury.[31] Assessment of lateral stability can trace which ligamentous structures are disrupted.

Greater than 20° of deformity in extension suggests complete collateral ligament disruption and at least 1 of the secondary stabilizers. Once lateral PIP joint dislocations are reduced, they are often stable by virtue of the double-column bony support.

Return to play
The athlete is allowed early movement with buddy taping for protection.[34] Open repair of the ruptured collateral ligaments has been performed in athletes to expedite return to play, although there is no significant evidence that it expedites healing or improves motion.[31] Occasionally, the collateral ligament becomes trapped in the joint and requires open reduction.[34] For unstable lateral dislocations and high-level sporting dislocations, return to play can include a ligament hinge brace with buddy taping (**Fig. 18**).

Volar Dislocations

Volar PIP joint dislocations are rare and usually occur from a sudden torque to the digit causing the base of the middle phalanx to dislocate volarly and rupture the central slip.[31] Even if the joint is reducible, clinicians should have a high index of suspicion for disruption of the extensor mechanism. Failure to immobilize the joint in extension to allow the central slip to heal can lead to a boutonnière deformity. Complex volar dislocations involve a rotatory component in which the condyle of the proximal phalanx buttonholes between the central slip and the lateral band (**Fig. 19**). Closed reduction can be attempted by relaxing the lateral bands through MCP joint and PIP joint flexion followed by gentle rotary manipulation. Most cases require open reduction because of failed reduction from the noose effect of the central slip and lateral band around the neck of the proximal phalanx. Less commonly, failed reduction can occur from

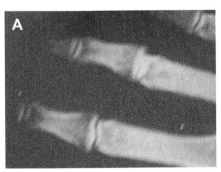
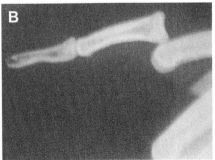

Fig. 16. Bayonet dislocation. (*A*) Anteroposterior and (*B*) lateral radiographs of a bayonet dislocation show the importance of obtaining a true lateral view for PIP joint fractures because the AP projection may look almost normal.

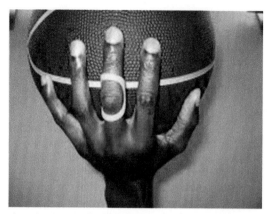

Fig. 17. Figure-of-eight splint. Murphy ring brace.

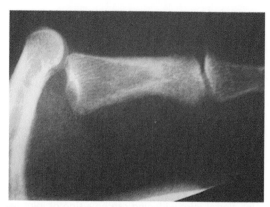

Fig. 19. Volar PIP dislocation. Volar PIP dislocations that are irreducible have a high likelihood of an interposed structure such as the fracture fragment.

interposition of the central slip, lateral band, or torn collateral ligament within the joint.[35]

Return to play

PIP joint dislocation can be seen as a complication of other digital injuries that are returned to play with limited immobilization. For instance, an athlete with a metacarpal fracture who is immobilized in an ulnar gutter with the PIP joint excluded is at high risk of volar PIP joint dislocation when coming in contact with balls or players (**Fig. 20**). With conservative management of volar plate dislocation, the athlete can return to play in a digital cast and buddy taping after 2 weeks. At 6 weeks with joint stability, the athlete can transition to buddy taping for an additional 6 to 8 weeks.

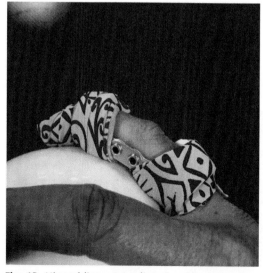

Fig. 18. Hinged ligament splint. Consider using tape under and over the brace to limit skin maceration and brace translation during play.

PROXIMAL INTERPHALANGEAL JOINT FRACTURE DISLOCATIONS

PIP joint fracture dislocations are categorized into 3 fracture patterns based on the morphology of the middle phalanx base fractures: palmar lip fracture, dorsal lip fracture, or pilon fracture.[33] Further classification is determined by joint stability (**Fig. 21**). Both lateral and volar to dorsal stability of the PIP joint are imparted largely by the locking articular buttressing surfaces. Fractures that involve sufficient size of the articulating joint facets are inherently unstable.

Palmar Lip Fractures

Palmar lip fracture stability depends on the degree of articular surface involvement. Fracture fragment involving less than 30% of the articular surface is considered stable because sufficient collateral ligament attachments are retained.[36] Treatment is targeted at maintaining joint congruity and encouraging early mobilization. Protected motion treatments allow the joint to move in an arc through which it remains concentrically reduced, but is restricted from unstable positions. Buddy taping is an option in cases requiring only prevention from hyperextension.[36] When a slight degree of flexion is required to maintain reduction, a figure-of-eight splint is a better choice. A dorsal blocking splint is appropriate when full active flexion is permitted but the last 10° to 15° of extension are blocked to promote palmar plate healing.[37]

Tenuous palmar lip fractures are those involving 30% to 50% of the articular surface and are considered unstable if reduction is not maintained with 30° of flexion.[33,36] The preferred treatment of stable tenuous palmar lip fractures is extension block splinting (**Fig. 22**). Bent aluminum splints are secured to the proximal and middle phalanges

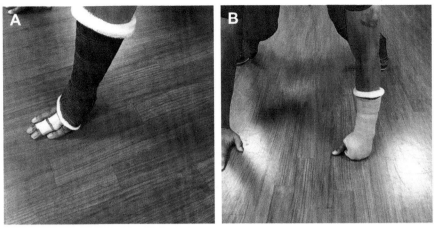

Fig. 20. Ulnar gutter splint. (*A*) Ulnar gutter splint or padded forearm-based orthosis with buddy taping of metacarpal fractures allows return to training. (*B*) Full-fist positioning should be considered for team practice and return to play because of risk of hyperextension injury to the digits.

in such a way that they allow PIP flexion but block extension beyond the point at which subluxation occurs.[36] Confirmation of proper splint placement with true lateral radiographs is recommended. Extension block pinning achieves a similar function to extension block splinting (**Fig. 23**). The K-wire is inserted retrograde into the proximal phalanx at a 30° angle to its long axis or at the angle that blocks unstable extension. Various methods of skeletal traction and dynamic external fixation have been used to treat unstable PIP fracture dislocations (**Fig. 24**). The advantage to these methods is that they allow for early motion and prevent joint stiffness. Athletes are not permitted to return to play while they have these devices in place.

Unstable palmar lip fractures involve more than 50% of the joint surface or involve 30% to 50% of the articular surface and require more than 30° of flexion to maintain reduction of the PIP joint.[33,36] Treatment is focused on restoring the palmar buttress. Open reduction and internal fixation

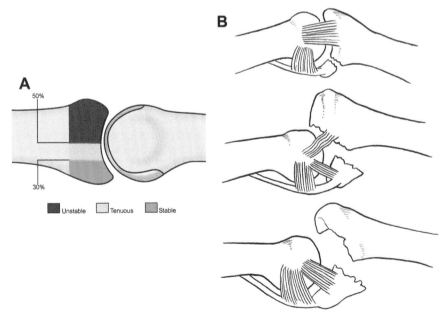

Fig. 21. PIP fracture dislocations. (*A*) PIP joint stability is classified based on the percentage of joint surface involvement. (*B*) The greater the percentage of articular surface involved, the more likely the ligamentous stabilizers are disrupted.

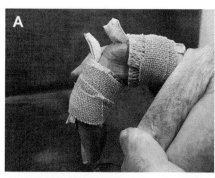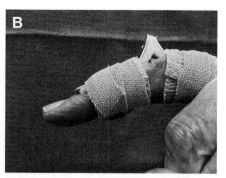

Fig. 22. Extension block splinting. (*A*) Full active flexion is permitted. (*B*) Extension is blocked beyond the point at which the joint becomes unstable.

with screws and K-wires is recommended for larger fracture fragments. For highly comminuted fractures of the base of the middle phalanx, cerclage wires can be used to stabilize the fragments by providing circumferential compression with wire tightening. When reconstructive procedures are required to restore or reconstruct the base of the middle phalanx, palmar plate arthroplasty or hamate osteochondral autograft arthroplasty are considered.

Dorsal Lip Fractures

Dorsal lip fractures commonly involve disruption of the central slip and are maximally stable in full extension.[36] Stable dorsal lip fractures are usually minimally displaced avulsion fractures involving less than 50% of the articular surface. Stable dorsal lip fractures with less than 2 mm of fragment displacement may initially be immobilized in extension by a splint or transarticular K-wire for 3 weeks. The PIP joint only should be immobilized and the DIP joint left free for active and passive range-of-motion exercises. The patient is then transitioned to a dynamic extension splint for 3 weeks to permit active flexion. At 6 weeks, passive flexion and strengthening exercises are started. Dorsal lip fractures with fragment displacement greater than 2 mm may have associated extensor lag and are best treated with open reduction and internal fixation with K-wires with or without a tension band wire, pullout suture, suture anchor, or lag screws.[36]

Dorsal lip fractures are categorized as unstable if there is any palmar subluxation or dislocation seen radiographically after closed reduction. Large fracture fragments are treated with open reduction and internal fixation. Highly comminuted fractures are better treated with closed reduction and percutaneous pinning of the PIP joint in full extension to allow the fragments to consolidate and the central slip to heal.

Pilon Fractures

Pilon fractures involve both palmar and dorsal lip fractures and are considered unstable. Traction is the treatment of choice because it provides alignment and permits early mobilization.[36] Open reduction and internal fixation is often not recommended because of an association with loss of reduction, stiffness, and infection.

Return to play

Professional athletes with stable PIP joint fracture dislocations who can function effectively with protected motion splints in place can return to play, although close observation and serial radiographic evaluation are needed to confirm maintenance of reduction.[33] Athletes with unstable PIP joint fracture dislocations are cautioned not to delay repair because it is associated with poorer outcomes and limited options. Return to play with functional protection is often permitted once stable fixation is obtained. Options for return-to-play immobilization include digital casting, taping, custom orthotics, or

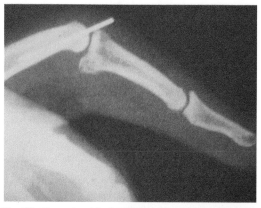

Fig. 23. Extension block pinning. Extension of the PIP joint is blocked with a K-wire advanced retrograde down the intramedullary canal of the middle phalanx.

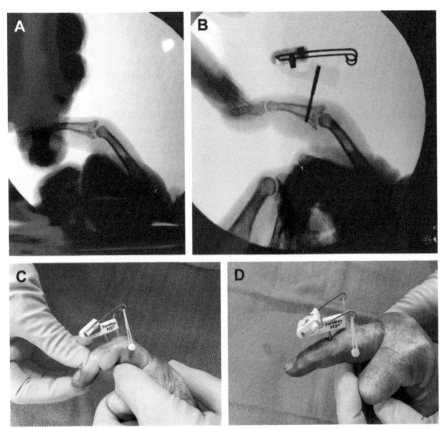

Fig. 24. Dynamic traction with TurnKey FCS device (Biomechanics Lab, Inc. Sacramento, CA). (*A*) A 54-year-old man with an unstable PIP joint fracture-dislocation on lateral radiograph. (*B*) After the device is installed, lateral radiograph confirmed joint realignment. (*C*) Active flexion and (*D*) extension exercises are performed during fracture healing.

reinforced personal protective equipment. All decisions regarding immobilization should be researched for compliance with the sports regulatory agency.

PROXIMAL INTERPHALANGEAL JOINT CONDYLAR FRACTURES

Condylar fractures of the PIP joint can be classified into 3 categories: type I is a stable fracture without displacement; type II is an unstable, unicondylar fracture; and type III is a bicondylar or comminuted fracture.[38] All 3 radiographic views are necessary for appropriate evaluation of joint stability. An anteroposterior (AP) radiograph can assess proximal migration and articular step-off, a lateral view can evaluate for volar displacement, and an oblique view can provide fracture geometry. Although type I PIP joint condylar fractures are considered stable, they should be treated with caution and with close follow-up because they are inherently unstable. Type II and III condylar fractures are highly unstable and nearly all require

operative intervention. Fixation requires at least 2 points of fixation to control rotation. For severe comminution, consider dynamic traction.

Return to Play

Depending on the stability of fixation, an athlete may be able to return to sports only if there is stable external bracing to the finger. Otherwise, it may be best to await fracture union. However, early PIP joint range of motion is always encouraged if fixation is secure enough in order to avoid joint stiffness.

SAGITTAL BAND INJURY

Sagittal band injury in athletes is more commonly known as boxer's knuckle, although it can occur in any sports that involve a direct blow to the MCP joint, such as football and rugby.[13] The middle finger is most susceptible to injury because of its prominent metacarpal head when making a fist. Athletes usually present with MCP joint swelling, tenderness, inability to initiate extension, and occasionally central tendon subluxation or dislocation. In addition to standard radiographic views, the Brewerton view may be helpful to identify collateral ligament avulsion injuries and occult fractures of the metacarpal head.[39] It is an AP view obtained with the MCP joint flexed 65° with the dorsal aspect of the fingers flat against the radiograph cassette and the beam angled 15° ulnar to radial. Rayan and Murray[40] classified closed sagittal band injuries into 3 types: type I, injury without extensor tendon instability; type II, injury with tendon subluxation; and type III, injury with tendon dislocation.[39]

Sagittal band injuries without extensor digitorum communis (EDC) subluxation can be managed with buddy taping to an adjacent digit for 4 weeks.[40] Acute injuries (<3 weeks) with EDC subluxation may be treated with an MCP joint flexion block splint, or sagittal band splint, for 8 weeks.[41] The splint is designed to hold the injured MCP joint in 25° to 35° of hyperextension relative to the adjacent digit, which allows for immediate active mobilization of the MCP joint with the splint in place. Catalano and colleagues[41] used the sagittal band splint to treat 10 patients with type III sagittal band injury. Eight patients had no pain, 3 patients had residual EDC subluxation, and 1 patient required sagittal band reconstruction.

For chronic sagittal band injuries (>3 weeks) or those who have failed nonsurgical treatment, there are several methods of sagittal band reconstruction that consist of sagittal band repair with realignment of the extensor tendon.[3] Carroll and colleagues[42] described a technique wherein a distally based radial slip of EDC is looped around the radial collateral ligament and sutured to itself for centralization. Postoperative rehabilitation may use a relative motion splint, as described by Merritt.[24] This method facilitates recovery and is less cumbersome than an outrigger orthosis with flexion block.

Return to Play

Athletes with acute sagittal band injury without subluxation can return to play with buddy taping within 10 days of injury. When EDC subluxation is present, the immobilization orthosis limits functional return to play and increases risk of injury to other joints in the hand. As such, return to play is discouraged for 8 to 12 weeks with chronic and postoperative sagittal band injuries. Once the athlete returns to play, buddy taping for 4 weeks is strongly encouraged. If the athlete returns to play before full tissue healing and return of strength, there is a significant risk of recurrent rupture of the sagittal band.

RADIAL COLLATERAL LIGAMENT RUPTURE OF THE METACARPOPHALANGEAL JOINT

Athletes with isolated radial collateral ligament (RCL) rupture of the MCP joint often present with persistent swelling and pain along the radial aspect of a previously injured finger.[25] RCL rupture of the MCP joint is typically caused by forced ulnar deviation while the MCP joint is flexed. A Brewerton radiographic view should be obtained to evaluate for avulsed bone fragments.[37] MRI may be required and can help differentiate partial from complete tears. Grade I injury is described as pain without laxity, grade II is laxity with an end point in 60° of flexion, and grade III has no end point. Treatment of grade I and II generally involves splinting the joint in 30° of flexion and reassessment for stability of the RCL in 3 weeks.[31] However, athletes are very active and may benefit from early surgical repair because it has been shown that most patients improve and have satisfactory results with surgery. Grade III injuries, when acute, can be managed nonoperatively initially with immobilization in radial deviation for 6 weeks. Surgical repair may be reserved for those who fail nonoperative treatment or is sometimes the primary treatment in an effort to return the player back to sports sooner.

Return to Play

Early management includes casting in 30° of MCP flexion for 4 weeks. During this period, athletes are not encouraged to return to play. This period is followed by taping and custom orthosis wear for an additional 4 weeks, at which time range-of-motion exercises begin (**Fig. 25**). Return to play at this point depends on the athlete's level of play, sport, and the digit involved. At 8 weeks after injury, athletes are encouraged to wean from the orthosis by taping during practice and then taping during play (**Fig. 26**).

METACARPAL OSTEOCHONDRAL FRACTURES

Professional ball sport players are susceptible to intra-articular metacarpal head fractures involving the index metacarpal because of it being an unprotected, border digit.[38] The middle finger may also be affected, being the longest finger and more susceptible to axial impact than the adjacent fingers. Radiographic evaluation requires the standard 3 views along with the Brewerton view to accurately evaluate the articular contour.[43] Displaced ligament avulsion fractures and

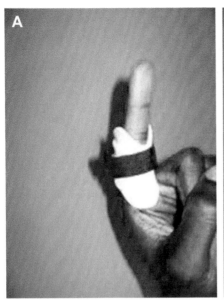
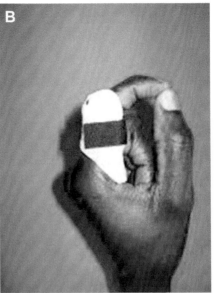

Fig. 25. Custom orthosis for MCP joint RCL rupture. (*A*) Lateral deviation and (*B*) MCP flexion can be restricted with a custom orthosis, which can be padded for return to play or taped for use in a glove.

osteochondral fracture should be managed with open reduction and internal fixation. Kumar and Satku[44] recommended that small osteochondral fragments should be reduced by approximating the capsule to trap and hold the fragments in place. Headless screws have facilitated intra-articular fracture fragment fixation.

Return to Play

Immobilization for metacarpal fracture healing includes ulnar gutter casting or custom orthosis for 10 to 21 days for callus formation. Although these types of immobilization are anatomically appropriate, care should be taken when immobilizing for return to practice or play in order to limit the risk of injury to other fingers.

THUMB ULNAR COLLATERAL LIGAMENT INJURY

Injury to the ulnar collateral ligament (UCL) of the thumb MCP joint was historically referred to as gamekeepers' thumb because of the chronic laxity

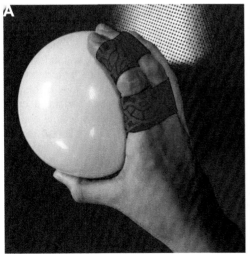
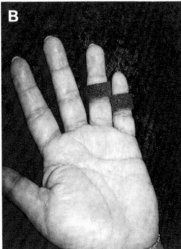

Fig. 26. Buddy taping for MCP joint RCL rupture. (*A*) Buddy taping permits early return to play and support. (*B*) For the small finger, a custom step-down strapping is required because of digital length discrepancy.

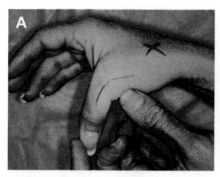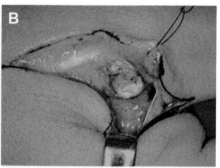

Fig. 27. Stener lesion. (*A*) A 35-year-old woman with unstable ulnar collateral ligament of the MCP joint of the thumb. (*B*) Distal insertion of the collateral ligament has avulsed and is blocked from reattachment to its insertion by the interposed adductor aponeurosis.

of UCL of the thumb observed in Scottish game-keepers.[45] It was later referred to as skier's thumb because this injury is frequently noted in skiers who fall on an outstretched hand strapped to the handle of a ski pole, causing forced abduction and extension of the thumb. Thumb MCP joint collateral ligament injuries are increasingly recognized in professional athletes who participate in ball-handling sports.[46]

Athletes typically describe a hyperabduction injury to the thumb and present with pain and swelling at the ulnar aspect of the thumb MCP joint. Radiographs may show an avulsion fracture at the attachment of the UCL to the base of the proximal phalanx or a widening of the ulnar aspect of the first MCP joint.[46] A local nerve block before valgus stress testing of the thumb MCP joint can be helpful to accurately assess stability. Tenderness without laxity indicates a partial tear. The criterion for joint instability is typically greater than 30° laxity with valgus stress or greater than 15° of increased radial deviation compared with the contralateral thumb.[47]

Acute partial ruptures of the thumb UCL can be treated with 4 weeks of continuous immobilization in a thumb spica cast or splint followed by protected range-of-motion exercises.[31] A complete tear generally warrants surgical repair with reattachment of the ligament to its bony insertion. However, large, avulsed, nondisplaced bone fragments may heal with immobilization alone. A Stener lesion is another indication for surgical repair. It occurs when the adductor aponeurosis is interposed between the distally avulsed UCL and its insertion at the base of the proximal phalanx.[48] Some clinicians are concerned that valgus stress testing of the thumb MCP joint can precipitate a Stener lesion that did not exist before (**Fig. 27**). Spontaneous ligament healing is inhibited because the ulnar ligament is not in contact with the bony insertion. Presence of a persistent firm mass on the ulnar aspect of the first metacarpal head is suspicious for a Stener lesion and should be confirmed with MRI or ultrasonography.

Return to Play

Return to play depends on the classification of the tear and the player's dominant hand. In baseball, early return to sport with a thumb spica splint is permitted for partial tears in the nonthrowing arm.[49] For partial tears in the throwing arm, 4 weeks of full-time immobilization followed by 2 to 4 weeks of protective splint during play is recommended. For complete tears that require operative repair, additional caution is taken to avoid reinjury with early return to play. It is advised to wait 6 to 8 weeks after surgery in the nonthrowing arm and 10 to 12 weeks in the throwing arm.

SUMMARY

Suggested orthoses, facilitations of return to play, and important considerations when returning an athlete to play are summarized in **Table 1**.[50] Although tissue healing is the primary consideration when treating finger injuries, in elite athletes there are several other factors to consider. The sport, position of play, level of play, hand dominance, age of athlete, financial considerations, and player compliance are all serious points to consider when determining the appropriate return-to-play style and timing. In addition, chronic use of performance-enhancing drugs, previous injury, and medical treatment to the area should be considered when determining healing time and prognosis for recovery. Communication between the athlete, surgeon, hand therapist, training staff, and coaches is often imperative for an informed decision-making process. These multifactorial considerations allow for great variance among injuries and athletes.

Table 1
Management of common finger injuries in ball sports

Injury	Orthosis	Return to Sport	Considerations
Mallet finger	• Full-finger cast or orthosis • Buddy tape to adjacent finger	• May return in orthosis based on edema and pain • Compliance with wearing and properly positioning the splint is necessary for a good outcome	• Hand dominance • Sport/equipment • Protect proximal and adjacent joints • Add tape under orthosis/cast to limit maceration and translation of orthosis
Swan neck deformity	• Full-finger cast/orthosis for 6 wk • Wean to figure-of-eight splint for 4 wk • Progress to PIP taping for 12 wk	• May return to training in figure-of-eight splint at 6 wk	• Consider full-finger cast with buddy tape for high-impact team sports • Add tape under orthosis/cast to limit maceration and translation of orthosis
Boutonnière deformity	• Closed injury: buddy tape • PIP extension orthosis for 6 wk at all times • Wean to nighttime splint for 6 additional weeks	• 0–10 d for closed injury based on comfort • May return with full-finger cast and buddy tape for nonoperative cases • For postoperative, 6–8 wk in cast	• Be sure to protect proximal and distal joints • Return to play in cast is based on sport and tissue integrity • Add tape/cohesive bandage under orthosis/cast to limit maceration and translation of orthosis
Pulley rupture	• Grade 1 and 2: tape support • Grade 3 and 4: pulley ring over tape	• Light sport activities such as training can be started after 4 wk • Full sport activities after 6 wk • At all times, use tape to support the pulley	• Confirm custom ring around sport equipment (bats, balls, rackets) and under protective devices (gloves). • Use tape under custom ring and over the fill finger to decrease ring translation during play
Dorsal PIP dislocations	• Buddy taping • Full-finger extension cast/orthosis • Figure-of-eight extension orthosis	• With stable joint and full range of motion, return to play immediately with buddy taping • If the joint is unstable, return to play at >4 wk with extension cast • Postoperative: return to play at 12–16 wk with buddy tape	• Joint stability and integrity • Position • Light vs heavy demands • Key player vs support player
Lateral PIP dislocations	• Buddy taping • Full-finger extension cast/orthosis • Hinged ligament splint	• Early movement with buddy taping for protection/deviation stability • 2–4 wk return to play with orthosis	• Joint stability and integrity • Position • Light vs heavy demands • Key player vs support player
Volar PIP dislocations	• Buddy taping • Full-finger flexion cast/orthosis • Figure-of-eight flexion orthosis	• In a digital cast and buddy taping after 2 wk • Continue buddy tape for 6–8 wk	• Joint stability and integrity • Position • Light vs heavy demands • Key player vs support player

REFERENCES

1. Rettig AC. Epidemiology of hand and wrist injuries in sports. Clin Sports Med 1998;17:401–6.
2. Yeh PC, Shin SS. Tendon ruptures: mallet, flexor digitorum profundus. Hand Clin 2012;28(3):425–30.
3. Strauch RJ. Extensor tendon injury. In: Wolfe SW, Hotchkiss RN, Pederson WC, et al, editors. Green's operative hand surgery. 6th edition. Philadelphia: Elsevier Churchill-Livingstone; 2011. p. 159–88.
4. Witherow EJ, Peiris CL. Custom-made finger orthoses have fewer skin complications than prefabricated finger orthoses in the management of mallet injury: a systematic review and meta-analysis. Arch Phys Med Rehabil 2015;96(10):1913–23.
5. Botero SS, Hidalgo Diaz JJ, Benaida A, et al. Review of acute traumatic closed mallet finger injuries in adults. Arch Plast Surg 2016;43(2):134–44.
6. Wehbe MA, Schneider LH. Mallet fractures. J Bone Joint Surg Am 1984;66(5):658–69.
7. Kalainov DM, Hoepfner PE, Hartigan BJ, et al. Nonsurgical treatment of closed mallet finger fractures. J Hand Surg Am 2005;30(3):580–6.
8. Shin SS. Baseball commentary–tendon ruptures: mallet, FDP. Hand Clin 2012;28(3):431–2.
9. Simpson D, McQueen MM, Kumar P. Mallet deformity in sport. J Hand Surg Br 2001;26(1):32–43.
10. Groth GN, Wilder DM, Young VL. The impact of compliance on the rehabilitation of patients with mallet finger injuries. J Hand Ther 1994;7(1):21–4.
11. Hovgaard C, Klareskov B. Alternate conservative treatment of mallet-finger injuries by elastic double-finger bandage. J Hand Surg Am 2005;30(3):580–6.
12. McMurtry JT, Isaacs J. Extensor tendon injuries. Clin Sports Med 2015;34:167–80.
13. Chauhan A, Jacobs B, Andoga A, et al. Extensor tendon injuries in athletes. Sports Med Arthrosc 2014;22(1):45–55.
14. Rozmaryn LM. Central slip tenotomy with distal repair in the treatment of severe chronic mallet fingers. J Hand Surg Am 2014;39(4):773–8.
15. Grundberg AB, Reagan DS. Central slip tenotomy for chronic mallet finger deformity. J Hand Surg Am 1987;12(4):545–7.
16. Houpt P, Dijkstra R, Storm van Leeuwen JB. Fowler's tenotomy for mallet deformity. J Hand Surg Br 1993;18(4):499–500.
17. Kleinman WB, Petersen DP. Oblique retinacular ligament reconstruction for chronic mallet finger deformity. J Hand Surg Am 1984;9(3):399–404.
18. Thompson JS, Littler JW, Upton J. The spiral oblique retinacular ligament (SORL). J Hand Surg Am 1978;3(5):482–7.
19. Shrewsbury MM, Johnson RK. A systematic study of the oblique retinacular ligament of the human finger: its structure and function. J Hand Surg Am 1977;2(3):194–9.
20. Marino JT, Lourie GM. Boutonniere and pulley rupture in elite athletes. Hand Clin 2012;28(3):437–45.
21. Aronowitz ER, Leddy JP. Closed tendon injuries of the hand and wrist in athletes. Clin Sports Med 1998;17(3):449–67.
22. Elson RA. Rupture of the central slip of the extensor hood of the finger. A test for early diagnosis. J Bone Joint Surg Br 1986;68(2):229–31.
23. Smith DW. Boutonniere and pulley rupture in elite basketball. Hand Clin 2012;28(3):449–50.
24. Merritt WH. Relative motion splint: active motion after extensor tendon injury and repair. J Hand Surg Am 2014;39(6):1187–94.
25. Dolphin JA. Extensor tenotomy for chronic boutonniere deformity of the finger; report of two cases. J Bone Joint Surg Am 1965;47:161–4.
26. Meadows SE, Schneider LH, Sherwyn JH. Treatment of the chronic boutonniere deformity by extensor tenotomy. Hand Clin 1995;11(3):441–7.
27. Curtis RM, Reid RL, Provost JM. A staged technique for the repair of the traumatic boutonniere deformity. J Hand Surg Am 1983;8(2):167–71.
28. McCue FC, Honner R, Johnson MC, et al. Athletics injuries of the proximal interphalangeal joint requiring surgical treatment. J Bone Joint Surg Am 1970;52(5):937–56.
29. Lourie GM, Hamby Z, Raasch WG, et al. Annular flexor pulley injuries in professional baseball pitchers: a case series. Am J Sports Med 2011;39(2):421–4.
30. Schoffl V, Hochholzer T, Winkelmann HP, et al. Pulley injuries in rock climbers. Wilderness Environ Med 2003;14(2):94–100.
31. Merrell G, Slade JF. Dislocations and ligament injuries in the digits. In: Wolfe SW, Hotchkiss RN, Pederson WC, et al, editors. Green's operative hand surgery. 6th edition. Philadelphia: Elsevier Churchill-Livingstone; 2011. p. 291–332.
32. Bindra RR, Foster BJ. Management of proximal interphalangeal joint dislocations in athletes. Hand Clin 2009;25(3):423–35.
33. Williams CS 4th. Proximal interphalangeal joint fracture dislocations: stable and unstable. Hand Clin 2012;28(3):409–16.
34. Vicar AJ. Proximal interphalangeal joint dislocations without fractures. Hand Clin 1988;4(1):5–13.
35. Boden RA, Srinivasan MS. Rotational dislocation of the proximal interphalangeal joint of the finger. J Bone Joint Surg Br 2008;90(3):385–6.
36. Kang R, Stern PJ. Fracture dislocations of the proximal interphalangeal joint. J Hand Surg Am 2002;2(2):47–59.
37. McElfresh EC, Dobyns JH, O'Brien ET. Management of fracture-dislocation of the proximal interphalangeal joints by extension-block splinting. J Bone Joint Surg Am 1972;54(8):1705–11.
38. Day CS, Stern PJ. Fractures of the metacarpals and phalanges. In: Wolfe SW, Hotchkiss RN,

Pederson WC, et al, editors. Green's operative hand surgery. 6th edition. Philadelphia: Elsevier Churchill-Livingstone; 2011. p. 239–90.

39. Kleinhenz BP, Adams BD. Closed sagittal band injury of the metacarpal joint. J Am Acad Orthop Surg 2015;23(7):415–23.

40. Rayan GM, Murray D. Classification and treatment of closed sagittal band injuries. J Hand Surg Am 1994; 19(4):590–4.

41. Catalano LW 3rd, Gupta S, Ragland R 3rd, et al. Closed treatment of nonrheumatoid extensor tendon dislocations at the metacarpophalangeal joint. J Hand Surg Am 2006;31(2):242–5.

42. Carroll CT, Moore JR, Weiland AJ. Posttraumatic ulnar subluxation of the extensor tendons: a reconstructive technique. J Hand Surg Am 1987;12(2): 227–31.

43. Lane CS. Detecting occult fractures of the metacarpal head: the Brewerton view. J Hand Surg Am 1977;2(2):131–3.

44. Kumar VP, Satku K. Surgical management of osteochondral fractures of the phalanges and metacarpals: a surgical technique. J Hand Surg Am 1995;20(6):1028–31.

45. Campbell CS. Gamekeeper's thumb. J Bone Joint Surg Br 1955;37(1):148–9.

46. Lee AT, Carlson MG. Thumb metacarpophalangeal joint collateral ligament injury management. Hand Clin 2012;28(3):361–70.

47. Heyman P. Injuries to the ulnar collateral ligament of the thumb metacarpophalangeal joint. J Am Acad Orthop Surg 1997;5(4):224–9.

48. Stener B. Displacement of the ruptured ulnar collateral ligament of the metacarpophalangeal joint of the thumb: a clinical and anatomical study. J Bone Joint Surg Br 1962;44:869–79.

49. Chhor KS, Culp RW. Baseball commentary "thumb ligament injuries: RCL and UCL". Hand Clin 2012; 28(3):371–2.

50. Goldie Staines K, Collins ED. The athlete. In: Jacobs MA, Austin NM, editors. Orthotic intervention for the hand and upper extremity: splinting principles and process. Baltimore (MD): Lippincott Williams & Wilkins; 2014. p. 544–65.

Flexor Tendon Pulley Injuries in Rock Climbers

Elizabeth A. King, MD[a], John R. Lien, MD[b],*

KEYWORDS

- Pulley rupture • Rock climbing • Pulley reconstruction

KEY POINTS

- Rock climbers have a greater incidence of closed traumatic pulley ruptures due to unique biomechanical demands on the hand.
- Dynamic ultrasound is a useful tool for diagnosis of pulley rupture.
- Isolated pulley ruptures can generally be treated conservatively with splinting and early functional therapy.
- Sequential pulley ruptures should be treated with surgical reconstruction; several successful techniques have been described.

INTRODUCTION

Closed traumatic flexor tendon pulley ruptures among rock climbers were first observed in the 1980s, recognizing that climbers are susceptible to certain injuries due to the unique biomechanical demands of grip positions.[1–3] Rock climbing has become increasingly popular in recent years, and hand and wrist injuries remain the most common injuries among competitive climbers. The predominant injury is to finger flexor tendons or pulleys, which account for 33% of all climbing injuries reported.[4] There is an estimated 19% to 26% incidence of pulley ruptures among competitive climbers.[5–8] These injuries are less common among the general population but can occur with a sudden force against a flexed digit.[9]

The goals of treatment are to restore biomechanics of the flexor pulley system and to allow patients to return to their previous activity level. This article discusses evaluation and treatment options for flexor tendon pulley ruptures in rock climbers.

ANATOMY AND BIOMECHANICS

The flexor tendon pulley system consists of 5 annular pulleys (A1–A5) and 3 cruciate pulleys (C1–C3), as depicted in **Fig. 1**. As described by Doyle and colleagues,[10,11] in early anatomic studies using methylene blue injections, the A2 and A4 pulleys are the largest, thickest, and most consistent in anatomic dissection studies, and are true fibro-osseous pulleys, arising from the periosteum of the proximal phalanx and middle phalanx, respectively. The A2 pulley measures 17 mm in length and is thickest distally. The A4 pulley measures 7 mm in length and is thickest at the midaspect.[11] A1, A3, and A5 pulleys are narrower and insert onto the volar plate. The A2 and A4 pulleys are the most significant biomechanically for flexor tendon function.[12] They act to maintain flexor tendons close to bone in flexion and extension, converting tendon excursion to rotation and torque at the metacarpophalangeal and interphalangeal joints.[12]

Grip positions used in rock climbing generate large forces on the flexor digitorum profundus

Disclosure Statement. The authors have nothing to disclose.
[a] Department of Orthopaedic Surgery, University of Cincinnati, TriHealth Hospital System, 538 Oak Street, Suite 200, Cincinnati, OH 45219, USA; [b] Section of Plastic Surgery, Department of Orthopaedic Surgery, University of Michigan, 2098 South Main Street, Ann Arbor, MI 48103, USA
* Corresponding author.
E-mail address: jlien@med.umich.edu

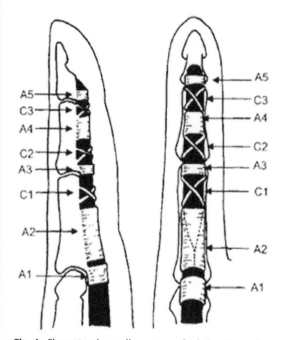

Fig. 1. Flexor tendon pulley system, depicting 5 annular pulleys (A1–A5) and 3 cruciate pulleys (C1–C3). (*From* Hauger O, Chung CB, Lektrakul N, et al. Pulley system in the fingers: normal anatomy and simulated lesions in cadavers at MR imaging, CT, and US with and without contrast material distention of the tendon sheath. Radiology 2000;217(1):201–12; with permission.)

and flexor digitorum superficialis tendons. In the crimp position, used to maintain a hold on a narrow ledge, the distal interphalangeal joints are hyperextended and proximal interphalangeal (PIP) joints are flexed 90° to 100°. Climbers may lock the thumb over the top of the index and middle fingers to decrease strain on the pulleys (**Fig. 2**). Tensile forces in tendons combined with joint flexion creates large demands on the annular pulleys, which is confirmed in biomechanical studies showing that forces acting on pulleys in the crimp position are 287 N at the A2 pulley and 226 N at the A4 pulley.[13] The force at the distal edge of the A2 pulley is 3 times the force at the fingertip in the crimp position.[14] Climbers typically load 380 N through their fingers, but a 70-kg climber shock loading a single finger would apply a force of 450N at approximately a right angle to the proximal phalanx, exceeding the failure force of the A2 pulley (400 N).[15,16]

In biomechanical studies evaluating load to failure in rock climbing grip positions, the A4 pulley most commonly failed first, followed by A2.[17] The A2 pulley failed from the distal to proximal edge, whereas the A4 pulley failed from proximal to distal, and ruptures occurred within intrasubstance collagen fibers rather than at the pulley insertion. Clinical bowstringing was not seen with isolated A2 or A4 pulley rupture. Subtle

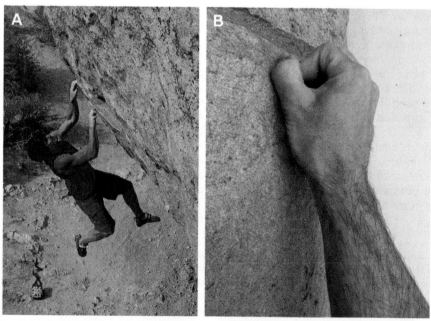

Fig. 2. (*A*) On narrow ledges, rock climbers may load their entire body weight through their fingers. (*B*) The crimp grip position, with PIP joints flexed and DIP joints hyperextended, stresses the pulleys. The thumb can be locked over top of the index/middle fingers to decrease strain on the pulleys. (*Courtesy of* S. Diamond, MD, Boston, MA.)

bowstringing occurred when A3 ruptured along with A2 or A4, and obvious bowstringing required rupture of A2, A3, and A4 pulleys sequentially.[17] An intact A3 pulley prevents bowstringing when A2 or A4 pulleys are ruptured.[18] In biomechanical studies, dividing A2 and A4 pulleys resulted in 30% increase in tendon excursion through a range of PIP joint motion, which clinically results in a motion deficit and increased work of flexion.[12,16] A1 and A5 pulleys did not affect tendon excursion in a cadaver model when cut in isolation.[19]

INJURY PATTERNS

A common mechanism for pulley injury among rock climbers is a slip in foot position, causing a sudden overload of the pulley system with the fingers in the crimp grip position.[2,6,15] Crimping a small edge seems to be the most dangerous position risking pulley injury.[8]

Clinically, patients present with acute onset of pain and swelling over the injured pulley. They may hear a pop or feel a sensation of giving way at the PIP joint. Local ecchymosis and hematoma formation can occur. When the finger is flexed against resistance, bowstringing occurs if there are multiple sequential pulley ruptures, usually including A2 and A4 pulleys.[18] In initial observational studies of rock climbers, A2 pulley injuries were most common, although in more recent studies A4 pulley injuries are more common, which may be due to grips used.[6,20] Patients with acute injuries typically present with loss of motion and strength, but patients with chronic pulley ruptures may also present in a delayed fashion with PIP joint flexion contracture.[21]

The ring and long fingers are most commonly injured.[1,7] In biomechanical studies, the greatest forces are at the middle and index fingers in crimp grip positions.[22] The tendon forces at the time of ring finger pulley rupture are lower than in the index and long fingers, which may explain the propensity for ring finger injuries.[17] Injuries range from pulley strain with no clinical bowstringing to complex injuries with multiple pulley ruptures.

DIAGNOSIS

Patients may present with bruising, swelling, and tenderness over the affected pulley and may report a snapping or popping sound at the time of injury. Clinically it may be difficult to differentiate between a pulley strain, partial tear, or complete rupture. Isolated A2 or A4 pulley ruptures present without clinical bowstringing, because bowstringing requires multiple sequential pulley ruptures.[17]

Imaging
- Radiographs should be performed to rule out fractures, volar plate avulsion injuries, and epiphyseal stress injuries, which are becoming more common in adolescent climbers.[20] These are frequently Salter-Harris III injuries on the dorsal aspect of the middle phalanx.
- MRI has been used to confirm isolated pulley rupture and rule out more complex injuries or other soft tissue pathology. Sagittal MRI in a flexed position provides measurement of increased distance from tendon to bone; a gap greater than 2 mm suggests a disrupted annular pulley, although some rock climbers do have an increased gap due to chronic repetitive trauma.[23,24]
- When available, ultrasound provides a dynamic assessment, to evaluate A2 and A4 pulleys, measure flexor tendon bowstringing, and assess the volar plate.[24] Dynamic ultrasound is highly accurate and is recommended rather than relying on clinical bowstringing to diagnose pulley ruptures.[25] In a study of 64 elite rock climbers, dynamic ultrasound has a 98% sensitivity and 100% specificity for diagnosis of pulley injuries and can be used to measure the distance between tendon and bone in forced flexion and extension.[5,26] Ultrasound has a significantly lower cost than MRI.[7]

Schoffl and colleagues[6] introduced a grading system for pulley injury severity in an attempt to guide treatment (**Table 1**).

Table 1 Grading system for flexor tendon pulley injuries		
Grade	**Injury**	**Treatment**
1	Pulley strain	Conservative
2	Complete rupture of A4 or partial rupture of A2 or A3	Conservative
3	Complete rupture of A2 or A3	Conservative
4	Multiple pulley ruptures (A2/A3, A2/A3/A4) or single rupture (A2 or A3) combined with lumbricalis muscles or collateral ligament injury	Surgical

Adapted from Schoffl V, Hochholzer T, Winkelmann HP, et al. Pulley injuries in rock climbers. Wilderness Environ Med 2003;14:94–100; with permission.

TREATMENT OPTIONS

In the earliest reports of pulley injuries among rock climbers, treatment was conservative, with taping at the base of the affected finger as needed.[15] Tropet and colleagues[3] reported primary repair of a pulley injury in a young rock climber with bowstringing tendon in 1990, and various surgical techniques have been described since then. Currently, conservative therapy is recommended for isolated pulley ruptures, and surgical reconstruction is reserved for more severe injuries with multiple pulley ruptures.

Conservative Treatment

Conservative treatment is recommended for an isolated pulley injury.[2,6,15] Conservative treatment consists of immobilization for 10 to 14 days with a palmar splint, with the metacarpophalangeal joint in flexion and interphalangeal joints in extension or slight flexion.[27] Early functional therapy should follow with pulley protection with taping or a soft ring splint.

For grade 3 injuries, easy sport-specific activities may resume after 6 to 8 weeks, with pulley protection (tape or ring) recommended. Patients may return to climbing when they can avoid grip positions that produce pain.[27] Patients typically may return to full sport activities after 3 months and should continue taping for at least 6 months. Grade 2 injuries can progress more rapidly. Long-term strength deficits were not observed in rock climbers treated following this algorithm.[8]

Taping has been used as a prophylactic and therapeutic intervention to reduce pulley load and can be applied over the base of the finger or in a figure-of-8 pattern over the center of rotation of the PIP joint (**Fig. 3**).[28] The H-taping figure-of-8 technique was shown by ultrasound to decrease the tendon to phalanx distance by 16%, and clinical gains in strength were observed, although this may be due to psychological benefit to taping. In a cadaveric climbing model, circumferential

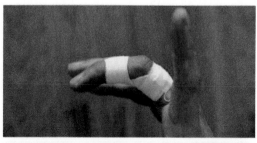

Fig. 3. Taping technique in a figure-of-8 pattern over the PIP joint center of rotation. (*Courtesy of* S. Diamond, MD, Boston, MA.)

taping at the base of the proximal phalanx did not increase load to failure for the A2 pulley, so there is not a definitive role for prophylactic taping, although it may increase comfort.[29]

Outcomes — Conservative Treatment

In a study of 21 rock climbers with grades 2 to 4 pulley injuries, clinical outcomes were excellent with conservative management; all regained their climbing level within 1 year, and there was no long-term strength deficit observed.[8] Repeat ultrasound showed no increase in flexor tendon–bone distance over baseline examination at an average follow-up of 3.5 years. The good results of five grade 4 pulley injuries treated conservatively suggest that a nonoperative approach is reasonable in the absence of clinical bowstringing or limited range of motion.

Schneeberger and Schweizer[30] recently reported a series of 47 cases of pulley ruptures in rock climbers treated conservatively with a pulley-protection thermoplast splint, worn continuously for 2 months. Tendon-phalanx distance in forced flexion was measured by ultrasound before and after treatment. After treatment in the splint, they showed decreases in tendon-phalanx distance from 4.4 mm to 2.3 mm for A2 pulley rupture and from 2.9 mm to 2.1 mm after A4 pulley rupture.[30] Of the 43 patients who responded to surveys, 38 had regained their climbing ability 8.8 months after injury, and only 1 reported reduced dexterity of the hand (while playing guitar).

Surgical Treatment

Multiple pulley ruptures (grade 4 injuries) generally require surgical repair. If left untreated, patients can develop a flexion contracture at the PIP joint secondary to flexor tendon bowstringing.[21] Moutet[31] advocates for surgical repair to allow elite climbers to return to their level of climbing; however, this is disputed by reports of successful return to climbing with conservative treatment.[8,30,32]

Techniques

Several techniques for surgical pulley reconstruction have been described, typically using palmaris longus tendon graft or extensor retinaculum in either a nonencircling or looped fashion (**Fig. 4**). Early active motion is typically permitted, because reconstruction of A2 and A4 pulleys restores near-normal tendon excursion and joint motion in a cadaver study.[16]

- Kleinert and Bennett (Weilby) technique: a nonencircling technique that uses a tendon graft (palmaris or slip of flexor digitorum

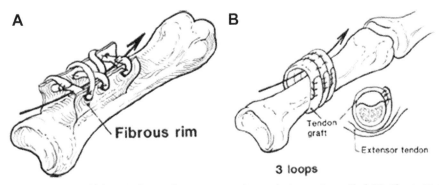

Fig. 4. (*A*) Nonencircling and (*B*) encircling pulley reconstruction techniques. *From* Clark TA, Skeete K, Amadio PC. Flexor tendon pulley reconstruction. J Hand Surg 2010;35A:1685–9. Used with permission of Mayo Foundation for Medical Education and Research. All rights reserved.

superficialis) woven into the residual end of flexor tendon sheath. This allows pulley tension to be set but does not have immediate strength.[33]

- Okutsu triple-loop reconstruction: encircling technique, modification of the Bunnell original loop reconstruction, uses a triple loop of free tendon graft (palmaris longus) passed around the phalanx subcutaneously.[34,35]
- Lister extensor retinaculum: encircling technique, uses a strip of extensor retinaculum graft harvested from over the fourth dorsal compartment, which is placed around the phalanx, overwrapped, and sutured. This provides a smooth gliding surface, and active and passive motion are permitted.[36]
- Loop-and-a-half technique: a tendon graft (palmaris longus) passes around phalanx and then through 1 limb of the tendon graft; suture 2 free ends, and then rotate away from the tendon graft. It is described by Widstrom and colleagues[37] and is the strongest in biomechanical cadaver studies (excluding the triple-loop technique).
- Karev belt loop technique: 2 transverse incisions are made in the volar plate, and the flexor tendon is passed through the belt loop created.[38] Because the flexor tendon must be passed through the loop, this technique can only be used in the setting of a flexor tendon repair and not for pulley reconstruction around an intact tendon.

Authors' Preferred Technique

The authors' preferred technique is the triple-loop technique for A2 pulley reconstruction, modified by passing the tendon graft between the extensor tendon and phalanx.[34,35]

The triple-loop pulley reconstruction is illustrated in **Fig. 5**. The finger is approached volarly via a standard Bruner incision. Scar is excised and tendon bowstringing is assessed. The reconstructed pulley should be placed where the original A2 pulley was located over the proximal phalanx. Palmaris tendon autograft is the preferred graft choice. After carefully dissecting the neurovascular bundles, the pulley graft is passed around the phalanx circumferentially, between the extensor tendon and the phalanx. The authors prefer to then weave the tendon through itself, because this allows easier tensioning of the graft. The graft is sutured to itself using 3-0 or 4-0 nonabsorbable suture. This is repeated twice for a total of 3 encircling loops. The sutured ends are rotated away from the flexor tendon surface and the loops are secured to one another.

For A4 pulley reconstruction, a single-loop reconstruction is used, passing the tendon graft between the subcutaneous tissue and terminal tendon.

Outcomes — Surgical Treatment

Surgical reconstruction usually allows climbers to return to their previous level of activity, although stiffness is a potential complication. Most published results are small case series, so it is difficult to compare clinical outcomes of reconstruction techniques.

In a retrospective comparison of 23 patients treated with 2 nonencircling techniques of pulley reconstruction, either using extensor retinaculum or free palmaris longus tendon grafts woven to the fibrous rim of the tendon sheath, all patients had unrestricted motion, with no difference between the 2 techniques in power or pinch grip.[39]

A group of 5 elite climbers were treated using the Weilby technique, which uses free palmaris longus graft sutured to the fibrocartilaginous

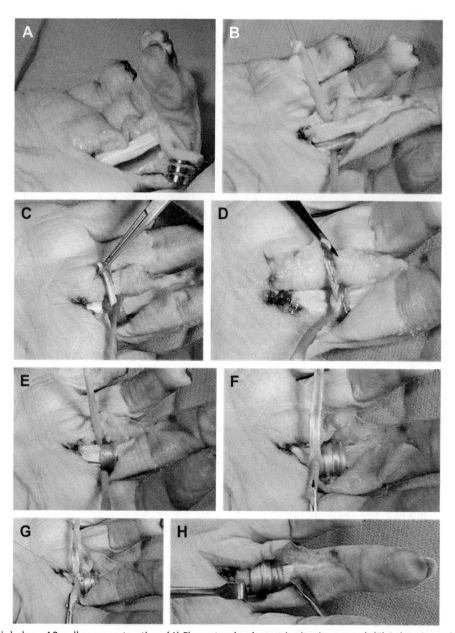

Fig. 5. Triple-loop A2 pulley reconstruction. (*A*) Flexor tendon bowstringing is assessed. (*B*) Palmaris tendon autograft is looped circumferentially, passing between the extensor tendon and the phalanx, ensuring that neurovascular bundles remain free. (*C*) Tendon graft is woven through itself, allowing tension to be set. (*D*) Graft is sutured to itself using 3-0 or 4-0 nonabsorbable suture. (*E–G*) This is repeated twice for a total of 3 encircling loops. (*H*) Rotate the sutured ends away so the flexor tendon glides freely.

remnants of the disrupted pulley. On average, they lost 4° of PIP joint motion and 12 N of grip strength, but all had resolution of bowstringing and returned to their previous level of climbing.[23]

Bouyer and colleagues followed 38 climbers with isolated or combined rupture of A2, A3, and A4 pulleys treated surgically with Lister encircling extensor retinaculum technique. At follow-up of minimum 6 months after returning to climbing, 30 had returned to their previous climbing level. No significant difference was seen in grip strength in crimp position between injured and noninjured sides. On follow-up ultrasound, 18 of 31 had bowstringing return to near normal. If bowstringing was corrected, climbers were more likely to return to their preinjury performance. Loss of PIP extension did occur in 7 patients and was believed due to scarring.[40]

SUMMARY

Pulley injuries are common injuries among rock climbers. Dynamic ultrasound is a useful tool to evaluate for pulley ruptures and displacement of the flexor tendons. Isolated pulley ruptures can be successfully treated conservatively with taping or splinting. Multiple pulley ruptures with bowstringing and limited active range of motion should be treated surgically, which typically involves an encircling tendon graft. Most climbers are able to return to their previous level of activity.

REFERENCES

1. Bollen S. Soft tissue injury in extreme rock climbers. Br J Sports Med 1988;22:145–7.
2. Bollen S. Upper limb injuries in elite rock climbers. J R Coll Surg Edinb 1990;35:S18–20.
3. Tropet Y, Menez D, Balmat P, et al. Closed traumatic rupture of the ring finger flexor tendon pulley. J Hand Surg 1990;15A(5):745–7.
4. Logan A, Makwana N, Mason G, et al. Acute hand and wrist injuries in experienced rock climbers. Br J Sports Med 2004;38:545–8.
5. Klauser A, Frauscher F, Bodner G, et al. Finger pulley injuries in extreme rock climbers: depiction with dynamic US. Radiology 2002;222:755–61.
6. Schoffl V, Hochholzer T, Winkelmann HP, et al. Pulley injuries in rock climbers. Wilderness Environ Med 2003;14:94–100.
7. Schoffl VR, Schoffl I. Injuries to the finger flexor pulley system in rock climbers: current concepts. J Hand Surg Am 2006;31(4):647–54.
8. Schoffl VR, Einwag F, Strecker W, et al. Strength measurement and clinical outcome after pulley ruptures in climbers. Med Sci Sports Exerc 2006;38(4):637–43.
9. Zafonte B, Rendulic D, Szabo RM. Flexor pulley system: anatomy, injury, and management. J Hand Surg Am 2014;39(12):2525–32 [quiz: 2533].
10. Doyle J. Anatomy of the flexor tendon sheath and pulley system: a current review. J Hand Surg Am 1989;14(2):349–51.
11. Doyle J. Anatomy of the finger flexor tendon sheath and pulley system. J Hand Surg Am 1988;13(4):473–84.
12. Peterson W, Manske PR, Bollinger BA, et al. Effect of pulley excision on flexor tendon biomechanics. J Orthop Res 1986;4(1):96–101.
13. Schoffl I, Oppelt K, Jüngert J, et al. The influence of the crimp and slope grip position on the finger pulley system. J Biomech 2009;42(13):2183–7.
14. Schweizer A. Biomechanical properties of the crimp grip position in rock climbers. J Biomech 2001;34:217–23.
15. Bollen S. Injury to the A2 pulley in rock climbers. J Hand Surg Br 1990;15:268–70.
16. Lin G, Amadio PC, An KN, et al. Biomechanical analysis of finger flexor pulley reconstruction. J Hand Surg Br 1989;14(3):278–82.
17. Marco R, Sharkey NA, Smith TS, et al. Pathomechanics of closed rupture of the flexor tendon pulleys in rock climbers. J Bone Joint Surg 1998;80(7):1012–9.
18. Tang JB, Xie RG. Effect of A3 pulley and adjacent sheath integrity on tendon excursion and bowstringing. J Hand Surg Am 2001;26(5):855–61.
19. Rispler D, Greenwald D, Shumway S, et al. Efficiency of the flexor tendon pulley system in human cadaver hands. J Hand Surg 1996;21A(3):444–50.
20. Schöffl V, Popp D, Küpper T, et al. Injury trends in rock climbers: evaluation of a case series of 911 injuries between 2009 and 2012. Wilderness Environ Med 2015;26(1):62–7.
21. Bowers W, Kuzma G, Bynum D. Closed traumatic rupture of finger flexor pulleys. J Hand Surg 1994;19A(5):782–7.
22. Quaine F, Vigouroux L, Martin L. Effect of simulated rock climbing finger postures on force sharing among the fingers. Clin Biomech 2003;18(5):385–8.
23. Gabl M, Rangger C, Lutz M, et al. Disruption of the finger flexor pulley system in elite rock climbers. Am J Sports Med 1998;26(5):651–5.
24. Chang CY, Torriani M, Huang AJ. Rock climbing injuries: acute and chronic repetitive trauma. Curr Probl Diagn Radiol 2015;45:205–14.
25. El-Sheikh Y, Wong I, Farrokhyar F, et al. Diagnosis of finger flexor pulley injury in rock climbers: a systematic review. Can J Plast Surg 2006;14(4):227–31.
26. Hauger O, Chung CB, Lektrakul N, et al. Pulley system in the fingers: normal anatomy and simulated lesions in cadavers at MR imaging, CT, and US with and without contrast material distention of the tendon sheath. Radiology 2000;217(1):201–12.
27. Kubiak E, Klugman J, Bosco J. Hand injuries in rock climbers. Bull NYU Hosp Jt Dis 2006;64(3–4):172–7.
28. Schoffl I, Einwag F, Strecker W, et al. Impact of taping after finger flexor tendon pulley ruptures in rock climbers. J Appl Biomech 2007;23(1):52–62.
29. Warme W, Brooks D. The effect of circumferential taping on flexor tendon pulley failure in rock climbers. Am J Sports Med 2000;28(5):674–8.
30. Schneeberger M, Schweizer A. Pulley ruptures in rock climbers: outcome of conservative treatment with the pulley-protection splint-a series of 47 cases. Wilderness Environ Med 2016;27:211–8.

31. Moutet F, Forli A, Vouilliaume D. Pulley rupture and reconstruction in rock climbers. Tech Hand Upper Extrem Surg 2004;8(3):149–55.

32. Voulliaume D, Forli A, Parzy O, et al. Réparation des ruptures de poulie chez le grimpeur. Chirurgie de la Main 2004;23(5):243–8.

33. Mehta V, Phillips CS. Flexor tendon pulley reconstruction. Hand Clin 2005;21(2):245–51.

34. Okutsu I, Ninomiya S, Hiraki S, et al. Three-loop technique for A2 pulley reconstruction. J Hand Surg Am 1987;12(5 Pt 1):790–4.

35. Clark TA, Skeete K, Amadio PC. Flexor tendon pulley reconstruction. J Hand Surg Am 2010;35(10):1685–9.

36. Lister G. Reconstruction of pulleys employing extensor retinaculum. J Hand Surg Am 1979;4(5):461–4.

37. Widstrom C, Doyle JR, Johnson G, et al. A mechanical study of six digital pulley reconstruction techniques: part II. Strength of individual reconstructions. J Hand Surg Am 1989;14(5):826–9.

38. Karev A. The "belt loop" technique for the reconstruction of pulleys in the first stage of flexor tendon grafting. J Hand Surg Am 1984;9(6):923–4.

39. Arora R, Fritz D, Zimmermann R, et al. Reconstruction of the digital flexor pulley system: a retrospective comparison of two methods of treatment. J Hand Surg Eur Vol 2007;32(1):60–6.

40. Bouyer M, Forli A, Semere A, et al. Recovery of rock climbing performance after surgical reconstruction of finger pulleys. J Hand Surg Eur Vol 2016;41(4):406–12.

Finger Injuries in Football and Rugby

Kate E. Elzinga, MD, FRCSC[a], Kevin C. Chung, MD, MS[b],*

KEYWORDS

- Rugby finger injuries • Football finger injuries • Jersey finger • Mallet finger • Return to play

KEY POINTS

- Football and rugby athletes are at increased risk of finger injuries owing to the full-contact nature of these sports.
- The timing of return to play is critically important for football and rugby athletes. The physical, emotional, and financial implications of time away from the field must be weighed against the risk of reinjury and the effects on long-term outcomes with an early return.
- Football players are permitted to wear playing casts. For nonskilled players, such as linemen who do not handle the ball, this can facilitate an early return to play. Skilled players, such as wide receivers, typically miss more games while recovering from a finger injury.
- Rugby players are not permitted to wear playing casts for the safety of their teammates and their opponents. Only taping can be used. This often leads to a delayed return to sport following a finger injury.

INTRODUCTION

In the United States, football is the most played sport and rugby is the fastest growing sport.[1] Football and rugby athletes are at increased risk of upper extremity injury because of the full-contact nature of these sports. A recent prospective cohort study found that collegiate rugby players sustained wrist and hand injuries 9.6 times more often than collegiate football players.[1] Hand injuries in rugby players occur most commonly during the tackle, the maul, and when handling the ball.[2] In football, injuries occur most commonly during tackling and in games rather than in practice.[3] Hand and finger injuries represent 12% of all football injuries.[4]

For the safety of a player's teammates and opponents, the only protective equipment that can be used in rugby is taping. Plastics and metals are prohibited. In football, padded playing splints and casts can be worn, facilitating an earlier return to play as the injured player's position permits.

For high school athletes, fracture rates are highest in football compared with other sports (4.37 per 10,000 athlete exposures; ie, 1 athlete participating in 1 practice or game).[5] Football players are the most likely to return to play immediately compared with other sports, in part because playing casts are permitted.[6] Fractures occur most commonly in the hand and fingers in football (36%).[5] Injuries result most commonly from contact with another player (63% of

Disclosure Statement: Research reported in this publication was supported by a Midcareer Investigator Award in Patient-Oriented Research (2K24 AR053120-06) to Dr K.C. Chung. The content is solely the responsibility of the authors and does not necessarily represent the official views of the National Institutes of Health. The authors do not have a conflict of interest to disclose.
a Section of Plastic Surgery, Division of Plastic Surgery, The University of Michigan Health System, University of Michigan, 1500 East Medical Center Drive, 2110 Taubman Center, SPC 5346, Ann Arbor, MI 48109-5346, USA;
b Section of Plastic Surgery, The University of Michigan Medical School, The University of Michigan Health System, 1500 East Medical Center Drive, 2130 Taubman Center, SPC 5340, Ann Arbor, MI 48109-0340, USA
* Corresponding author.
E-mail address: kecchung@med.umich.edu

Hand Clin 33 (2017) 149–160
http://dx.doi.org/10.1016/j.hcl.2016.08.007
0749-0712/17/© 2016 Elsevier Inc. All rights reserved.

fractures).[6] Fractures are most commonly sustained during running plays while being tackled (27%), tackling (22%), or blocking (14%).[6]

A study by Goldfarb and colleagues[3] of hand, thumb, and finger injuries in National Football League (NFL) players over a 10-year period found that 48% of injuries involved the fingers, 30% involved the thumb, and 22% involved the hand. Hand injuries were most common in lineman, whereas wide receivers and defensive secondary players (safeties and cornerbacks) sustained the most finger injuries.[3] The fewest injuries were seen in tight ends for hand, thumb, and finger injuries, followed by quarterbacks.[3] Metacarpal fractures (80% of hand injuries) and proximal interphalangeal (PIP) joint dislocations were the most common injuries.[3] The most days missed from play resulted from hand bursitis (41 days), PIP subluxations (41 days), thumb sprains (35 days), tendon lacerations (30 days), and Bennett fractures (30 days).[3]

For physicians caring for athletes, the most challenging treatment decision is when to permit the athlete to return to play. The risks and benefits should be discussed with the player and his or her family, coach, athletic therapist, trainer, and agent. The risks of reinjury and long-term morbidity with early return to play must be weighed against the professional and financial consequences incurred if return to play is delayed. Factors to consider are the player's hand dominance, stage of career, future playing career, position, and ability to play with a protective splint. The amount of time left in the season, the level of play, and the timing of contract negotiations are also important factors. A young player's potential college and professional careers must be considered because the injury could greatly affect his or her livelihood. A study surveying 37 consultant hand surgeons for teams in the NFL, National Basketball Association, and Major League Baseball demonstrated considerable variability for the initial management and return to protected and unprotected play for professional athletes, highlighting the need for individualized management for each injured athlete.[7]

In football, injuries to the dominant hand are most limiting for quarterbacks and centers.[8] Skilled position players tend to have a delayed return to play compared with nonskilled position players. Skilled players include quarterbacks, running backs, wide receivers, and tight ends. Nonskilled players include offensive and defensive linemen and linebackers who do not require ball-handling skills.

Athletes tend to recover more quickly and more completely than the general population. Their superior baseline health, absence of comorbidities,

motivation, and access to physicians and therapists improve their outcomes. Twice daily hand therapy with skilled hand or athletic therapists helps accelerate recovery compared with the general public.

A thorough history and physical examination is important for every injured athlete. Although rare, it is important not to miss a second injury that may be masked by the first due to pain, swelling, or a physical examination that is overly focused. For example, Bhargava and Jennings[9] describe a ulnar collateral ligament (UCL) tear that occurred simultaneously with a carpometacarpal dislocation of the thumb in a football player. The consequences of continued play with a missed injury can have serious long-term effects on rugby and football players. Comparison with the contralateral uninjured hand is particularly important for assessment of ligamentous laxity and tears, as well as rotational deformity of the digits secondary to fractures. Digit or wrist block anesthesia can facilitate a throughout examination.[10]

SOFT TISSUE INJURIES
Mallet Finger

The most common closed tendon injury in athletes is a mallet injury of the finger.[11] Forced flexion during active extension of the distal interphalangeal (DIP) joint or direct strikes of the football or rugby ball to the tip of the finger can result in this injury. The extensor tendon is torn at its insertion on the dorsal base of the distal phalanx. In rugby, back row forwards, full backs, and wingers most frequently sustain a mallet finger injury.[2]

An untreated mallet finger can progress to a swan-neck deformity of the finger with hyperextension of the PIP joint due to tendon imbalances. Early recognition and treatment are important for optimal recovery of DIP joint extension and finger strength.

Isolated tendinous injuries can be treated with extension splinting of the DIP joint or with buried, percutaneously placed Kirschner wires (K-wires) for 6 weeks (**Fig. 1**). The effectiveness of splinting can be confirmed with high-resolution ultrasound (US) but this technology is seldom needed.[12] To be successful, the extension splint must permit the ruptured end of the extensor tendon to be in contact with the bone for secondary healing. If there is a gap between the bone insertion and the terminal tendon despite DIP joint extension, open surgical repair is necessary.[13]

When there is an associated fracture, treatment may require splinting, K-wires, or open reduction and internal fixation, depending on the fracture

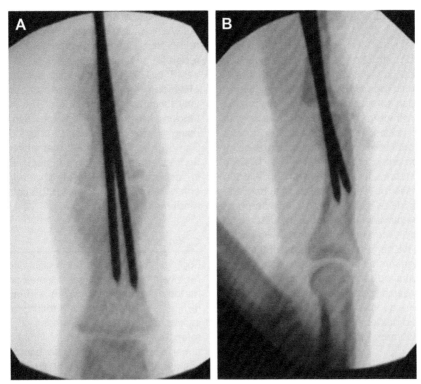

Fig. 1. (*A*) Posteroanterior and (*B*) lateral radiographs showing 2 buried, percutaneously placed K-wires used to treat a mallet finger. The DIP joint is held in extension for 6 weeks. If the player returns to play with the K-wires in place, a DIP extension splint is recommended for additional protection.

pattern and the degree of articular surface involvement. Restoration and maintenance of a concentric DIP joint is important for range of motion, prevention of a painful joint, and mitigating the risk of post-traumatic arthritis.

K-wires are preferred to lessen the risk of splint dislodgement during sport, which would require the period of immobilization to be restarted. Burying the K-wires lessens the risk of pin site infection, osteomyelitis, pin migration, and skin breakdown. Two K-wires should be used to prevent rotation of the distal phalanx relative to the middle phalanx and to increase stability of the DIP joint.

Typically, the athlete can continue training and game play with the appropriate splint or fixation with K-wires. If tolerated by the athlete's position requirements, a splint is worn for play with K-wires in place for further protection. The skin is monitored for maceration and breakdown daily. However, some think that athletes should wait 6 weeks for K-wire removal before return to play, given the risk of pin breakage, migration, and infection.[14] After 6 weeks, the K-wires are removed. All athletes, whether treated nonsurgically or surgically, are advised to continue splinting for an additional 6 weeks at night and during sports.[15]

Jersey Finger

Rupture of the flexor digitorum profundus (FDP) occurs more commonly during contact sports than during noncontact sports.[11] The FDP is avulsed from its insertion on the volar base of the distal phalanx and retracts a variable distance depending on the presence of an avulsion fracture and the integrity of the vincula system. This is known as a jersey or rugger finger. Closed FDP ruptures are uncommon in young healthy athletes.[16] Football and rugby players are at risk of this injury when the DIP joint is forced into extension while actively flexed. This occurs most commonly while pulling on a loose jersey. Jersey finger can affect all fingers but injuries to the ring finger account for 75% of cases.[15]

FDP injuries require surgery to restore active flexion of the DIP joint. They cannot be adequately treated with splinting alone. Controlled, guided physiotherapy is required postoperatively for 3 to 6 months to maximize range of motion and strength outcomes. A dorsal blocking splint is worn for 6 weeks after surgical repair. Strengthening exercises begin 8 weeks postoperatively if full range of motion is present. For athletes who require the full use of their affected hand for their position, return to play may take 4 to 6 months.[15]

The timing of surgical repair varies based on the level of tendon retraction and the presence of a fracture. Based on the Leddy and Packer classification and Smith modification, type I (retraction of the FDP tendon to the palm) and IV (associated volar avulsion fracture of the distal phalanx with simultaneous avulsion of the FDP from the fracture fragment, retraction of the FDP tendon to the palm) injuries require early surgical repair within 10 days of the injury to prevent tendon retraction.[17] If the athlete chooses not to be treated during the season, his or her overall outcome will be compromised and the player must be properly counseled on the options. A tenodesis or arthrodesis of the DIP joint can be performed at the end of the season. Or 2-stage tendon reconstruction can be performed in a delayed fashion; however, the athlete must be counseled that this technique requires 2 surgeries and extensive physiotherapy both preoperatively and postoperatively to maximize range of motion outcomes. Full return of range of motion is unusual.

Early surgical repair can be done using a variety of techniques, including a transverse intraosseous suture, Z-lengthening of the retracted tendon stump, or a pull-though suture over button repair (**Fig. 2**).[18] Bone anchor techniques or lag screw fixation are also commonly used.[19]

With a type II (retraction of the FDP tendon to the PIP joint) or III (associated volar avulsion fracture of the distal phalanx that limits retraction of the FDP tendon to the DIP joint) jersey finger, repair can generally be delayed 6 weeks if the tendon gap is less than 1 cm.[20] However, there have been reports of marked tendon retraction following a type II injury that have required tendon lengthening to facilitate repair.[21] Athletes must be

counseled that there may be additional risk with delayed repair compared with early surgical treatment. Some authors recommend timely surgical repair for all types of jersey finger.[15]

MRI or US of a tendon can quantify the amount of tendon retraction to guide treatment, particularly for type II jersey fingers. The integrity of the tendon sheath and pulleys can also be assessed using these noninvasive imaging modalities. Some investigators think that physical examination is inaccurate and that imaging is more helpful in determining the level of tendon retraction compared with palpating for the point of maximal tenderness.[18]

Collateral Ligament Tears

Football, rugby, and other tackling sports result in repetitive radial and ulnar directed stresses to the metacarpophalangeal (MCP) and interphalangeal (IP) joints of the hand. As a result, radial and UCL injuries are common. Coaches and athletes often refer to a collateral ligament injury as a jammed finger. Centers, wingers, and back row forwards sustain the most collateral ligament injuries in rugby.[2]

On lateral stress testing, incomplete collateral ligament tears maintain a firm endpoint and have less than 20° of joint opening compared with the contralateral uninjured finger. These injuries can be treated with buddy taping to the adjacent finger. Alternatively, the injured digit alone may be taped to permit for flexion and extension while maximizing radial and ulnar support (**Fig. 3**).[22] Early hand therapy is important to minimize adhesions and to maximize range of motion.[22]

Complete tears lack a firm endpoint and demonstrate more than 20° of joint opening on lateral

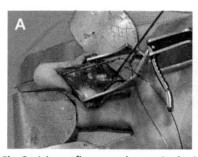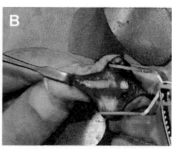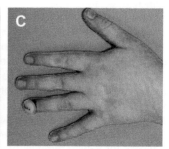

Fig. 2. A jersey finger can be repaired using a pull-through suture button technique. (*A*) The distally avulsed FDP tendon is reattached to its insertion on the volar base of the distal phalanx using a nonabsorbable suture. Two Keith needles are drilled through the distal phalanx obliquely to pass the suture tails from the volar distal phalanx base to the dorsal distal phalanx, through the nail distal to the germinal matrix. (*B*) The pulleys are maintained. (*C*) The suture is tied over a button dorsally and remains in place for 6 weeks following repair of a jersey finger. Early hand therapy, with the button in place, is critical to allow tendon gilding to optimize the range of motion of the injured finger.

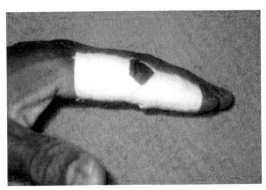

Fig. 3. Individual finger taping can be used to allow early return to play for collateral ligament injuries. (*From* Singletary S, Geissler WB. Bracing and rehabilitation for wrist and hand injuries in collegiate athletes. Hand Clin 2009;25(3):447; with permission.)

stress testing. These injuries can be treated closed with buddy taping or open using suture anchors.[23] Following suture anchor repair, active motion can be started 2 weeks postoperatively and return to play is permitted 6 weeks postoperatively.[24]

Ulnar collateral ligament injuries of the thumb metacarpophalangeal joint

Thumb UCL injuries occur in rugby and football from falls on an outstretched hand or with forced abduction of the thumb MCP joint. These injuries can lead to joint instability, an abduction deformity of the MCP, chronic pain, decreased pinch strength, joint incongruity, and post-traumatic arthritis. When a compete tear is present, stress testing of the thumb MCP joint with a distal radially directed force reveals more than 30° of joint space opening, more than 15° of increased UCL laxity compared with the contralateral, uninjured thumb; and the loss of a firm endpoint. Stress radiographs, US, or MRI can help establish the diagnosis when the clinical findings are equivocal.

Partial UCL tears of the thumb MCP joint are treated with joint immobilization. A thumb spica splint or cast is worn to prevent further damage, particularly with repeated abduction forces to the thumb. A partial tear with no ligamentous laxity can be splinted until pain and tenderness resolve.[15] Pain can persist for months, often noted with gripping activities; prolonged immobilization may be required with splinting or taping techniques.[25] Partial tears with ligamentous laxity on abduction stress testing require splinting for 4 to 6 weeks.[15]

Football players who are able to play with a cast may do so early. They must be aware of the risk of progression to a complete tear with a repeat injury that could lead to the need for surgery, MCP joint

instability, and post-traumatic arthritis.[25] Skilled players with dominant hand injuries may require 12 weeks away from play until the ligament is healed and the MCP joint is stable.

Complete UCL tears typically mandate surgical repair. In uncertain cases, US or MRI can be used to look for a Stener lesion, confirming the need for surgical intervention. Some investigators think that casting alone for 6 weeks may lead to favorable outcomes, eliminating the need for surgical intervention.[15] However, if the MCP joint remains unstable after 6 weeks of immobilization, surgery is required. Depending when the injury occurs, ball handling players may prefer early acute surgical repair to avoid the possibility of surgery later in the season. The opposite may apply to nonskilled players who are able to complete their season in a playing cast and can consider surgery in the off-season if joint instability persists.

If surgery is performed, the player can consider return to play with a protective cast 2 weeks postoperatively once the soft tissues are healed.[25] The MCP joint is immobilized for 6 to 8 weeks. Abduction and adduction stresses are avoided. Strengthening exercises are started 6 weeks postoperatively. Once the player is back playing, protective taping can be used for the rest of the season.[25]

Common surgical options include direct ligament repair with a nonabsorbable suture for intraligamentous ruptures and suture anchors when the ligament is avulsed from its insertion on the base of the proximal phalanx (**Fig. 4**). Pull-out buttons can also be used to reinsert the ligament into bone. Cadaveric studies suggest that pull-out buttons have greater resistance to force compared with suture anchor techniques.[26] Chhabra and colleagues[27] reported quick return to play and

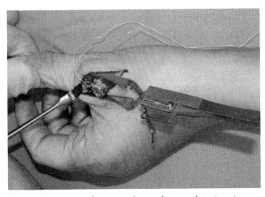

Fig. 4. Suture anchor repair can be used to treat complete tears of the thumb MCP UCL. The ligament is more commonly avulsed from its distal insertion on the base of the proximal phalanx than from its origin on the metacarpal head.

excellent long-term results in their study of 18 college football players following UCL repair with a suture anchor. The average time to surgery was 12 days for skilled players and 43 days for non-skilled players.[27] Skilled players returned to play 7 weeks postoperatively, whereas nonskilled players returned 4 weeks after surgery. All athletes returned to the same level of play and there was no difference in clinical outcomes between the skilled and nonskilled player groups over a 2-year follow-up period.[27] Of consultant hand surgeons surveyed by Carlson and colleagues,[7] 64% recommended waiting 12 weeks before return to unprotected play for NFL players.

Finger interphalangeal joint dislocations

IP joint dislocations are common in contact sports. PIP joint dislocations are the most common finger injury sustained by football players.[3] The ulnar 2 digits are injured in 66% of cases.[3] Preventive taping or bracing can be considered for the PIP joints of the ring and small fingers of wide receivers, safeties, cornerbacks, and linemen who are most prone to injury.[3] Taping techniques can also be used to help prevent IP joint dislocations of the thumb.[22]

Many IP joint dislocations are treated with closed reduction on the field. It is important for the player to be evaluated as soon as possible following the injury. If the player remains in the game, he or she should be evaluated at half time or immediately after the game. Radiographs are performed to ensure the joint is congruent and to assess for associated fractures. The volar plate, ulnar and radial collateral ligaments, and extensor tendon (central slip for PIP dislocations, terminal tendon for DIP dislocations) are examined. The range of motion of the reduced joint is tested actively and passively, and joint stability is assessed.

Stable IP joints may be immobilized for 2 to 3 days for comfort then range-of-motion exercises are begun.[15] Others investigators think that athletes may return immediately to play if the joint is stable following reduction.[7] Buddy taping or protective splinting, as permitted by league rules, is used to protect the digit when the athlete returns to play. Buddy taping decreases the incidence of recurrent hyperextension and lateral displacement.[28] Zinc oxide, self-adhesive tape, and commercially available straps can be used for buddy taping.[29]

Bowers[30] reported that virtually all pure hyperextension injuries of the PIP joint result in rupture of the distal insertion of the volar plate from the base of the middle phalanx. These injuries can be treated with buddy taping. PIP joint

fracture-dislocations occur based on the angle of the PIP joint at the time of injury. Axial stress on the middle phalanx can result in volar, dorsal, or a combination of fractures, depending on the angle of the PIP joint.[31]

Stable dorsal fracture-dislocations of the IP joints are treated with dorsal blocking splinting and early range-of-motion exercises. The joint is flexed and blocked at the angle in which joint stability and congruency are maintained. The splint prevents further extension beyond this angle and reduces the chance of repeat dislocation or subluxation. Often, 20° to 30° of flexion is used for 3 weeks and the angle is decreased by 10° every week thereafter. Joint stability must be assured at all times with repeat clinical examination and radiograph imaging. Protective static splinting can enable early return to play for football athletes; dorsal block splinting is used when not playing.

Unstable dislocations and fracture-dislocations require operative intervention. Instability often results from PIP fracture-dislocations involving more than 40% of the volar base of the middle phalanx. Dynamic traction, open reduction, and fixation with K-wires or screws; hemihamate or volar plate arthroplasty; or cerclage and tension band wiring techniques can be used to treat these injuries. Players should be counseled about the increased severity of these injuries compared with purely ligamentous PIP injuries and the increased likelihood of residual stiffness, decreased flexion, and post-traumatic arthritis.

Boutonniere Deformity

Volar PIP joint dislocations are far less common than dorsal dislocations. Following closed reduction, the integrity of the central slip must be assessed. If closed reduction fails, open reduction is required. Following either a volar PIP joint dislocation or an isolated central slip injury, the player is examined using an Elson test to evaluate the integrity of the central slip. The player's PIP joint is flexed over the end of an examination table with the palm and proximal phalanx on the table. The player is asked to extend his or her middle phalanx joint against resistance. If the central slip is injured, PIP extension is absent or weak; instead, DIP extension occurs as the extension force is transmitted through the lateral bands to the distal phalanx. If the athlete is unable to maintain extension of his or her PIP joint, he or she should be treated as an acute Boutonniere injury with 6 weeks of full-time extension splinting of the PIP joint with the DIP joint free.[23,32] An additional 6 weeks of night-time splinting is often recommended, particularly if a mild, residual PIP hypertension deformity persists. Range of motion of the DIP joint is encouraged to maintain the dorsal location of the lateral bands.

Football players can return to sport if they are able to play their position while wearing a splint. Buddy taping is also performed to further protect the injured digit.[14] Players requiring the use of their digit for their position are unable to return to play for a minimum of 6 weeks until the tendon has healed.

If a skilled football player or rugby player is unable to take time off from the sport, secondary Boutonniere reconstruction can be performed after the season. Often an extensor tenotomy is required to correct the PIP hyperextension deformity.[14]

An open central slip injury requires open tendon repair. If there is an associated fracture requiring fixation, K-wires or screws can be used. If K-wires are used, these players may be unable return to play until the K-wires are removed in 6 weeks unless they can be adequately protected in a playing cast. If stable screw fixation is achieved, players can often return to play in 2 weeks with a playing cast once the skin and soft tissues are healed.

BONE INJURIES
Fractures

Hand fractures account for up to a third of all fractures sustained by athletes.[33] Most are low energy and result in minimally displaced, extra-articular fractures with limited soft tissue injury.[34] Football has the highest rate of hand fractures, accounting for 50% of all hand fractures sustained playing sport.[22] In rugby, the centers, back row forwards, and scrum halves sustain hand fractures most frequently.[2] Anatomic, stable fracture restoration and early range of motion are critical to maximizing outcomes following a fracture.[34,35] Percutaneous techniques can reduce soft tissue dissection, edema, and fibrosis while ensuring stable fracture fixation and limiting fragment devascularization.[35]

Nondisplaced, stable fractures of the hand can be treated with a playing cast for 4 to 6 weeks.[36] Displaced fractures are treated with closed reduction to convert an unstable fracture to a stable pattern. Displaced fractures that are stable following closed reduction can be treated nonoperatively.[37] If a displaced fracture cannot be converted to a stable fracture, operative intervention is indicated. Unstable fractures are treated surgically and then protected with a cast. Range-of-motion exercises with protective splinting are started 7 to 10 days postoperatively.[36]

Timing of return to play depends on the position of the player. Because playing casts are permitted in football but not in rugby, earlier return is possible for football athletes. Return to play in football with a playing cast occurs at 1 to 2 weeks for a lineman, linebacker, or kicker with a nonsurgical fracture. If open reduction internal fixation is performed, 2 to 4 weeks away from contact play may be required for these positions, depending on the fixation stability. Once the soft tissues are healed, play may be resumed in a protective playing cast. Six to 10 weeks may be required for a running back, receiver, or quarterback in football and for all rugby players before return to contact practices and games. These players can return to play once normal (85% of contralateral) strength has been reestablished in the injured hand and splinting has been weaned.[36] Fractures in the throwing hand and in those requiring a strong power grip for tackling typically have the most delayed return to play.

Metacarpal fractures

An axial force (eg, a fall on a clenched fist), a direct blow to the hand (from another player or the ball), a fall, getting the hand twisted in a jersey, and being stepped on are mechanisms that result in metacarpal fractures in football or rugby.[38] Fractures occur most commonly in the mid-diaphysis of the metacarpal; the long finger is most commonly injured.[38] In athletes, 80% of metacarpal fractures are minimally or nondisplaced, 5% remain stable after reduction and can be maintained with functional bracing, and the remaining 15% require surgical treatment.[39]

Of consultant hand surgeons, 38% let professional football, baseball, and basketball players return to protected play with a nondisplaced metacarpal fracture immediately; 57% waited 3 to 4 weeks after injury[7]; and 73% permitted unprotected play 4 to 8 weeks after injury.[7] For collegiate and high school football athletes, protective splints were used for an average of 21 days.[38] Glove casts can be used to immobilize a stable metacarpal fracture, permitting continued range of motion and use of the wrist.[10]

Surgical intervention is recommended for metacarpal shaft fractures with more than 5 mm of shortening and more than 30° of dorsal angulation, displacement, or rotational malignment.[10] Articular incongruency is another indication for operative fixation. Minimal rotation deformity is accepted in athletes who require their hands to grasp and throw to maintain maximal grip strength.[40] If surgical intervention is required to restore alignment or stability following a fracture, techniques that provide the greatest strength with the least amount of tissue dissection are preferred.[37,39]

If surgical intervention is needed, plate fixation or lag screws are often used. Geissler and McCraney recommend using a 2.0 mm cage plate and subsequent return to protected play in 2 weeks.[41] Fufa and Goldfarb[40] also recommend time for wound healing and suture removal with return to play at 2 weeks followed by 6 weeks of protective play. Other experts report return to play in less than 10 days following surgery for a metacarpal fracture for high school athletes and in less than 3 days for college football players with no additional incidence of postoperative hardware failure or wound complications.[38]

Unstable metacarpal fracture patterns, such as undisplaced intra-articular head and base fractures, are often treated prophylactically with internal fixation in athletes to prevent later displacement.[42] Plate and screw fixation are preferred, facilitating return to play in 14 days compared with 36 days with K-wires.[43] Lag screws provide excellent fixation for long spiral metacarpal fractures. Geissler recommends considering the use of plate fixation for border digit metacarpal fractures in contact athletes.[35]

Phalangeal fractures

Phalangeal fractures are the most common fracture of the hand in athletes, as well as the general population.[37] The metacarpals are more protected and less prone to injury. In the hand, the distal phalanx is the least well protected. Consequently, distal phalanx fractures constitute almost half of all hand fractures.[44]

Some hand surgeons authorize players with stable phalangeal fractures in good anatomic position to participate in sports immediately after injury in a protective cast. Others prefer to wait until there is evidence of radiographic healing around 3 weeks after injury.[42] Unstable fractures include those with displaced articular fragments, rotational deformity, more than 15° of angulation, and more than 6 mm of shortening.[37] For these unstable fractures, play can be resumed in 1 to 2 weeks after surgery with a playing cast; 6 to 8 weeks is required before unprotected play.[8]

Open reduction with internal fixation with plates is most commonly used for unstable phalangeal shaft fractures.[37] Rigid fixation permits immediate range-of-motion exercises and earlier return to play.[37] A dorsal or midaxial surgical approach is used. Plates are placed on the dorsal or lateral surface of the phalanx. Lateral placement is preferred by Geissler[35] to decrease extensor tendon adhesions. Alternatively, percutaneous techniques can be used. Geissler[45] described the use of headless cannulated mini screws for intraarticular unicondylar and bicondylar fractures.

Stable proximal and middle phalanx fractures are treated with buddy taping and protective splinting for 4 to 6 weeks.[37] Unstable proximal and middle phalangeal shaft fractures are stabilized with K-wires, screws, or plates.[37] Plates and screws are preferred over K-wires in athletes to increase biomechanical strength, minimize soft tissue irritation, minimize the incidence of pin site infection, minimize the risk of hardware breakage or migration, and to facilitate earlier range of motion.

Long oblique fractures, with a fracture length more than twice the diameter of the bone shaft, can be fixed percutaneously or open with 3 lag screws to achieve the same biomechanical torsion strength as plate fixation.[37] Intraarticular unicondylar fractures are most commonly treated operatively in athletes owing to their high propensity for displacement.[42] Even if these fractures appear undisplaced initially, there is a tendency for later loss of reduction due to the unstable nature of this fracture pattern. Percutaneously placed headless compression screws are often used (**Fig. 5**).[35,37] Bicondylar fractures may require a plate in addition to lag screws across the condyles for adequate stability.[37] Unstable intraarticular phalangeal base fractures are treated with screws via a percutaneous or open approach.[37] If screw placement is not possible, K-wires can be used.

Stable distal phalanx fractures are treated with protective splinting for 2 to 3 weeks with the PIP joint free.[37] Unstable fractures are treated with K-wires or single screw fixation.[37]

Proximal interphalangeal joint fractures

Outcomes after a PIP joint fracture tend to be better with primary intervention rather than delayed reconstruction.[28] Stable dorsal fractures (eg, a reducible volar lip fracture-dislocation) can be treated with buddy taping and early return to play.[28] Splints can be worn outside of sports. Close follow-up and range-of-motion exercises are required to aid in the return of full motion. Stable lateral fracture-dislocations, both ulnar and radial, can be treated with buddy taping and protective splinting if the avulsion fracture is displaced less than 2 mm.[37]

Unstable dorsal fracture-dislocations with a tendency toward recurrent dorsal subluxation require dorsal block splinting to maintain joint congruency while permitting early range of motion to prevent joint stiffness and permanent limitations in range of motion. PIP joint flexion is maintained at all times; dorsal block splinting is used when the player is not playing and protective casting is used when participating in practices and games.

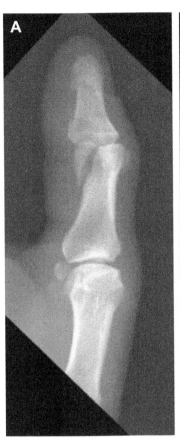
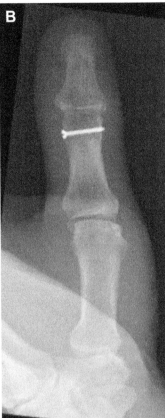

Fig. 5. A percutaneously placed screw can be used for fixation of unicondylar phalangeal fractures. This minimally invasive technique minimizes tissue trauma and is preferred for athletes. (*A*) Preoperative and (*B*) postoperative radiographs are shown for an ulnar unicondylar fracture of the proximal phalanx of a thumb.

Close observation with repeat clinical examinations and radiographs is required, predominantly during the first 3 weeks after injury.[28]

Unstable volar fracture-dislocations with dorsal lip fractures are typically treated with extension splinting. If football players' positions permit, they may return to play early in a protective cast. For a rugby player or skilled football player, return to play is delayed. Alternatively, the fracture can be treated surgically. Nonomura and colleagues[46] reported good results with open reduction and internal fixation of a bony central slip dorsal middle phalanx fracture using a mini hook plate.

Unstable volar fractures (eg, a volar lip fracture involving more than 50% of the articular surface) should be treated acutely to optimize the player's long-term result.[28] An open shotgun approach to the PIP joint enables placement of screws if the fracture fragment is of adequate size.[37] Return to play following surgical intervention can occur 1 week postoperatively for football players able to play in a cast and 4 to 6 weeks postoperatively for players requiring their hands to tackle. For the latter, buddy taping and thermoplastic splint reinforcement are advised when play is resumed.[28]

HAND THERAPY

In general, hand therapy is started 2 to 3 days after injury with range-of-motion exercises. Noninvolved joints of the hands should be mobilized immediately. Early range-of-motion exercises are important in achieving optimal outcomes.[34]

Edema control is imperative for all finger injuries. Elevation, compression gloves, sleeves, taping, retrograde massage, antiinflammatory medications, and icing can be used. Fingers should be monitored daily and therapy exercises should be adjusted if causing worsening edema. Controlled, noncontact athletic training can be resumed with the hand properly protected once the initial injury edema has subsided.[8]

Protective Equipment

In rugby, no plastic and metal can be worn, even if covered by padding or tape. Only soft braces or neoprene sleeves are permitted. Full-finger gloves are not permitted, only rugby-specific unpadded gloves with open fingers can be worn.[47] Gloves can be used in football at all levels, including compression gloves for edema management.

Taping is permitted in both rugby and football and can be used to prevent injuries or to stabilize digits after injury when play is resumed.[48]

In football, playing casts are permitted to facilitate early return to game play (**Fig. 6**).[35] Playing casts must be padded to protect the player, his or her teammates, and his or her opponents. High-density, slow-recovery, closed-cell polyurethane foam is commonly used. Padded gloves, a bivalved padded cast, a padded club cast, and a padded splint may also be worn.[38] Skilled position players often use padded gloves when they return to protected play. Nonskilled position players can return sooner with greater protective offered by padded casts.

High school athletes have been able to wear playing casts since 1994.[49] The National Federation of State High School Associations states in 1.5.3b1:

ILLEGAL: Hard substance in its final form such as leather, rubber, plastic, plaster or fiberglass when worn on the hand, wrist, forearm or elbow unless covered on all exterior surfaces with no less than 1/2 inch thick, high-density, closed-cell polyurethane, or an alternate material of the same minimum thickness, and with similar physical properties to protect an injury.[50]

For football, National Collegiate Athletic Association athletes must also wear 0.5 inch closed-cell polyurethane padding. For NFL athletes, 0.25 inch padding is required.[22] Protective splinting for fractures should include the joint above and below the fracture site.[37]

To prevent injuries, shorts with pockets should not be worn while playing rugby.[19] When pockets are worn, catching a finger in the pocket of an opponent's shorts is the most common mechanism of jersey finger injuries.[51]

Off the field, continuous splitting can be stopped 4 to 6 weeks after injury if the player demonstrates radiographic evidence of fracture healing and the fracture site is no longer tender with palpation or with use.[39]

RETURN TO PLAY

Early return to controlled conditioning exercises is safe for most athletes. Stationary bikes, incline treadmill walking, trunk and abdominal exercises, and lower body strengthening can be performed.

In general, return to contact drills and games after an open surgical procedure should be no sooner than 1 to 2 weeks postoperatively for skin and soft tissue healing and suture removal.[14,52] In a study by Kodama and colleagues,[52] 2 rugby players were not compliant with their postoperative instructions and suffered a wound dehiscence when they returned to play the day after their open reduction and internal fixation of their hand fractures.

Players are most prone to injury during tackling, blocking, and other contact.[3] The act of tackling or

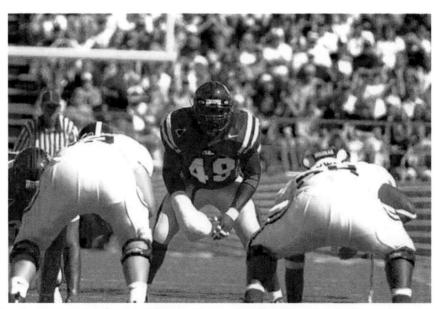

Fig. 6. A closed-cell polyurethane padded club cast can be worn to protect a hand injury during football practices and games. (*From* Geissler WB. Operative fixation of metacarpal and phalangeal fractures in athletes. Hand Clin 2009;25(3):417; with permission.)

blocking results in more injuries than being tackled or blocked.[3] Protective splinting is very important when these activities are resumed. Return to unprotected play can be permitted when the player no longer has pain with impact.[39] For players with injuries to their nondominant hand or who play nonskilled positions, the protective splint may be continued for the rest of the season during play.[39]

SUMMARY

Physicians may feel pressure to permit athletes, particularly high-level players with professional aspirations, an early return to play by the athlete, as well as by his or her coach, family, agent, and trainer. The risks and benefits should be discussed and documented and an informed decision should be reached. The risk of reinjury and long-term morbidity must be carefully considered by all involved parties.

It is important to set aside adequate time for a comprehensive consultation with an athlete. There are many factors to consider when treating football and rugby players, including the decision for nonoperative versus operative intervention, the use of casts, splints, and taping both off and on the field; the timing of return to protected and unprotected play; and the creation of weekly hand therapy goals. Typed instructions can be helpful in guiding a player's treatment. Athletes are goal-oriented individuals and having weekly recovery milestones can help them stay on track and engaged in their treatment plan.

Athletes' aspirations for their playing career and for their life after sport must be thoroughly discussed. Players' long-term life ambitions should not be compromised for their short-term playing careers. Obtaining a second and even a third opinion from other hand surgeons can be helpful for athletes as they consider their treatment options following a finger injury.

REFERENCES

1. Willigenburg NW, Borchers JR, Quincy R, et al. Comparison of injuries in American Collegiate Football and Club Rugby: a prospective cohort study. Am J Sports Med 2016;44(3):753–60.
2. Shewring DJ, Matthewson MH. Injuries to the hand in rugby union football. J Hand Surg Br 1993;18(1):122–4.
3. Mall NA, Carlisle JC, Matava MJ, et al. Upper extremity injuries in the National Football League: part I: hand and digital injuries. Am J Sports Med 2008;36(10):1938–44.
4. Culpepper MI, Niemann KM. High school football injuries in Birmingham, Alabama. South Med J 1983;76(7):873–5, 878.
5. Swenson DM, Henke NM, Collins CL, et al. Epidemiology of United States high school sports-related fractures, 2008-09 to 2010-11. Am J Sports Med 2012;40(9):2078–84.
6. Swenson DM, Yard EF, Collins CL, et al. Epidemiology of US high school sports-related fractures, 2005–2009. Clin J Sport Med 2010;20(4):293–9.
7. Dy CJ, Khmelnitskaya E, Hearns KA, et al. Opinions regarding the management of hand and wrist injuries in elite athletes. Orthopedics 2013;36(6):815–9.
8. Gaston RG. Football commentary: phalangeal fractures–displaced/nondisplaced. Hand Clin 2012;28(3):407–8.
9. Bhargava A, Jennings AG. Simultaneous metacarpophalangeal joint ulnar collateral ligament injury and carpometacarpal dislocation of the thumb in a football player: a case report. Hand Surg 2009;14(1):23–4.
10. Toronto R, Donovan PJ, Macintyre J. An alternative method of treatment for metacarpal fractures in athletes. Clin J Sport Med 1996;6(1):4–8.
11. Yeh PC, Shin SS. Tendon ruptures: mallet, flexor digitorum profundus. Hand Clin 2012;28(3):425–30, xi.
12. Soni P, Stern CA, Foreman KB, et al. Advances in extensor tendon diagnosis and therapy. Plast Reconstr Surg 2009;123(2):52e–7e.
13. McKenna SM, Eames MH. Unusual mechanism of injury to the extensor pollicis longus tendon in a professional rugby player. J Hand Surg Eur Vol 2014;39(7):781–2.
14. Lourie GM. Boutonniere and pulley rupture football commentary. Hand Clin 2012;28(3):451–2.
15. Kovacic J, Bergfeld J. Return to play issues in upper extremity injuries. Clin J Sport Med 2005;15(6):448–52.
16. Kelly EG, Collins AM, Imran FH, et al. Double trouble: rugby associated simultaneous rupture of flexor digitorum profundus tendon in zones I and III. J Plast Reconstr Aesthet Surg 2013;66(12):1795–7.
17. Leddy JP, Packer JW. Avulsion of the profundus tendon insertion in athletes. J Hand Surg 1977;2(1):66–9.
18. Goodson A, Morgan M, Rajeswaran G, et al. Current management of Jersey finger in rugby players: case series and literature review. Hand Surg 2010;15(2):103–7.
19. O'Keeffe ME, Conroy FJ, Kelly J, et al. Tag rugby: a safe alternative? A review of hand injuries sustained playing tag rugby (2007 season). Emerg Med J 2011;28(7):599–600.

20. Brody GA. Tendon ruptures: mallet, FDP in football. Hand Clin 2012;28(3):435.

21. Sawaya ET, Choughri H, Pelissier P. One-stage treatment of delayed 'jersey finger' by Z-step lengthening of the flexor digitorum profundus tendon at the wrist. J Plast Reconstr Aesthet Surg 2012;65(2):264–6.

22. Singletary S, Geissler WB. Bracing and rehabilitation for wrist and hand injuries in collegiate athletes. Hand Clin 2009;25(3):443–8.

23. Wolfe SW, Hotchkiss RN, Pederson WC, et al. Green's Operative Hand Surgery. 6th edition. Philadelphia: Elsevier; 2011.

24. Kato H, Minami A, Takahara M, et al. Surgical repair of acute collateral ligament injuries in digits with the Mitek bone suture anchor. J Hand Surg Br 1999;24(1):70–5.

25. Williams CS 4th. Thumb metacarpophalangeal joint ligament injury: football commentary. Hand Clin 2012;28(3):377–8.

26. Latendresse K, Dona E, Scougall PJ, et al. Cyclic testing of pullout sutures and micro-mitek suture anchors in flexor digitorum profundus tendon distal fixation. J Hand Surg 2005;30(3):471–8.

27. Werner BC, Hadeed MM, Lyons ML, et al. Return to football and long-term clinical outcomes after thumb ulnar collateral ligament suture anchor repair in collegiate athletes. J Hand Surg 2014;39(10):1992–8.

28. Williams CS 4th. Football commentary: PIP fracture. Hand Clin 2012;28(3):423–4.

29. Devitt BM, Baker JF, Fitzgerald E, et al. Website malfunction: a case report highlighting the danger of using electrical insulating tape for buddy strapping. BMJ Case Rep 2010;2010. Available at: http://www.ncbi.nlm.nih.gov/pubmed/?term=Website+malfunction 3A+a+case+report+highlighting+the+danger+of+using+electrical+insulating+tape+for+buddy+strapping.

30. Bowers WH. The proximal interphalangeal joint volar plate. II: a clinical study of hyperextension injury. J Hand Surg 1981;6(1):77–81.

31. Akagi T, Hashizume H, Inoue H, et al. Computer simulation analysis of fracture dislocation of the proximal interphalangeal joint using the finite element method. Acta Med Okayama 1994;48(5):263–70.

32. Elson RA. Rupture of the central slip of the extensor hood of the finger. A test for early diagnosis. J Bone Joint Surg Br 1986;68(2):229–31.

33. Amadio PC. Epidemiology of hand and wrist injuries in sports. Hand Clin 1990;6(3):379–81.

34. Cotterell IH, Richard MJ. Metacarpal and phalangeal fractures in athletes. Clin Sports Med 2015;34(1):69–98.

35. Geissler WB. Operative fixation of metacarpal and phalangeal fractures in athletes. Hand Clin 2009;25(3):409–21.

36. Evans P, Pervaiz K. Sport-specific commentary on Bennett and metacarpal fractures in football. Hand Clin 2012;28(3):393–4.

37. Gaston RG, Chadderdon C. Phalangeal fractures: displaced/nondisplaced. Hand Clin 2012;28(3):395–401, x.

38. Etier BE, Scillia AJ, Tessier DD, et al. Return to play following metacarpal fractures in football players. Hand (N Y) 2015;10(4):762–6.

39. Singletary S, Freeland AE, Jarrett CA. Metacarpal fractures in athletes: treatment, rehabilitation, and safe early return to play. J Hand Ther 2003;16(2):171–9.

40. Fufa DT, Goldfarb CA. Fractures of the thumb and finger metacarpals in athletes. Hand Clin 2012;28(3):379–88, x.

41. Geissler WB, McCraney WO. Fractures of the hand and wrist. Operative management of metacarpal fractures. New York: Informa Healthcare USA, Inc; 2007.

42. Robertson GA, Wood AM. Fractures in sport: optimising their management and outcome. World J Orthop 2015;6(11):850–63.

43. Rettig AC, Ryan R, Shelbourne KD, et al. Metacarpal fractures in the athlete. Am J Sports Med 1989;17(4):567–72.

44. Schneider LH. Fractures of the distal phalanx. Hand Clin 1988;4(3):537–47.

45. Geissler WB. Cannulated percutaneous fixation of intra-articular hand fractures. Hand Clin 2006;22(3):297–305, vi.

46. Komura S, Yokoi T, Nonomura H. Mini hook plate fixation for palmar fracture-dislocation of the proximal interphalangeal joint. Arch Orthop Trauma Surg 2011;131(4):563–6.

47. Rugby U. Protective equipment and clothing guidelines. 2015. Available at: https://assets.usarugby.org/docs/refereeing/protective-equipment-clothing-guidelines.pdf. Accessed May 29, 2016.

48. Marshall SW, Waller AE, Loomis DP, et al. Use of protective equipment in a cohort of rugby players. Med Sci Sports Exerc 2001;33(12):2131–8.

49. DeCarlo M, Malone K, Darmelio J, et al. Casting in sport. J Athl Train 1994;29(1):37–43.

50. Football Highlights. 2013. Available at: https://www.iahsaa.org/football/2013%20Football%20Information/2013%20FOOTBALL%20HIGHLIGHTS.pdf. Accessed June 12, 2016.

51. Barton N. Sports injuries of the hand and wrist. Br J Sports Med 1997;31(3):191–6.

52. Kodama N, Takemura Y, Ueba H, et al. Operative treatment of metacarpal and phalangeal fractures in athletes: early return to play. J Orthop Sci 2014;19(5):729–36.

Thumb Injuries in Athletes

Tiffany R. Kadow, MD, John R. Fowler, MD*

KEYWORDS

- Thumb • Ulnar collateral ligament • Phalanx fracture • Bennett • Rolando

KEY POINTS

- A thorough clinical and radiographic assessment is important clinically for an accurate diagnosis to prevent delays in appropriate treatment and return to sport.
- Anatomic reduction and internal fixation of thumb metacarpal base fractures gives the greatest chance of return to sport.
- Ulnar collateral ligament tears are common in athletes and complete tears are commonly treated with surgical repair.

Acute injuries of the hand and thumb in athletes present a challenge for physicians. Physicians must remain committed to preventing harm and keep the best interests of the athlete's health in mind while navigating financial implications, self-esteem issues, and coaching and/or administrative pressures. Treating physicians must tailor the treatment based on the sport and position played, the level of competition, and future requirements both with sport, rehabilitation, and the potential to use protective devices to hasten return to sport. A thorough assessment both clinically and radiographically is important for an accurate diagnosis to prevent delays in appropriate treatment and return to sport.

EPIDEMIOLOGY

Hand injuries are common among athletes both in contact and noncontact sports, accounting for 9% of sports injuries in athletes overall and 15% of the injuries in football.[1,2] Thumb and finger injuries are the most common upper extremity injury in competitive team sports.[1] Despite the hand being the most active portion of the upper extremity, it is the least protected and is at high risk for injury.[3]

THUMB CARPOMETACARPAL JOINT INJURIES

Thumb carpometacarpal (CMC) injuries include dislocations, Bennett fractures, Rolando fractures, and extraarticular fractures of the base of the thumb metacarpal.[4,5]

ANATOMY OF THE THUMB CARPOMETACARPAL JOINT

The trapeziometacarpal (TM) joint is a double saddle that moves in 3 planes: flexion/extension, abduction/adduction, and pronation/supination.[4] The stability of the joint comes from its bony geometry, ligaments, and joint capsule.[4,5] The specific anatomic structures of the TM joint that contribute to stability are debated in the literature but include the beak of the thumb metacarpal, the recess in the trapezium into which the volar beak inserts, the volar beak (anterior oblique) ligament, the intermetacarpal ligament, and the dorsal ligament complex.[6,7] Bettinger and colleagues[8] identified 16 individual ligaments of the TM joint. However, understanding of the dorsal ligament complex, the volar beak ligament, and the intermetacarpal ligament are the most critical for understanding the stability of the TM joint.[9]

Disclosure Statement: The authors have nothing to disclose.
Department of Orthopaedics, University of Pittsburgh, Suite 911, Kaufmann Building, 3471 Fifth Avenue, Pittsburgh, PA 15213, USA
* Corresponding author.
E-mail address: fowlerjr@upmc.edu

Hand Clin 33 (2017) 161–173
http://dx.doi.org/10.1016/j.hcl.2016.08.008
0749-0712/17/© 2016 Elsevier Inc. All rights reserved.

The biconcave structure of the TM joint has been reported to provide as much as 47% of the stability of the joint while in opposition.[10] The bony volar beak of the thumb metacarpal permits locking into the trapezium recess as part of a cantilever force couple. The other portion of this cantilever force couple is the tension of the dorsal ligament complex, which provides compression to convert a lax, unstable incongruous joint into a rigidly stable and congruous TM joint. The dorsal ligament complex is the widest, thickest, and shortest ligament spanning the TM joint. Some authors argue that this ligament complex is the key stabilizer in power pinch and grip and the primary stabilizer against dorsal dislocation.[6,11–14] The volar beak ligament has been referred to as the "palmar beak" ligament,[15] anterior oblique ligament,[16] ulnar ligament,[17] or the palmar ligament.[18] This ligament originates on the trapezium and inserts onto the volar beak of the thumb metacarpal. Some studies suggest that the volar beak ligament is thin and weak and does not play an important role in stabilizing the TM joint in power pinch and grasp,[6] whereas others describe it as crucial for TM joint stability. It provides approximately 40% of the resistance to pronation.[10] The intermetacarpal ligament tethers the thumb metacarpal to the index metacarpal and resists supination forces as well as acts as a pivot point if the dorsal ligament complex and beak ligament fail, preventing a completely free dislocation.

THUMB CARPOMETACARPAL JOINT DISLOCATIONS

Thumb CMC joint dislocations are rare.[19] The majority of thumb CMC dislocations occur owing to an axial load with the thumb flexed, resulting in dorsal dislocation. However, there have been reports of volar dislocations in children and adolescents.[4,5,11,20] Strauch and colleagues[11] performed an anatomic study to determine the specific ligamentous injury that occurs with acute thumb CMC dislocations by progressively dividing the ligaments of the thumb CMC joint and found the primary restraint to dorsal dislocation was the dorsoradial ligament of the dorsal ligamentous complex. This has been confirmed by other anatomic and biomechanical studies. After reduction, the authors noted that the joint was most stable in pronation and extension, which tightened the anterior oblique ligament.[11]

Imaging

Standard hand radiographs including anteroposterior (AP), oblique, and lateral views should be obtained. Additional views can be obtained to gain more information about the injury. The Roberts view is a true AP view of the thumb CMC joint and is performed with hyperpronation of the forearm with the dorsum of the thumb placed against the radiograph plate and the beam directed 90° to the plate. The Betts view is obtained with the palm overpronated 20° from flat against the radiograph plate and the beam directed 15° proximal to distal.[21,22] Stress radiographs can be performed by pressing the radial border of the thumbs together, parallel to the film, on an AP view. This may demonstrate subluxation of the metacarpal base radially on the trapezium.[4,16] Traction radiographs may be useful to determine the benefit of ligamentotaxis on the reduction.[23]

Treatment

Pure dislocations of the thumb CMC joint result in an unstable injury with most authors recommending surgical reconstruction.[4,19,24,25] Closed reduction and percutaneous pinning of these injuries has a high rate of persistent symptomatic instability.[25] Reconstruction of the anterior oblique ligament using a flexor carpi radialis autograft has been reported and may offer added stability.[26,27] Because of the risk of persistent instability, ligamentous reconstruction is preferred for athletes to increase the likelihood of return to play. If athletes do not participate in a sport that requires strong grip, pinch, or opposition, it is reasonable to consider initial treatment of an acute dislocation of the thumb CMC joint with reduction and cast application. The athlete is monitored closely with serial radiographs to ensure a congruent reduction. In the setting of a chronic dislocation, ligament reconstruction is performed.[14]

THUMB METACARPAL FRACTURES

Thumb metacarpal fractures account for approximately 25% of all metacarpal fractures, with 80% of those occurring at the metacarpal base. Fractures at the base of the thumb metacarpal can be divided into extraarticular, Bennett, and Rolando fracture patterns. Bennett and Rolando fractures occur by an axial load directed through a partially flexed metacarpal shaft.

Anatomy

The surrounding soft tissue attachments determine the direction deforming forces for both extraarticular and intraarticular fractures of the thumb metacarpal. Extraarticular fractures become angulated dorsally owing to extension of the metacarpal base by the abductor pollicis longus and flexion of the distal shaft by thenar muscles.

A Bennett fracture is an avulsion fracture of the volar/ulnar portion of the metacarpal base. This volar/ulnar fragment is held to the trapezium by the volar beak (anterior oblique) ligament.[9,28] The metacarpal shaft is pulled dorsal, proximal, and radially by the abductor pollicis longus, extensor pollicis longus, extensor pollicis brevis, and adductor pollicis longus.[23]

Rolando fractures are Y-shaped intraarticular fractures of the base of the thumb metacarpal. The beak ligament prevents displacement of the volar fragment but the dorsal fragment displaces via the abductor pollicis longus with the shaft displaced by the adductor and extensor pollicis longus.[23]

Extraarticular metacarpal fractures

Treatment principles for extraarticular metacarpal fractures of the thumb remain similar to those for the finger metacarpals. Angulation up to 30° is acceptable for extraarticular thumb metacarpal fractures owing to the compensatory motion at the thumb CMC joint and little deficit in function is typically noted.[29] However, apex dorsal angulation of more than 30° will narrow the thumb webspace and cause compensatory metacarpophalangeal (MCP) joint hyperextension, which is poorly tolerated.

The majority of extraarticular thumb metacarpal fractures can be treated with immobilization in a thumb spica cast or splint. If an acceptable reduction cannot be maintained with immobilization alone, these fractures are most commonly approached with closed reduction and crossed Kirschner wire (K-wire) fixation.[23,30] Open reduction and internal fixation can be performed and may be favored because it provides a more stable construct than K-wires and may permit earlier motion and return to sport after surgery. Athletes may return to sport in a protective splint or cast once the wound has healed.

Bennett fractures

Bennett fractures were described initially by E.H. Bennett in 1882 as an intraarticular 2-part fracture at the base of the thumb metacarpal.[31] Contemporary description of a Bennett fracture refers to an intraarticular fracture separating the volar, ulnar aspect of the metacarpal base from the remaining thumb metacarpal (**Fig. 1**).[7] The Bennett fracture is the most common fracture pattern at the base of the thumb metacarpal.[32]

Radiographs

Bennett fractures have been classified into 3 types by Gedda[33]: (1) a fracture with a single large ulnar fragment and subluxation of the metacarpal base,

(2) impaction fracture without subluxation of the metacarpal, and (3) fracture with small ulnar avulsion fragment in association with a metacarpal dislocation (**Box 1**). Bennett fractures may be associated with fractures of the trapezium and/or concomitant collateral ligament injuries of the MCP joint.[34] Suspicion and careful evaluation of all radiographs is critical to avoid missing these concomitant injuries.

Treatment

A preliminary closed reduction of Bennett fractures should be performed and is accomplished with axial traction, palmar abduction, and pronation while applying pressure over the metacarpal base.[7] Palmar abduction of the thumb and pronation of the metacarpal base theoretically tightens the dorsal ligament complex.[7] Hyperextension of the thumb should be avoided because it can cause further fracture displacement.[7]

A debate remains in the literature regarding the amount of articular incongruity that is acceptable in nonathlete populations. Some authors have found no correlation between the quality of articular reduction and radiologic or subjective outcomes (**Fig. 2**).[35,36] Biomechanical studies demonstrate that 2 mm of persistent displacement at the articular surface does not alter the contact pressures at the area of the step off. Therefore, bony apposition of the fragments within 2 mm and correction of any joint subluxation will be tolerated without increasing the risk of posttraumatic arthritis when compared with anatomic reduction.[37]

Despite biomechanical evidence that articular step-off may be well-tolerated, several clinical studies have suggested that anatomic reduction is preferred.[38,39] Kjaer-Peterson and colleagues[40] reported on the treatment of 41 Bennett fractures with a variety of techniques, including closed reduction and casting, pinning, or open reduction internal fixation (ORIF). The authors found a correlation between the quality of the reduction and patient reported outcomes with 86% of patients who had an anatomic or near-anatomic reduction (<1 mm step off) reporting no residual symptoms but only 46% of patients with a step off of greater than 1 mm remaining asymptomatic. The specific fixation for displaced Bennett fractures is also debated in the literature. Lutz and colleagues[41] reported no difference in outcomes between type I Bennett fractures treated with closed reduction and K-wire fixation compared with ORIF at the 7-year follow-up.

A small amount of articular step off (1–2 mm) may be well-tolerated if the subluxation of the thumb metacarpal base is reduced. Additionally, the size of the fragment is important. Large fragments of

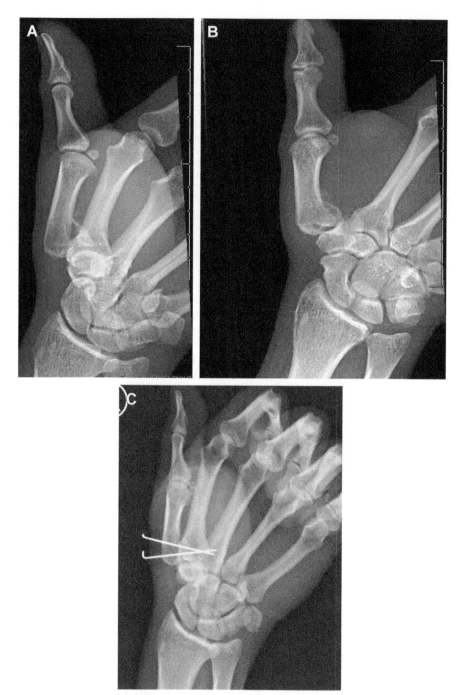

Fig. 1. (*A*) Anteroposterior and (*B*) oblique radiographs demonstrating a Bennett fracture of the thumb metacarpal base. (*C*) Postoperative radiograph demonstrating reduction and pinning of the volar–ulnar fragment.

greater than 30% of the articular surface are unlikely to achieve an acceptable closed reduction that restores articular congruity. Smaller fragments often reduce well with ligamentotaxis. Our algorithm for treatment starts with closed reduction in the operating room using traction, palmar abduction, and pronation with direct pressure on the base of the thumb metacarpal. If the joint is reduced under fluoroscopy and there is less than 1 mm of articular step off, a K-wire is placed from the thumb metacarpal base into the index metacarpal.[42] A second K-wire can be placed into the index metacarpal or the trapezium to add stability. If an acceptable closed reduction cannot be achieved and/or maintained with closed means, a Wagner approach between the glabrous and non-glabrous skin is used to visualize the reduction. We take care to not strip the volar–ulnar fragment. It is reduced with the help of a clamp or K-wire used as a joystick. The fragment is then fixed to the metacarpal base using mini-fragment screws or K-wires. Large fragments are more amenable to screw fixation.[43] The joint is then reduced and held by placing K-wires from the thumb metacarpal base into the index metacarpal. Range of motion exercises can begin at 5 to 10 days with screw fixation or after 4 weeks with pinning (after pins are

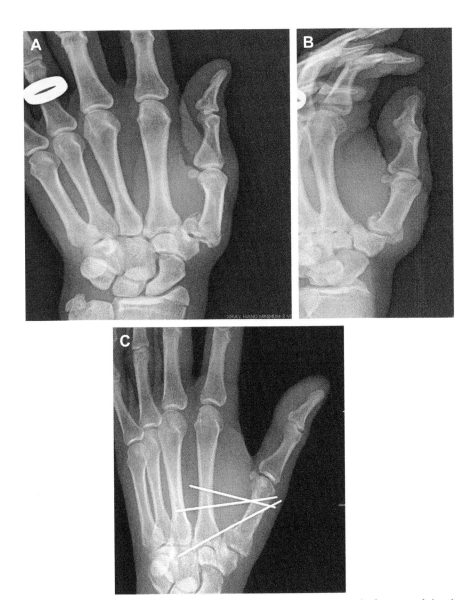

Fig. 2. (*A*) Anteroposterior and (*B*) oblique radiographs demonstrating a Rolando fracture of the thumb metacarpal base. (*C*) Postoperative radiograph demonstrating reduction and pinning.

removed). Nonthrowing athletes can return to sport in 2 to 3 weeks with protective devices, whereas throwing/grasp/pinch requiring athletes often do not return for 6 to 10 weeks.[43]

Rolando fractures

In 1910, Silvio Rolando published a report of 3 cases of a Y-shaped fracture of the metacarpal base.[44] Currently, a Rolando fracture refers to a Y- or T-shaped pattern that involves the volar–ulnar Bennett fragment and a dorsal radial fragment, but it is often used to refer to comminuted fractures of the thumb metacarpal base (see **Fig. 2**). Rolando fractures maintain an intact volar carpal ligament, which prevents displacement of the volar fragment, whereas the dorsal fragment is displaced by the abductor pollicis longus. The shaft is displaced by the adductor and extensor pollicis longus.[23] This fracture pattern is more difficult to treat than a Bennett fracture and has a worse prognosis.[45,46] If 2 large fragments exist, ORIF through a Wagner approach is performed. For severely comminuted injuries, distraction and reliance on ligamentotaxis may be required. This procedure can be performed with oblique traction pinning[47] or external fixation.[48]

Long-term outcome studies of Rolando fractures are lacking. Langhoff and colleagues[49] followed Rolando fractures that were treated with ORIF (11 of 14 patients). Follow-up at 6 years noted arthritic changes in 6 patients, but the authors were unable to correlate the quality of reduction with late symptoms or long-term osteoarthritis.[46,49] Our algorithm for treatment of Rolando fractures depends on the size and number of fragments. Rolando fractures with 2 large fragments are treated with ORIF to restore articular congruity. Comminuted fractures are treated with distraction pinning, sometimes supplemented with a mini external fixator. Patients are immobilized for 6 weeks for fracture consolidation.

INJURIES TO THE METACARPOPHALANGEAL JOINT
Anatomy

The thumb MCP joint is a diarthrodial condyloid joint that allows for flexion, extension, abduction, and adduction.[50,51] The thumb MCP joint remains stable through the flexion–extension arch, which is different from the finger MCP joints that are stable in flexion and lax in extension. Radially and ulnarly, the MCP joint is stabilized by a strong collateral ligament system with both proper and accessory collateral ligaments. The proper collateral ligaments are taut in flexion, whereas the accessory collateral ligaments are taut in extension. The MCP joint is also stabilized by the static dorsal capsule and volar plate. The MCP joint is stabilized dynamically by the extrinsic and intrinsic musculature of the thumb including the adductor pollicis and flexor pollicis brevis. The adductor pollicis inserts on the ulnar sesamoid, whereas the flexor pollicis brevis inserts on the radial sesamoid.[51]

The ulnar collateral ligament (UCL) and radial collateral ligament (RCL) provide dorsal as well as radial and ulnar support to the MCP joint.[51,52] The UCL and RCL are approximately 4 to 8 mm wide and 12 to 14 mm in length.[53] The collateral ligaments originate from the dorsal metacarpal head and course distally and palmarly to the proximal phalanx.[53] The proper collateral ligaments attach directly to the proximal phalanx based whereas the accessory collateral ligaments attach to the volar plate.

The metacarpal origin of the UCL has been termed the dorsal condyle[54] or posterior tubercle[55] of the metacarpal head and is located 4.2 mm from the dorsal surface and 5.3 mm from the articular surface. The phalangeal insertion[56] is 3.4 mm distal to the articular surface and 2.8 mm dorsal to the volar edge of the phalanx.[51] The RCL origin on the metacarpal is 3.5 mm volar to the dorsal edge of the metacarpal and 3.3 mm proximal to the articular surface. The phalangeal insertion of the RCL[57] is 2.6 mm distal to the articular surface and 2.8 mm dorsal to the volar edge of the phalanx.[51] The exact location of the origin and insertion sites permits anatomic repair and/or reconstruction of the collateral ligaments, more closely replicating normal anatomy.

The adductor pollicis aponeurosis lies superficial to the UCL as it blends into the extensor hood of the thumb.[58,59] The abductor pollicis aponeurosis extends more proximally than the adductor pollicis aponeurosis and lies superficial to the RCL.[59] There is a net flexion moment on the MCP joint and volar pull of the proximal phalanx owing to stronger force of the flexor pollicis longus and thenar muscles compared with the extensor pollicis longus and extensor pollicis brevis.[60] Dorsal support to the MP joint is provided by the dorsal capsule as well as the RCL and UCL, and when this support is lost, the flexor tendons cause volar subluxation rather than flexion at the joint.[61]

ULNAR AND RADIAL COLLATERAL LIGAMENT INJURIES
Acute Ulnar and Radial Collateral Ligament Injuries

Injuries to the UCL are common during contact sports as well as skiing owing to hyperabduction and forceful radial deviation of the thumb MCP joint.[43] An acute injury to the UCL carries the eponym "skier's thumb" owing to the prominence of this injury among skiers, because the pole maintains the thumb in an abducted position and puts the thumb at risk for excessive radial deviation. Hyperabduction and radial deviation injuries typically damage both the proper and accessory collateral ligaments. The vast majority of injuries (90%) result in a distal avulsion of the UCL[62] and 50% of all UCL injuries will have an associated fracture at the base of the proximal phalanx.[47]

Patients typically complain of difficulty or pain with pinching and gripping activities. Ligament sprain, partial, and complete injuries can be clarified on physical examination. Greater than 30° of joint angulation with valgus stress of the flexed MCP signifies a complete tear of the proper collateral ligament, whereas greater than 30° of MCP joint opening with valgus stress in full MCP extension signifies complete tear of the accessory collateral ligament. Joint opening/angulation of 15° greater than the contralateral thumb in full MCP extension and/or 30° of MCP flexion is also an indication of compete accessory collateral and proper collateral ligaments, respectively.[63,64] Malik and colleagues[65] found a greater than 10° variation on MCP testing in uninjured individuals, prompting the authors to recommend the lack of a firm endpoint with stress testing to be more determinant of injury than relative instability of greater than 15°.

The location of the adductor pollicis aponeurosis plays an important role in the treatment of UCL tears. When the UCL ruptures, it may retract and allow the adductor pollicis aponeurosis, which usually lies superficial to the UCL, to become interposed between the ligament and its insertion on the proximal phalanx. This injury was described by Stener in 1962 and is clinically important, because the soft tissue interposition prevents healing of the UCL back to its bony attachment.[58] Stener lesions are common with complete UCL ruptures, occurring in more than 80% of cases.[63] A Stener lesion is an indication for UCL repair; however, diagnosis can be challenging, even with advanced imaging. Some investigators have described a palpable mass proximal to the MCP joint as a sign of a Stener lesion and occasionally an associated avulsion fracture with the fragment proximal to the location of the adductor hood will indicate a "bony Stener" lesion.[64,66] Some have advocated avoiding stressing the UCL or RCL if radiographs reveal a nondisplaced avulsion fracture to prevent displacement. Others advocate for stress testing, even if a fracture exists as the UCL/RCL can sustain a 2-level injury pattern with

an avulsion fracture occurring with a concomitant midsubstance tear,[67,68] causing a loss of stability and the formation of a Stener lesion despite an aligned avulsion fragment.

RCL injuries are caused by an abrupt, ulnar-directed stress. Patients with RCL injuries complain of pain and weakness with similar activities as those with UCL injuries.[62] Additionally, patients will have pain with activities that cause ulnar stress such as pushing a door or opening a jar. Compared with UCL injuries, RCL injuries are more variable, occurring proximally in 55% of patients, distally in 29%, and midsubstance in 16%.[62] A radial-sided Stener-equivalent lesion is rare owing to the position of the abductor aponeurosis, which lies dorsal to the RCL.[62] Joint subluxation is more common with RCL injuries owing to the adductor pollicis insertion on the proximal phalanx and ulnar sesamoid. These insertions lie volar to the MP axis of rotation, causing a volar and ulnar deforming force on the proximal phalanx.[69]

Imaging

Standard radiographs of the thumb (AP and lateral) are obtained to determine if there is a fracture, subluxation, or dislocation of the thumb MCP joint. If there is suspicion for a complete collateral ligament tear, consideration may be given to advanced imaging to confirm a complete tear and to determine if a Stener lesion is present. Advanced imaging may also be beneficial because it can demonstrate the location (proximal/distal) of the tear, thus guiding surgical exploration and fixation. Advanced imaging for thumb collateral ligament tears includes ultrasound imaging and MRI. Ultrasound imaging is the less expensive and faster modality; however, the diagnostic accuracy is highly dependent on examiner skill and experience and the examination may be painful for patients with acute injuries. The sensitivity and specificity of ultrasound imaging for the diagnosis of a Stener lesion is 76% and 81%, respectively.[70,71] MRI is a highly sensitive (100%) and specific (94%) test for thumb ulnar collateral injuries.[72,73]

Treatment

Stable UCL sprains or partial tears can be treated with 4 weeks of immobilization in a thumb spica cast with the interphalangeal joint left free. After 4 weeks of immobilization, a removable thermoplastic hand based thumb spica splint can be used to allow for the initiation of a range of motion program for the thumb and wrist. After full range of motion has been achieved, sport-specific training can be initiated. Depending on the sport and position, athletes may be permitted to return to sport with casting. Acute complete tears of the UCL and RCL are typically addressed with surgical repair. Ulnar and RCL avulsion fractures have been treated with[68,74] or without surgery[66,75] in nonathletic populations with both options well-supported in the literature if the fracture is minimally displaced. Kuz and colleagues[66] performed a retrospective study of 30 UCL avulsion fractures. No patient had a change in recreational activities or employment owing to their thumb and no pain. However, 3 patients had persistent instability and 25% were found to have a nonunion.[66] ORIF for a thumb collateral avulsion fracture is indicated for:

1. At least 20% of articular surface involvement
2. Considerable displacement of the fragment, or
3. Instability on stress testing of the UCL/RCL.

Rigid fixation of fragment can be performed with a tension band construct or a 1.5-mm interfragmentary screw. If there are multiple small fragments, excision of those fragments with reattachment of the insertion of the UCL/RCL can be performed.[74]

Our treatment algorithm in athletes is more proactive than in the general population. Any athlete with a soft endpoint on examination is studied with advanced imaging (usually an MRI). Complete tears are treated with surgical repair to prevent instability and to return athletes to play in a timely fashion (**Fig. 3**). It is the senior

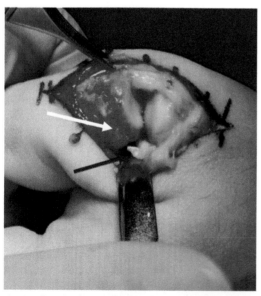

Fig. 3. Thumb ulnar collateral ligament (*black arrow*) and its insertion on the proximal phalanx (*white arrow*).

author's opinion that, although nonoperative treatment of collateral ligament tears without Stener lesions results in resolution of symptoms in most patients in a nonathletic population, the quality of the tendon–bone attachment is not strong enough to allow high-level athletes to return to sport reliably without symptoms. Therefore, we offer nearly all athletes with complete thumb collateral ligament injuries surgical repair. The presence of a Stener lesion is an absolute indication for surgery. In the case of avulsion fragments, these authors believe that bone–bone healing is superior to bone–tendon healing and therefore attempt to fix the avulsion fragment whenever possible.

Chronic Ulnar Collateral Ligament Injuries

Chronic UCL injuries have been referred to as "gamekeeper's thumb" based on the mechanism of injury identified in Scottish gamekeepers by Campbell. The chronic ligament insufficiency was the sequelae from the method used to break the necks of rabbits between the thumb and index finger.[76]

The workup for chronic UCL injuries is similar to that of acute injuries. Standard radiographs are obtained to document joint alignment and the presence of any degenerative changes. Significant degenerative changes are a contraindication to ligament reconstruction and should be assessed carefully.[63] The radiographs may also identify nonunion of a ligament avulsion fracture. The physical examination is similar to the examination for acute injuries, but may be better tolerated by the athlete because acute swelling and inflammation are not typically present. The thumb is tested in full extension and 30° of flexion. Greater than 30° of joint angulation/opening with varus/valgus stress and/or greater than 15° of increased angulation over the contralateral side are indications for ligament reconstruction.

Chronic UCL injuries in the nonathletic population are often not able to be primarily repaired owing to poor tissue quality and therefore reconstruction is required. However, Pai and colleagues[77] were able to primarily repair chronic UCL injuries as late as 2 years after injury using suture anchors by releasing the contracted volar plate and mobilizing the UCL from the surroundings scar tissue. We recommend that treatment be individualized for each patient based on intraoperative findings of native ligament quality and excursion. In our experience, young athletes have more robust tissue that can be mobilized and primarily repaired, even in the chronic setting. Primary repair is preferable in this setting.

In the setting of poor tissue quality or a midsubstance tear, a ligament reconstruction is performed using palmaris longus autograft or one-half of the flexor carpi radialis tendon if the palmaris is not present. Drill holes are placed at the isometric points on the proximal phalanx and metacarpal and the tendon autograft weaved through the holes and sutured back on itself.[61,78,79] Postoperatively, patients are placed into a thumb spica splint for 2 weeks and then a short arm thumb spica cast for 4 weeks to protect the reconstruction. Athletes may return to sport once range of motion and grip strength reaches 80% of the contralateral side.[80]

PHALANGEAL INJURIES
Anatomy

The thumb interphalangeal joint is stabilized by the volar plate, collateral ligaments, flexor pollicis longus and extensor pollicis longus.[81] The head of the proximal phalanx has 2 condyles with an intercondylar notch that confer stability while articulating with the ridge on the base of the distal phalanx. The dorsal aspect of the distal phalanx base has a central flare and dorsal tubercle, which is the insertion site for the terminal extensor tendon. On each side of this dorsal tubercle are lateral tubercles, which are the attachment sites for the collateral ligaments of the distal interphalangeal joint.[82] The volar lip/tubercle is the insertion site for the volar plate and the flexor digitorum profundus tendon inserts onto a flat area just distal to the volar plate.[82] The tuft of the distal phalanx is crescent shaped and provides support for the nail complex, including septa from the tuft to the skin to support the pulp and structural support to the germinal matrix, which lies on the dorsal surface of the distal phalanx just distal to the insertion site of extensor pollicis longus.

Distal phalanx fractures
The thumb distal phalanx, similar to the other digits, is divided into the base, shaft, and tuft. Distal phalanx fractures are often owing to direct trauma and are less common than thumb metacarpal fractures.[83] Distal phalanx fractures are often divided into tuft, mallet, and transverse shaft fractures.

Tuft Fractures

Tuft fractures in the thumb are caused by a similar mechanism as in the lesser digits, often a crush injury, causing damage to the nail matrix, digit pulp, or both. Subungal hematomas should be drained and the injured area should be evaluated for injury to the nail matrix and repaired if necessary. These injuries are treated with splint immobilization for 3 to 4 weeks, but athletes with minimal throwing can typically return to play with protective splints.[83]

Mallet Thumb

Although mallet finger injuries are quite common in sports, mallet thumb injuries account for only 2% to 3% of all mallet injuries.[80] Similar to mallet fingers, mallet thumbs are the result of a flexion force directed to an actively extended finger with an avulsion fracture of the dorsal base of the distal phalanx. In pediatric patients, the extensor tendon avulses a fragment of the physis, which causes an intraarticular fracture that may extend into the metaphysis and thus should be identified as a Salter Harris III or IV type fracture.

Treatment principles for both children and adults are similar. Fractures involving less than 30% of the joint are typically stable and can be treated with extension splinting; however, fractures with persistent volar subluxation, joint incongruity, or greater than 50% involvement of the joint should be addressed surgically.[84] For fractures involving less than 30% of the joint, extension splinting can be used, but this requires a long duration of splint use and excellent patient compliance. If athletes understand the commitment on their part for nonoperative treatment, nonthrowing athletes can attempt extension splinting and can continue to play with the splint in place. It is especially useful to address these injuries early; Miura and colleagues[85] found 84% satisfactory results with extension splining of mallet thumbs but noted that better results were obtained by those treated less than 2 weeks from injury. Given the prolonged compliance required, many athletes will prefer operative treatment, especially those requiring intricate use of their hands which prevents them from playing with protective devices in place. Din and Meggitt[86] recommended open repair because they noted a gap in the terminal extensor tendon of the thumb that prevented adequate healing.

Transverse Distal Phalangeal Fractures

Transverse distal phalangeal shaft fractures often present with a pseudomallet appearance to the digit as the fracture line is often just distal to the insertion of the extensor tendon. Seymour fractures are open fractures of the distal phalanx that occur in children owing to a fracture at the physis of the distal phlanx causing the distal fragment to protrude through the dorsal surface entrapping the nail matrix under the distal fracture segment.[83] These injuries are often missed because careful evaluation of the nail bed is required.[87] A pseudomallet finger with blood at the nail fold should be considered an open fracture through the distal phalanx physis (Salter Harris I) and/or metaphysis (Salter Harris II) until proven otherwise. Seymour fractures require operative irrigation and debridement, as well as removal of the proximal nail plate from the site of incarceration. Often, after the nail plate is removed, the fracture can be easily reduced and maintained.[87,88]

Fractures of the proximal phalanx

Proximal phalanx fractures at the head or neck are treated by the same principles as in the digits (**Fig. 4**). If fractures are displaced with spiral or oblique patterns, they can be treated with percutaneous pinning versus open reduction and internal fixation with screws or pins. Similar to transverse proximal phalanx fractures, transverse distal fractures will develop an apex volar deformity. Angulation of greater than 20° in the sagittal plane will result in an extensor lag of the interphalangeal joint and should be treated with percutaneous pinning versus open reduction and internal fixation.[83]

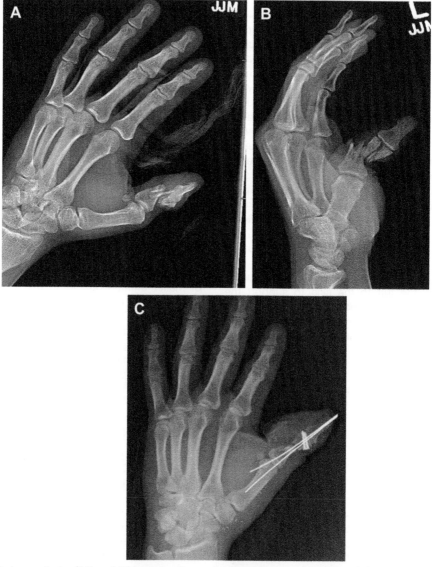

Fig. 4. (*A*) Anteroposterior (AP) and (*B*) lateral radiographs demonstrating a fracture of the thumb proximal phalanx. Postoperative (*C*) AP radiograph demonstrating open reduction and internal fixation.

SUMMARY

Thumb injuries are common in athletes and present a challenging opportunity for upper extremity physicians. This review, although not exhaustive, has highlighted some of the most common thumb injuries in athletes. The treating physician must balance pressure from athletes, parents, coaches, and executives to expedite return to play with the long-term well-being of the athlete. Operative treatment may expedite return to play; however, one must carefully weigh the added risks involved with surgical intervention.

REFERENCES

1. Retting AC. Epidemiology of hand and wrist injuries in sports. Clin Sports Med 1998;17:401–6.
2. Retting AC. Athletic injuries of the hand and wrist. Part 1: traumatic injuries of the wrist. Am J Sports Med 2003;31:1038–48.
3. Patel D, Dean C, Baker JR. The hand in sports: an update on the clinical anatomy and physical exam. Prim Care 2005;32:71–89.
4. Glickel S, Barron A, Catalano L. Dislocations and ligament injuries in the digits. In: Green D, Hotchkiss R, Pederson W, et al, editors. Green's operative hand surgery. 5th edition. Philadelphia: Churchill Livingstone; 2005. p. 382–6.
5. Sawalha S. Volar dislocation of the thumb carpometacarpal joint: a case report. Injury Extra 2008; 39(10):332–4.
6. Edmunds JO. Current concepts of the anatomy of the thumb trapeziometacarpal joint. J Hand Surg 2011;36A:170–82.
7. Edunds JO. Traumatic dislocations and instability of the trapeziometacarpal joint of the thumb. Hand Clin 2006;22(3):365–92.
8. Bettinger PC, Smutz WP, Linscheid RL, et al. Material properties of the trapezial and trapeziometacarpal ligaments. J Hand Surg 2000;25A: 1085–95.
9. Bettinger PC, Linscheid R, Berger RA, et al. An anatomic study of the stabilizing ligaments of the trapezium and the trapezio-metacarpal joint. J Hand Surg 1999;24A:786–98.
10. Imaeda T, An KN, Cooney WP III. Functional anatomy and biomechanics of the thumb. Hand Clin 1992;8:9–15.
11. Strauch RJ, Behrman MJ, Rosenwasser MP. Acute dislocation of the carpometacarpal joint of the thumb: an anatomic and cadaver study. J Hand Surg Am 1994;19(1):93–8.
12. Van Brenk B, Richards RR, Mackay MB, et al. A biomechanical assessment of ligaments preventing dorsoradial subluxation of the trapeziometacarpal joint. J Hand Surg 1998;23A:607–11.
13. Colman M, Mass DP, Draganich LF. Effects of the deep anterior oblique and dorsoradial ligaments on trapeziometacarpal joint stability. J Hand Surg 2007;32A:310–7.
14. Bosmans B, Verhofstad MHJ, Gosens T. Traumatic thumb carpometacarpal joint dislocations. J Hand Surg 2008;33A:438–41.
15. Pellegrini V. The ABJS Nicolas Andry Award: osteoarthritis and injury at the base of the human thumb: survival of the fittest? Clin Orthop Relat Res 2005; 438:266–76.
16. Eaton RG, Lane LB, Littler JW, et al. Ligament reconstruction for the painful thumb carpo-metacarpal joint: a long term assessment. J Hand Surg 1984; 9A:692–9.
17. Spinner M. Kaplan's functional and surgical anatomy of the hand. 3rd edition. Philadelphia: Lippincott Williams & Wilkins; 1984. p. 121–4.
18. Zancolli EA, Cozzi EP. Atlas of surgical anatomy of the hand. New York: Churchill Livingstone; 1992. p. 432–561.
19. Pizon AF, Wang HE. Carpometacarpal dislocation of the thumb. J Emerg Med 2010;38(3):376–7.
20. Henry M. Hand fractures and dislocations. In: Bucholz R, Court-brown C, Heckman J, editors. Rockwood and green's fractures in adults. 7th edition. Philadelphia: Lippincott Williams & Wilkins; 2010. p. 600–709.
21. Billing L, Gedda KO. Roentgen examination of Bennett's fracture. Acta Radiol 1952;38:471–6.
22. Fufa DT, Goldfarb CA. Fractures of the thumb and finger metacarpals in athletes. Hand Clin 2012;28: 379–88.
23. Soyer AD. Fractures of the base of the thumb metacarpal: current treatment options. J Am Acad Orthop Surg 1999;7:403–12.
24. Lahiji F, Zandi R, Maleki A. Thumb carpometacarpal joint dislocation and review of literatures. Arch Bone Jt Surg 2015;3(4):300–3.
25. Simonian PT, Trumble TE. Traumatic dislocation of the thumb carpometacarpal joint: early ligamentous reconstruction versus closed reduction and pinning. J Hand Surg Am 1996;21(5):802–6.
26. Khan AM, Ryan MG, Teplitz GA. Bilateral carpometacarpal dislocations of the thumb. Am J Orthop 2003;32:38–41.
27. Jeong C, Huoung-Min K, Lee SU, et al. Bilateral carpometacarpal joint dislocations of the thumb. Clin Orthop Surg 2012;4(3):246–8.
28. Bettinger PC, Berger RA. Functional ligamentous anatomy of the trapezium and trapeziometacarpal joint (gross and arthroscopic). Hand Clin 2001;17:151–68.
29. Huang JI, Fernandez DL. Fractures of the base of the thumb metacarpal. Instr Course Lect 2010;59: 343–56.
30. Stern PJ. Fractures of the metacarpals and phalanges. In: Green DP, Hotchkiss RN, editors.

Operative hand surgery. 3rd edition. New York: Churchill-Livingstone; 1993. p. 695–758.

31. Bennett EH. Fractures of metacarpal bone of the thumb. Br Med J 1886;2:12–5.

32. Gedda KO, Moberg E. Open reduction and osteosynthesis of the so-called Bennett's fracture in the carpometacarpal joint of the thumb. Acta Orthop Scand 1953;22:249–57.

33. Gedda KO. Studies on Bennett's fracture; anatomy, roentgenology and therapy. Acta Chir Scand Suppl 1954;193:1–114.

34. McGuigan FX, Culp RW. Surgical treatment of intraarticular fractures of the trapezium. J Hand Surg 2002;27A:697–703.

35. Cannon SR, Dowd GS, Williams DH, et al. A long-term study following Bennett's fracture. J Hand Surg 1986;11B:426–31.

36. Demir E, Unglaub F, Wittemann M, et al. Surgically treated intraarticular fractures of the trapeziometacarpal joint-a clinical and radiological outcome study. Unfallchirurg 2006;109:13–21.

37. Cullen JP, Parentis MA, Chinchilli VM, et al. Simulated Bennett fracture treated with closed reduction and percutaneous pinning. A biomechanical analysis of residual incongruity of the joint. J Bone Joint Surg Am 1997;79A:413–20.

38. Oosterbos CJ, de Boer HH. Nonoperative treatment of Bennett's fracture: a 13-year follow-up. J Orthop Trauma 1995;9:23–7.

39. Thurston AJ, Dempsey SM. Bennett's fracture: a medium to long term review. Aust N Z J Surg 1993;63:120–3.

40. Kjaer-Petersen K, Langhoff O, Andersen K. Bennett's fracture. J Hand Surg 1990;15B:58–61.

41. Lutz M, Sailer R, Zimmermann M, et al. Closed reduction transarticular Kirschner wire fixation versus open reduction internal fixation in the treatment of Bennett's fracture dislocation. J Hand Surg 2003;28B:142–7.

42. Baltera RM, Hastings H, Sachar K, et al. Fractures and dislocations: hand. In: Hammert WC, Calfee RP, Bozentka DJ, et al, editors. Manual of hand surgery. Philadelphia: Lippincott Williams & Wilkins; 2010. p. 186–215.

43. Retting AC. Athletic injuries of the hand and wrist. Part II: overuse injuries of the wrist and traumatic injuries to the hand. Am J Sports Med 2004;32(1):262–73.

44. Rolando S. Fracture of the base of the thumb metacarpal and a variation that has not yet been described: 1910. [Trans. Roy A. Meals]. Clin Orthop Relat Res 2006;445:15–8.

45. Buchler U, McCollam SM, Pooikofer C. Comminuted fractures of the basilar joint of the thumb. Combined treatment by external fixation, limited internal fixation and bone grafting. J Hand Surg 1991;16:L556–60.

46. Foster RJ, Hastings H. Treatment of Bennett, Rolando and vertical intraarticular trapezial fractures. Clin Orthop 1987;214:121–9.

47. Carlsen BT, Moran SL. Thumb trauma: Bennett fractures, Rolando fractures, and ulnar collateral ligament injuries. J Hand Surg 2009;34A:945–52.

48. Bruske J, Bednarski M, Niedzwiedz Z, et al. The results of operative treatment of fractures of the thumb metacarpal base. Acta Orthop Belg 2001;67:368–73.

49. Langhoff O, Andersen K, Kjaer-Petersen K. Rolando's fracture. J Hand Surg 1991;16B:454–9.

50. Barmakian JT. Anatomy of the joints of the thumb. Hand Clin 1992;8:683–91.

51. Carlson MG, Warner KK, Meyers KN, et al. Anatomy of the thumb metacarpophalangeal ulnar and radial collateral ligaments. J Hand Surg 2012;37A:2021–6.

52. Loebig TG, Anderson DD, Baratz ME, et al. Radial instability of the metacarpophalangeal joint of the thumb. A biomechanical investigation. J Hand Surg 1995;20B:102–4.

53. Melone CP Jr, Beldner S, Basuk RS. Thumb collateral ligament injuries. An anatomic basis for treatment. Hand Clin 2000;16:345–7.

54. Fraser B, Veitch J, Firoozbakhsh K. Assessment of rotational instability with disruption of the accessory collateral ligament of the thumb MCP joint: a biomechanical study. Hand (N Y) 2008;3:224–8.

55. Frank WE, Dobyns J. Surgical pathology of collateral ligamentous injuries of the thumb. Clin Orthop Relat Res 1972;83:102–14.

56. Ebrahim FS, De Maeseneer M, Jager T, et al. US diagnosis of UCL tears of the thumb and Stener lesions: technique, pattern-based approach, and differential diagnosis. Radiographics 2006;26:1007–20.

57. McDermott TP, Levin LS. Suture anchor repair of chronic radial ligament injuries of the metacarpophalangeal joint of the thumb. J Hand Surg 1998;23B:271–4.

58. Stener B. Skeletal injuries associated with rupture of the ulnar collateral ligament of the metacarpophalangeal joint of the thumb. A clinical and anatomical study. Acta Chir Scand 1963;125:583–6.

59. Schroeder NS, Goldfarb CA. Thumb ulnar collateral and radial collateral ligament injuries. Clin Sports Med 2015;34:117–26.

60. Posner MA, Retaillaud JL. Metacarpophalangeal joint injuries of the thumb. Hand Clin 1992;8(4):713–32.

61. Smith RJ. Post-traumatic instability of the metacarpophalangeal joint of the thumb. J Bone Joint Surg Am 1977;59(1):14–21.

62. Coyle MP Jr. Grade III radial collateral ligament injuries of the thumb metacarpophalangeal joint: treatment by soft tissue advancement and bony reattachment. J Hand Surg Am 2003;28(1):14–20.

63. Heyman P, Gelberman RH, Duncan K, et al. Injuries of the ulnar collateral ligament of the thumb metacarpophalangeal joint. Biomechanical and prospective clinical studies on the usefulness of valgus stress testing. Clin Orthop Relat Res 1993;292:165–71.

64. Thirkannad S, Wolff TW. The "two fleck sign" for an occult Stener lesion. J Hand Surg 2008;33E:208–11.

65. Malik AK, Morris T, Chou D, et al. Clinical testing of ulnar collateral ligament injuries of the thumb. J Hand Surg Eur Vol 2009;34(3):363–6.

66. Kuz JE, Husband JB, Tokar N, et al. Outcome of avulsion fractures of the ulnar base of the proximal phalanx of the thumb treated nonsurgically. J Hand Surg 1999;24A:275–82.

67. Giele H, Martin J. The two-level ulnar collateral ligament injury of the metacarpophalangeal joint of the thumb. J Hand Surg 2003;28B:92–3.

68. Hintermann B, Holzach PJ, Schutz M, et al. Skier's thumb—the significance of bony injuries. Am J Sports Med 1993;21:800–4.

69. Tang P. Collateral ligament injuries of the thumb metacarpophalangeal joint. J Am Acad Orthop Surg 2011;19(5):287–96.

70. Spaeth HJ, Abrams RA, Bock GW, et al. Gamekeeper thumb: differentiation of nondisplaced and displaced tears of the ulnar collateral ligament with MR imaging. Work in progress. Radiology 1993;188:553–6.

71. Papandrea RF, Fowler T. Injury at the thumb UCL: is there a Stener Lesion? J Hand Surg 2008;33A:1882–4.

72. Ahn JM, Sartoris DJ, Kang HS, et al. Gamekeeper thumb: comparison of MR arthrography with conventional arthrography and MR imaging in cadavers. Radiology 1998;206:737–44.

73. Hergan K, Mittler C, Oser W. Ulnar collateral ligament: differentiation of displaced and nondisplaced tears with US and MR imaging. Radiology 1995;194:65–71.

74. Dinowitz M, Trumble T, Hanel D, et al. Failure of cast immobilization for thumb ulnar collateral ligament avulsion fractures. J Hand Surg 1997;22A:1057–63.

75. Landsman JC, Seitz WH Jr, Froimson AI, et al. Splint immobilization of gamekeeper's thumb. Orthopedics 1995;18:1161–5.

76. Campbell CS. Gamekeeper's thumb. J Bone Joint Surg Am 1955;37B:148–9.

77. Pai S, Smit A, Birch A, et al. Delayed anatomical repair of the ruptured ulnar collateral ligament injuries of the thumb using a dissolvable polylatctic acid bone anchor. J Trauma 2008;65:1502–6.

78. Glickel SZ, Malerich M, Pearce SM, et al. Ligament replacement for chronic instability of the ulnar collateral ligament of the metacarpophalangeal joint of the thumb. J Hand Surg Am 1993;18(5):930–41.

79. Glickel SZ. Thumb metacarpophalangeal joint ulnar collateral ligament reconstruction using a tendon graft. Tech Hand Up Extrem Surg 2002;6(3):133–9.

80. Doyle JR. Extensor tendons-acute injuries. In: Green DP, editor. Operative hand surgery. New York: Churchill Livingstone; 1982. p. 2045–72.

81. Cooney WP, An KN, Daube JR, et al. Electromyographic analysis of the thumb: a study of isometric forces in pinch and grasp. J Hand Surg Am 1985;10:202–10.

82. Panchal-Kildare S, Malone K. Skeletal anatomy of the hand. Hand Clin 2013;29(4):459–71.

83. Day CS, Stern PS. Fractures of the metacarpals and phalanges. In: Wolfe, Hotchkiss, Pederson, et al, editors. Green's operative hand surgery. Philadelphia: Elsevier; 2011. p. 239–90. Chapter 8.

84. Pegoli L, Toh S, Arai K, et al. The Ishiguro extension block technique for the treatment of mallet finger fracture: indications and clinical results. J Hand Surg Br 2003;28:15–7.

85. Miura T, Nakamura R, Torii S. Conservative treatment for a rupture extensor tendon of the dorsum of the proximal phalanges of the thumb (mallet thumb). J Hand Surg 1986;11A:229–33.

86. Din KM, Meggitt BF. Mallet thumb. J Bone Joint Surg Am 1983;65B:606–7.

87. Nellans KW, Chung KC. Pediatric hand fractures. Hand Clin 2013;29(4):569–78.

88. Al-Qattan M. Extra-articular transverse fractures of the base of the distal phalanx in children and adults. J Hand Surg Br 2001;26:201–6.

Upper Extremity Injuries in Tennis Players
Diagnosis, Treatment, and Management

Kevin C. Chung, MD, MS[a],*, Meghan E. Lark, BS[b]

KEYWORDS

- Upper extremity • Tennis • Shoulder • Wrist • Elbow • Treatment

KEY POINTS

- Common upper extremity tennis injuries involve soft tissue and are usually a result of overuse.
- Tennis injuries have a complex association with biomechanical properties of tennis strokes and serves.
- Injury profile of tennis injuries varies by injury site, mechanism of injury, athlete experience level, and presence of known risk factors.
- Diagnosis can be a challenge and depends on a thorough understanding of current research topics.

INTRODUCTION

Tennis is one of the most popular sports in the world, owing to the unique combination of aerobic and anaerobic activity that is enjoyable for all ages and skill levels. At the competitive level, tennis is showcased through the dynamic exchange of intricate strokes and serves by some of the world's most versatile athletes. However, the physical demands of this sport are known to put athletes at risk for a variety of musculoskeletal injuries.[1] A recent study of professional tennis competitions found that more than 50% of men's and women's departures from competition could be attributed to injury.[2] Although specific injury incidence varies by age, sex, and experience level, studies of the general tennis population report that incidence can range from 0.05 to 2.9 injuries per player per year.[1] This observed high prevalence of injury has led many researchers to study how tennis mechanics contribute to the profiles of various musculoskeletal injuries.

Descriptive epidemiologic studies of tennis injuries have found that injuries occur most frequently in the lower extremity, followed by the upper extremity, then trunk.[1–3] Although the upper extremities are not the most prevalent injury site, a recent study investigating the epidemiology of the National Collegiate Athletic Association (NCAA) men's and women's tennis injuries suggested that tennis has a higher proportion of upper extremity injuries than other NCAA sports.[3] Additionally, distinct patterns of injury are observed among sites of occurrence. Lower extremity tennis injuries are mostly acute and result from traumatic events, whereas upper extremity injuries are mostly chronic and result from repetitive overuse. To better understand these findings, risk factors for upper extremity overuse injuries have been widely

Disclosure: Research reported in this publication was supported by a Midcareer Investigator Award in Patient-Oriented Research (2K24 AR053120-06) to Dr K.C. Chung. The content is solely the responsibility of the authors and does not necessarily represent the official views of the National Institutes of Health. The authors do not have a conflict of interest to disclose.

a Section of Plastic Surgery, University of Michigan Medical School, University of Michigan Health System, 2130 Taubman Center, SPC 5340, 1500 East Medical Center Drive, Ann Arbor, MI 48109-5340, USA; b Section of Plastic Surgery, Department of Surgery, University of Michigan Health System, Ann Arbor, MI, USA
* Corresponding author.
E-mail address: kecchung@umich.edu

Hand Clin 33 (2017) 175–186
http://dx.doi.org/10.1016/j.hcl.2016.08.009
0749-0712/17/© 2016 Elsevier Inc. All rights reserved.

hand.theclinics.com

presented in the literature for the overhead-throwing and striking athlete population. These studies proposed that the excessive loading of upper extremity contributes significantly to soft tissue problems,[4] revealing the important role that technique modification of joint biomechanics can have in both injury prevention and treatment.

Physicians are confronted with a variety of challenges in the management of injuries sustained in the upper extremity joints of the wrist, elbow, and shoulder. These challenges are intensified in the overhead athlete, as the complex anatomic interactions of these joints often produce a spectrum of pathology.[5] This article aims to review concepts related to the biomechanical origin, diagnosis, treatment, and prevention of common upper extremity tennis injuries in an effort to guide clinical decision-making. With knowledge of tennis biomechanics and their relation to injury, physicians can provide patients with informed opinions and make treatment recommendations that fit the individual needs and expectations of each athlete.

BIOMECHANICS

Similar to other racket sports, tennis is composed of diverse strokes and serves, each consisting of different biomechanical factors that could contribute to the spectrum of upper extremity injury. The tennis serve is the most energy-demanding tennis motion, and has been shown to comprise nearly 45% to 60% of all strokes performed in a tennis match.[6] The serve is characterized by 5 different phases of motion:

1. Wind-up
2. Early cocking
3. Late cocking
4. Acceleration
5. Follow through

Other stroke types include the forehand or backhand groundstroke, which each have 3 different phases of motion:

1. Racket preparation
2. Acceleration
3. Follow through

Specific and dynamic upper extremity positioning can account for large amounts of the speed at impact and varies by stroke type.

When investigating the production of high-energy tennis strokes and their contribution to tennis injury etiology, the kinetic chain concept of motion cannot be ignored. The kinetic chain describes the route and direction of energy flow in tennis strokes and serves. In this process, musculoskeletal joints, such as the knee, shoulder, and elbow, serve as links in the kinetic chain by absorbing, generating, and transmitting energy to the next link, completing a cycle of energy from the ground to the tennis ball at impact with the racket. In a single tennis match, this cycle is repeated numerous times and relies heavily on an athlete's strength, endurance, flexibility, and technique.[6,7] If energy transfer in one joint is not efficiently coordinated, subsequent joints can easily become overloaded. For example, a biomechanical study of the tennis serve found that the mechanical loads transmitted to the shoulder and elbow increased by 17% and 23% in the absence of proper knee flexion when attempting to produce a velocity similar to that of a serve performed with correct knee flexion.[8,9] Additionally, a tennis player's ability to use the kinetic chain is often dependent on experience level. Several studies have found that advanced players are more efficient at manipulating the kinetic chain to reduce the impact forces transmitted to upper extremity joints. In turn, novice or recreational tennis players often use excessive and uncoordinated strength in the absence of efficient technique, which does not translate into increased ball velocity and rather overload the joint and increases risk of injury.[10,11] These results imply that optimal technique can contribute immensely to maximizing injury prevention and minimizing loads placed on each joint.

WRIST INJURIES

In tennis, wrist injuries are most commonly experienced as ulnar pathology related to the extensor carpi ulnaris (ECU) tendon and occur during forehand groundstrokes. The forehand stroke is the most frequently used groundstroke in tennis and is performed with the dominant forearm in full supination and the wrist flexed in ulnar deviation.[6] Wrist flexion and extension are important components of ball velocity after ball-racket impact. For example, a study by Seeley and colleagues[12] determined that increasing tennis ball velocity from medium to fast during the forehand stroke required 31% greater angular velocity of the wrist joint at impact. Therefore, dynamic repetition of this stroke depends largely on the integrity of the ECU and its ability to contribute to wrist flexion and extension.

Injury risk to both the ECU tendon and its fibro-osseous sheath increases when the tendon is overloaded by strong forces transmitted to the wrist at impact. A major component of the forehand stroke that is associated with wrist extensor and flexor overload is the generation of top-spin, which can be accomplished through using specific racket grip techniques. The contribution of grip techniques to wrist injury was studied by Tagliafico and colleagues[13] in 370 nonprofessional tennis players. These investigators found that utilization of Western and semi-Western grip types, which are most effective in generating top-spin rotation in the forehand stroke, were associated with ulnar-sided wrist injuries that almost exclusively pertained to ECU tendinopathy. Additionally, the nondominant wrist in the 2-handed backhand stroke can be subjected to the same harmful forces as that of the forehand stroke. This observation is most likely attributed to the extensive ulnar deviation experienced by the nondominant wrist at stroke impact.[14] These studies indicate that athletes using the Western or semi-Western grip types of the forehand stroke, as well as those using the 2-handed backhand stroke, are at higher risk of experiencing ulnar wrist symptoms and can benefit from prevention exercises aimed at strengthening the wrist extensor and flexor units of both arms.

Although less prevalent than ECU tendinitis, tennis players can also experience acute ECU injury as a result of traumatic subsheath rupture or attenuation. Disruption of the ECU subsheath leads to a loss of tendon stabilization and can result in painful subluxation or snapping of the ECU tendon over the ulnar groove.[15] Specifically, acute ECU subluxation is connected with performance of the low forehand stroke. In this stroke, sudden hyper-supination of the forearm occurs with the wrist in flexion and ulnar deviation, generating a traumatic force capable of disrupting subsheath integrity. Physicians treating tennis players with ECU pathology should distinguish between these chronic and acute injuries to make informed treatment decisions.

Diagnosis

In many cases of ECU subluxation, patients may report painful snapping over the ulnar styloid of the wrist that limits athletic participation. A detailed physical examination starts with discussion of both mechanism of injury and symptom history. Next, physicians should carefully palpate the dorsoulnar wrist, specifically assessing the scapholunate, triquetrolunate, distal radio-ulna, and ulnocarpal joints. Additionally, the hook of the hamate, flexor, and extensor tendons are examined and the Finkelstein test for DeQuervain tenosynovitis is performed. Plain radiographs in 3 views should be ordered to rule out osseous pathologies, such as fractures or distal radio-ulna joint arthritis.

Although various physical tests for ECU pathology exist, the intricate structures of the wrist are often difficult to isolate. For this reason, results of clinical maneuvers often can be elusive and contradictory, further complicating the diagnostic process. Recently, in an effort to better distinguish ECU tendinitis from ECU subluxation, Ruland and Hogan[16] developed the ECU synergy test. This key provocative maneuver relies on synergistic muscle activity to achieve isometric contraction of the ECU tendon and discern between intra-articular and extra-articular ECU pathology (Table 1). This test has proven useful in clinical settings and should be used before imaging studies. In the case of an ambiguous diagnosis or recurrent symptoms, MRI and dynamic ultrasound studies can supplement physical examination. MRI can be useful for visualization of ECU tendinitis or confirmation of other soft tissue abnormalities, such as scapholunate ligament or triangular fibrocartilage complex tears.[17] Dynamic ultrasound is an effective method for identification of ECU subluxation.[18–20] These differing findings highlight the clinical importance of performing the ECU synergy test before selecting an imaging modality, in an effort to gain information about injury type and minimize the unnecessary use of imaging studies.

Treatment

ECU tendinitis is treated with nonoperative methods such as rest, nonsteroidal anti-inflammatory drugs (NSAIDs), splinting, and technique modification. If symptoms are persistent, corticosteroid injections into the ECU sheath may be useful. For the treatment of ECU subluxation, cast immobilization with the wrist pronated and extended for 6 weeks can be considered before operative treatment.[15] If symptoms persist after conservative treatment, surgical reconstruction of the fibro-osseous tunnel of the sixth extensor compartment is recommended. Typically, this reconstruction can be performed by wrapping a strip of the extensor retinaculum around the ECU and suturing the tendon in place. A recent study by MacLennan and colleagues[18] investigating outcomes of ECU tendon sheath reconstruction in 21 patients diagnosed with ECU subluxation observed a significant improvement in postoperative grip strength, flexion-extension, pronation-supination, and Disabilities of the Arm, Shoulder, and Hand (DASH) scores at long-term follow-up. Another study that evaluated surgical outcome in a sample consisting of 10 professional athletes (7 tennis players) found that the athletes were able to return to previous levels of play after an average of 8 months (range 3–21).[21] These study results indicated that excellent surgical outcomes

Table 1
A summary of physical tests useful for the diagnosis of common upper extremity tennis conditions

Condition	Physical Test	Description	Positive Result
Extensor carpi ulnaris (ECU) tendinitis/subluxation	ECU synergy test	• Patient rests arm on table with elbow flexed at 90° • With forearm in full supination, examiner palpates the ECU tendon • Ensuring that wrist is neutral, use other hand to grasp patient's long finger and resist patient's radial abduction of the thumb	Pain experienced along the dorsal ulnar wrist
Lateral epicondylitis	Cozen test	• Patient elbow is stabilized by palpation of examiner's thumb over lateral epicondyle • Patient is asked to make a fist and pronate forearm with radial deviation and extension • Examiner resists patient movement	Pain experienced at the lateral epicondyle
	Mill test	• Patient arm in passive pronation with wrist flexed and elbow extended • Examiner palpates the lateral epicondyle with thumb	Pain experienced at lateral epicondyle
	Maudsley test	• Resisted middle digit extension • Specifically target resistance of the middle extensor digitorum communis (EDC) tendon	Pain experienced in elbow region above lateral epicondyle
Labral pathology	Modified dynamic labral shear test	• Patient stands • Examiner flexes elbow 90°, then abducts into scapular plane above 120° and externally rotated to maximum ability • Guide arm into maximal horizontal abduction, and shear load to joint maintaining this position	Pain experienced along posterior joint line with or without clicking
	O'Brien test	• Patient stands • Examiner places arm at 90° forward flexion, 10° horizontal adduction with internal rotation • Place hand over elbow and ask patient to resist downward pressure • Ask patient to externally rotate palms up, place hand over palm and ask patient to resist downward pressure	Pain experienced at joint line during internal rotation, yet pain improves with external rotation
Rotator cuff pathology	Neer test	• Patient stands with arm passive at side of body with elbow extended • Examiner internally rotates arm through full forward flexion	Pain experienced at anterior-lateral area of shoulder
	Hawkin test	• Patient stands • Examiner places shoulder in 90° of shoulder and elbow flexion, then rotates internally	Pain experienced with internal rotation

facilitating a return to previous level of play are achievable in both operative and nonoperative treatments for ECU wrist pathology.

ELBOW INJURIES

Elbow pathology in tennis players frequently differs by level of play. Less-experienced or recreational tennis players typically experience elbow injury as a result of incorrect technique or equipment, whereas professional tennis players may injure the elbow as a result of more subtle incorrect technique. With this, physicians can tailor medical treatment and recommendations to fit the tennis player's experience level for both the treatment and prevention of elbow injury.

Lateral Epicondylitis

One of the most prevalent tennis injuries presenting to general and specialty clinicians is lateral epicondylosis, commonly termed "tennis elbow." Epidemiologic studies estimated that up to 50% of tennis players will develop lateral elbow symptoms throughout their tennis career, with a primary population consisting of recreational tennis players.[22,23] Consensus on cause of lateral epicondylitis does not exist; however, many different etiologies have been proposed. In addition to anatomic predisposition of the extensor carpi radialis brevis (ECRB) tendon to irritation, overloading of wrist extensors during the backhand tennis stroke is thought to be a key contributor to the prevalence of the condition.[24–26] Despite lower utilization compared with forehand strokes and serves, the backhand stroke is an important skill for tennis players. It can be performed using a 1-handed or 2-handed approach; however, the 1-handed approach is more commonly associated with elbow pathology. This stroke is accomplished with the elbow extended and the wrist supinated, applying stress to the forearm extensor unit and transmitting particularly large forces to the ECRB at the lateral epicondyle. Numerous studies have identified both intrinsic technical skill factors and extrinsic equipment variations that contribute to the high prevalence of this condition in the recreational tennis player.

Differences in the backhand technique of experienced and recreational tennis players can be observed in kinematic studies of forearm muscle coordination during backhand stroke production. Grip tightness is a key feature of a powerful backhand stroke; however, it must be coordinated appropriately with phases of the backhand serve to prevent injury to the elbow. For example, a kinematic study of the backstroke performed by Wei and colleagues[10] found that experienced tennis

players use a tight grip at ball-racket impact, then immediately decrease their grip tightness in the follow-through phase. This study found that use of this quick-release grip reduced 89.2% of the impact force transmitted to the lateral epicondyle region of the elbow. However, when grip force was quantified in recreational players, these researchers found that the tight grip was incorrectly retained throughout both ball impact and follow-through phase, resulting in reduction of only 61.8% of impact force transmitted to the elbow. Electromyography studies of the same test groups revealed similar results when forearm muscle activity was quantified, finding that the wrist extensors of recreational players exceeded maximal contraction levels at both ball impact and follow-through phase, whereas those of experienced players reached maximal activity at ball impact and were submaximal in the follow-through phase. From this, physicians and rehabilitation specialists should communicate the importance of decreasing grip strength and relaxing forearm muscles in the follow-through phase of the backhand stroke. These modifications have serious implications for lateral epicondylitis prevention in recreational tennis players.

Overloading of the elbow joint also can occur as a result of equipment-dependent factors, such as racket size or quality. Incorrect grip size of the racket handle has recently been associated with increased force transmission to the elbow. A study by Rossi and colleagues[27] quantified the forces acting on the dominant tennis arm with varying racket handle grip sizes, finding that grip size significantly influenced the impact forces transmitted to the forearm extensor muscles, particularly when the grip was too small or large. These researchers observed that when racket handles were not the appropriate size for a tennis player's hand, the players increased grip force on the racket, which in turn increased harmful force transmission to the elbow. This study highlights the benefits of properly fitting equipment, of which less-experienced tennis players may not be familiar with.

Diagnosis

Patients with lateral epicondylitis typically present with pain and tenderness over the lateral epicondyle, which may radiate distal to the forearm throughout the extensor muscle area. Patients usually experience discomfort with passive flexion and resisted wrist extension, as well as pain with grasping objects firmly. A variety of physical tests can be performed to aid diagnosis, including the Cozen test, Mill test, and Maudsley test (see **Table 1**). The differential diagnosis includes radial tunnel syndrome and posterior interosseous nerve entrapment. In cases in which the diagnosis is unclear, MRI can be used to confirm and plan treatment; however, clinical tests and physical examination are typically sufficient for diagnosis.[28]

Treatment

There is no standard protocol for treatment of lateral epicondylitis. Nonoperative therapy is recommended before operative intervention. In most cases, symptoms will resolve without treatment within 6 to 12 months. In the tennis athlete, the wait-and-see approach is not always a realistic option, as athletes often need to return to play quickly. When conservative treatment is selected by the patient and physician, NSAIDs are typically the first approach and are often recommended with splinting, stretching, and strengthening exercises. Additionally, physiotherapy that combines elbow manipulation and strengthening exercises targeting the extensor muscles of the forearm have proven to provide short-term symptom relief.[29] If symptoms do not improve with NSAIDs or therapy, corticosteroid or platelet-rich plasma injections may be considered, although there is a lack of evidence supporting the use of injections over other nonoperative treatments. A recent randomized control trial conducted by Coombes and colleagues[30] compared 1-year postoperative outcome measures of 3 groups of lateral epicondylitis patients: those receiving physiotherapy with corticosteroid injection, those receiving physiotherapy only, and those receiving injection only. These researchers did not observe a clear benefit when comparing these groups with control patients with lateral epicondylitis, and in turn found that corticosteroid treatment resulted in less improvement and greater 1-year recurrence. Similar studies of conservative treatments have failed to find long-term benefits.[29,31–35]

In the case of nonoperative treatment failure, surgical release of the ECRB at the lateral epicondyle can be performed with an arthroscopic or open approach, and provides safe and effective relief of symptoms with minimal complications.[36–38] Recent literature has focused on exploring outcomes of arthroscopic release and has contributed to the growing support of arthroscopy as a viable method of ECRB release for recalcitrant cases.[39–42] Studies of functional recovery after surgical ECRB release indicated that patients can typically return to play within 3 to 6 months after surgery.[43]

Medial Epicondylitis

Medial epicondylitis involves tendinopathy of the pronator teres and flexor carpi radialis muscles in the attachment of the flexor-pronator tendon to the medial epicondyle. This condition is found in 10% to 20% of epicondylitis cases and is believed to be a result of repetitive eccentric loading of the flexor and pronator muscles of the forearm.[44] Contrary to the incidence of lateral epicondylitis, medial epicondylitis is most common among higher-level tennis players, and can result from advanced technical deficits, such as open-stance hitting, short-arming strokes, and excessive wrist snapping during serves and forehand strokes.[9]

Diagnosis

Patients with medial epicondylitis present with persistent pain and tenderness over the medial epicondyle, which may radiate distal to the forearm throughout the flexor-pronator muscle area. Specifically, patients experience pain during the early acceleration phase of serves and forehand strokes, in which the forearm is pronated with wrist flexion. In this position, the elbow joint is in valgus stress and the flexor-pronator muscles are maximally contributing to elbow stabilization.

Physical examination reveals tenderness with resisted wrist flexion and forearm protonation. Possible differential diagnoses include medial collateral ligament tear, ulnar neuropathy, and medial elbow instability. Similar to lateral epicondylitis, a medial epicondylitis diagnosis is usually achieved clinically through physical examination and MRI is useful in diagnosis confirmation in cases of ambiguity.[45] A recent retrospective review of surgical patients with medial epicondylitis conducted by Vinod and Ross[46] emphasized the utility of clinically evaluating pronator strength to quantify weakness of the forearm and clinically track pathologic changes in flexor-pronator tendon injury. This aspect is useful in monitoring the clinical course and making treatment decisions for recalcitrant medial epicondylitis in the tennis player.

Treatment

Nonoperative approaches to treatment, such as NSAIDs, strength and flexibility programs, and rest, are used before operative treatment. Steroid injections may provide short-term symptom relief, yet fail to display significant long-term benefits when compared with control patients.[47] Conservative treatment is typically effective in symptom alleviation in 88% to 96% of cases.[48] If symptoms persist after 3 to 6 months of conservative treatment, operative intervention is considered. Surgical methods can be implemented earlier in athletes with MRI indicating tendon disruption. Open methods of surgical debridement of the common flexor tendon have continually demonstrated successful in symptom alleviation.[49] Additionally, recent investigations have suggested that suture anchor fixation of the flexor-pronator mass can also be a method of symptom relief.[50] Contrary to lateral epicondylitis, an arthroscopic approach is typically not recommended in surgical management of medial epicondylitis, owing to the close proximity of both the ulnar collateral ligament and the ulnar nerve to the medial epicondyle. Postoperative rehabilitation is centered on the strengthening and stretching of the flexor-pronator muscles and athletes can return to play in 3 to 6 months as tolerated.[50]

SHOULDER INJURIES

The shoulder joint is the most mobile joint in the body and balances both stabilization and rotational range of motion. In tennis players, this delicate equilibrium is manipulated to create powerful serves and groundstrokes through external rotation and abduction of the shoulder. Overuse injuries to the shoulder are prevalent among tennis players of all skill levels and have been shown to contribute to nearly 4% to 17% of all tennis injuries.[3,51] In a recent study investigating the causes of professional tennis player departures from competition, Okholm Kryger and colleagues[2] found that shoulder injuries were the second most frequent cause of departure for both sexes. For these reasons, it is not only important that clinicians are familiar with the intricate pathology, diagnosis, and treatment of athletic shoulder injuries, but also aware of the mechanical origin of these injuries and how they relate to tennis-specific movements.

Risk Factors

The scapula plays a key role in stabilizing glenohumeral joint mobility during arm motion by frequently changing positions to promote shoulder movements. In the tennis serve, the scapula follows distinct patterns of motion, characterized by retraction/protraction as the serve progresses from early to late cocking stage and upward rotation during the acceleration phase.[52] These fine movements are orchestrated by surrounding rotator cuff muscles that attach to the scapula and other surrounding capsular structures. If shoulder structures become weak or dysfunctional as a result of chronic overload, tennis players may develop scapular dyskinesis. This condition is characterized by an imbalance of the scapula, leading to alterations in scapular movement, which produces pain and functional deficiency during overhead serving motions. In some cases, the affected scapula may demonstrate a drooping appearance or inferior medial border prominence at rest when compared with the unaffected shoulder, a condition commonly referred to as SICK (Scapular malposition, Inferior medial border prominence, Coracoid pain, and dysKinesis of scapular movement) scapula.[53] In most tennis athletes, the presence of scapular dyskinesis or SICK scapula has been found to be associated with shoulder injuries,[53–57] although the exact interactions of these conditions with shoulder injuries are largely undefined.[58] The scapula's role in optimal shoulder performance indicates that an assessment of scapular function is crucial in both preparticipation athletic evaluations and evaluation of tennis athletes presenting with shoulder pain or dysfunction. Once identified, scapular abnormalities can be corrected with rehabilitative stretching programs that successfully target the restoration of muscular and capsular strength and flexibility in the shoulder.[59,60]

In tennis, internal rotation of the shoulder is considered one of the most important positive contributors to ball velocity, especially during the serve.[8] However, repetition of the abduction-extension motion of tennis serves and other overhead strokes can alter the rotational arc of the shoulder, producing an increased degree of external rotation at the expense of posterior capsule tightening. Although increased external rotation produces a more powerful serve, posterior tightening decreases the degree to which the athlete's shoulder can internally rotate and can eventually lead to the development of glenohumeral internal-rotation deficit (GIRD). GIRD is quantitatively characterized by a >18° loss of internal rotation in the athlete's dominant shoulder compared with the nondominant shoulder, as measured during clinical evaluation.[61] The presence of this deficit changes the glenohumeral kinematics of the tennis serve and has also been found to be associated with higher risks of shoulder injury.[62,63] Athletes with GIRD typically present with deep posterior shoulder pain that is accompanied with a decrease in degrees of internal rotation and increase in external rotation, as compared to the nondominant arm and measured by a goniometer. The progression of GIRD can be reversed by stretching programs that target the posteroinferior capsule, which have proven to successfully increase internal and total rotation and reduce GIRD in high-level tennis players.[5,64]

Internal impingement is another condition that is related to shoulder injury development. It is defined as the abnormal mechanical impingement of rotator cuff tendons against the superior glenoid rim and labrum. Internal impingement occurs in healthy shoulders of athletes[65]; however, it can be injured from increased posterior capsule compression. Continual compressive forces in the posterior shoulder capsule can cause a shift of the glenohumeral joint axis.[5] Similar to GIRD and scapular dyskinesis, these compressive loads are experienced during exaggerated external rotation in the late cocking stage of the tennis serve and patients will present with posterosuperior pain and dysfunction. Posterior internal impingement has been shown to occur alongside both GIRD and scapular dyskinesis, and may become increasingly pathologic when associated with these risk factors.[55,66]

Labral Injury

The labrum is a common site of injury for overhead athletes, as it is a key contributor to optimizing capsular tension in the shoulder. Labral pathology in athletes has been studied extensively in literature and is often associated with both GIRD and scapular dyskinesis conditions.[55,57,62,67] Superior labral anterior-to-posterior (SLAP) lesions are the most common labral injuries experienced by athletes. They are characterized by fraying or tearing of the superior labrum at the site of biceps tendon attachment, disrupting the underlying interaction with the glenoid. Although different classifications of severity exist, the most common SLAP lesion involves the detachment of both the superior labrum and the biceps tendon from the glenoid.[68] Biomechanical studies investigating athletic labral injuries have indicated that the mechanics of the late cocking stage of overhead throws and serves play the largest role in the etiology of SLAP lesions.[69,70]

Diagnosis

The diagnosis of the SLAP lesion is notoriously difficult for physicians and requires detailed knowledge of shoulder pathology and careful clinical examination. Athletes with SLAP lesions will present with deep pain that is accompanied by shoulder weakness or dysfunction experienced during the external rotation of the cocking stage of the overhead motion. Some athletes may also report the experience of a popping sensation.[67] There are many clinical tests to aid in the diagnosis of an SLAP lesion; however, a single test with optimal specificity does not exist.[61] Despite these diagnostic limitations, recent explorations have indicated that a combination of the modified dynamic labral shear test and O'Brien active compression test yields the most accurate diagnosis (see **Table 1**).[71] MRI has also proven to be a useful modality to rule out the diagnosis of an SLAP lesion, but is not an accurate clinical diagnostic tool when used alone.[72]

Treatment

Similar to other chronic soft tissue injuries, nonoperative treatment is used before consideration of surgical[46] repair for SLAP lesions. Conservative treatment typically encompasses the use of NSAIDs with the same specialized physical therapy programs that strengthen, stabilize, and increase flexibility of scapular and posterior capsule structures. Surgical treatment of SLAP lesions is usually deployed if symptoms are not relieved after 4 to 6 months. Depending on the severity of the SLAP lesion, patients may benefit from either arthroscopic debridement or repair. However, arthroscopic repair is the standard treatment for SLAP lesions, especially those that involve the detachment of both the posterior labrum and the biceps tendon from the glenoid. The arthroscopic approach typically involves placing multiple suture anchors on the glenoid to secure the attachment of the labrum. A recent prospective study evaluating this technique found that 87% of patients reported a good or excellent outcome at a 2 year follow-up.[73] Similar studies on pain and functional outcome improvement in overhead athlete populations have also supported these findings.[74,75] Alternatively, recent literature has described the utility of biceps tenodesis in the surgical treatment of SLAP lesions, but outcomes studies have indicated that this procedure is most effective for an older, nonathletic population.[76] The results of these evaluations indicate that the athletic status of a patient may have a large role in guiding the treatment decisions being made for SLAP lesions.

It is undisputed that athletic activity contributes heavily to the etiology of labral injury in tennis players. It is also a significant factor in evaluating postoperative outcome, as an athlete's perception of treatment success is largely based on the ability to return to play. Functional outcomes and return to play period of both nonoperative and operative SLAP lesion treatments continue to be a source of controversy in athletic literature. Studies of overhead athletes have reported inconsistent results regarding return to previous level of play, reporting successful return in anywhere from 20% to 94%[61,77,78] of overhead athlete patients. Additionally, literature suggested that the likelihood of overhead athletes returning to previous levels of play is significantly lower than that of nonthrowing athletes.[79] These studies have strong implications for clinicians, in that they suggest postoperative return to play cannot be guaranteed in the overhead athlete. This observation highlights the necessity for sufficient physician communication with tennis players about realistic treatment outcomes that may not satisfy the patient's athletic expectations.

Rotator Cuff Injury

Rotator cuff injury is frequent in the general population, with a degenerative etiology seen mostly in older patients. However, these injuries are also prevalent in younger populations of overhead-throwing athletes, occurring as a result of repetitive, high-energy loading of the shoulder joint. In energetic overhead motions, the muscles and tendons comprising the rotator cuff are the most important components of dynamic shoulder stabilization. In athletes, rotator cuff tendinopathy is most often associated with posterior internal impingement, which can cause fraying or tearing of the rotator cuff tendons with repetition. Additionally, scapular dyskinesis has been shown to contribute to rotator cuff pathology, as the rotator cuff muscles synchronicity is disrupted by abnormal scapular range of motion.

Diagnosis

Patients with rotator cuff injury typically present with pain experienced during throwing and dysfunction that inhibits peak performance of tennis serves and other overhead motions, similar to other soft tissue shoulder pathology. If the injury is the result of posterior internal impingement, the supraspinatus and infraspinatus tendons will be most affected, and pain will be experienced in the late cocking phase of the tennis serve. Diagnosis can be achieved during a careful clinical examination that assesses rotator cuff muscle strength, range of motion, and posterior instability supplemented with imaging studies. In many cases, tests that evaluate impingement, such as the Neer or Hawkin test, can be useful for diagnosis (see **Table 1**). MRI has proven to be a successful supplement to clinical examination and can aid in rotator cuff tear identification, although ultrasound has also proven to be an effective diagnostic tool when used correctly.

Treatment

As a mainstay of chronic soft tissue injury, conservative treatment of rest, NSAIDs, and physical therapy programs focusing on strengthening and stretching of the rotator cuff muscles are used before the consideration of surgery. Minor injuries to the rotator cuff usually respond well to treatment, and often permit return to athletic overhead activity within approximately 3 months.[80] If nonsurgical treatment fails after 3 to 6 months, operative treatment is considered via arthroscopy or open methods. Surgical treatment methods depend on the thickness and location of the muscle tear, as surgical approach is typically altered to fit individual patient needs. Surgery can be accomplished through open or arthroscopic methods, offering either debridement or

repair to improve symptoms. For partial thickness tears, repair is recommended if the tear comprises greater than 50% of the tendon, whereas debridement is recommended in cases below 50%. For full-thickness tears, a suture anchor approach has increasingly emerged as viable option for firm restoration of rotator cuff tendons to the proper anatomic position. These strengths were demonstrated in a cadaver study conducted by Burkhart and colleagues[81] that tested the cyclic loading capabilities of suture anchor fixation compared with transosseous bone tunnel fixation. The long-term outcomes of rotator cuff debridement and repair in the overhead athlete are not well defined in the literature. However, the few studies that have investigated outcomes in this population reported that satisfactory result of debridement is achieved in anywhere from 66% to 76% of athletes, with roughly 45% to 85% being able to return to play.[82–84] Whereas debridement results are somewhat promising, outcomes of surgical partial- and full-thickness repair are increasingly dismal, with some studies observing an inability to return to play in more than half of patients.[84,85] These suboptimal results suggest that physicians should approach surgical repair of rotator cuff tears with caution when considering overhead athletes. Similar to outcomes of SLAP repair, it is imperative that physicians discuss the realities of surgical intervention in shoulder pathology and prepare athletes for potential inability to return to previous levels of play.

SUMMARY

Tennis is a complex and physically demanding sport that can produce a wide range of similarly complex injuries. Upper extremity injuries occur from repetitive overloading of joints, and diagnosis is frequently challenging for physicians, owing to the complex interaction between soft tissue anatomy and biomechanics of the kinetic chain. Diagnosis and treatment of common tennis injuries vary by the location of the injury and can depend on the mechanism of injury, experience level of the athlete, and the presence of physical risk factors that are affected by muscular strength, flexibility, and coordination. Operative management is considered after trying conservative treatment, yet should be approached with caution, in that favorable outcomes may not be realistic and a return to previous level of play may not be achievable.

REFERENCES

1. Pluim BM, Staal JB, Windler GE, et al. Tennis injuries: occurrence, aetiology, and prevention. Br J Sports Med 2006;40(5):415–23.

2. Okholm Kryger K, Dor F, Guillaume M, et al. Medical reasons behind player departures from male and female professional tennis competitions. Am J Sports Med 2015;43(1):34–40.

3. Lynall RC, Kerr ZY, Djoko A, et al. Epidemiology of National Collegiate Athletic Association men's and women's tennis injuries, 2009/2010-2014/2015. Br J Sports Med 2016;50(19):1211–6.

4. Anz AW, Bushnell BD, Griffin LP, et al. Correlation of torque and elbow injury in professional baseball pitchers. Am J Sports Med 2010;38(7):1368–74.

5. Burkhart SS, Morgan CD, Kibler WB. The disabled throwing shoulder: spectrum of pathology Part I: pathoanatomy and biomechanics. Arthroscopy 2003;19(4):404–20.

6. Johnson CD, McHugh MP, Wood T, et al. Performance demands of professional male tennis players. Br J Sports Med 2006;40(8):696–9 [discussion: 699].

7. Kovacs MS. Applied physiology of tennis performance. Br J Sports Med 2006;40(5):381–5.

8. Elliott B. Biomechanics and tennis. Br J Sports Med 2006;40(5):392–6.

9. Elliott B, Fleisig G, Nicholls R, et al. Technique effects on upper limb loading in the tennis serve. J Sci Med Sport 2003;6(1):76–87.

10. Wei SH, Chiang JY, Shiang TY, et al. Comparison of shock transmission and forearm electromyography between experienced and recreational tennis players during backhand strokes. Clin J Sport Med 2006;16(2):129–35.

11. Lo KC, Hsieh YC. Comparison of ball-and-racket impact force in two-handed backhand stroke stances for different-skill-level tennis players. J Sports Sci Med 2016;15(2):301–7.

12. Seeley MK, Funk MD, Denning WM, et al. Tennis forehand kinematics change as post-impact ball speed is altered. Sports Biomech 2011;10(4):415–26.

13. Tagliafico AS, Ameri P, Michaud J, et al. Wrist injuries in nonprofessional tennis players: relationships with different grips. Am J Sports Med 2009;37(4):760–7.

14. Rettig AC. Wrist problems in the tennis player. Med Sci Sports Exerc 1994;26(10):1207–12.

15. Burkhart SS, Wood MB, Linscheid RL. Posttraumatic recurrent subluxation of the extensor carpi ulnaris tendon. J Hand Surg Am 1982;7(1):1–3.

16. Ruland RT, Hogan CJ. The ECU synergy test: an aid to diagnose ECU tendonitis. J Hand Surg Am 2008; 33(10):1777–82.

17. Kuntz MT, Janssen SJ, Ring D. Incidental signal changes in the extensor carpi ulnaris on MRI. Hand (N Y) 2015;10(4):750–5.

18. MacLennan AJ, Nemechek NM, Waitayawinyu T, et al. Diagnosis and anatomic reconstruction of extensor carpi ulnaris subluxation. J Hand Surg Am 2008;33(1):59–64.

19. Sole JS, Wisniewski SJ, Newcomer KL, et al. Sonographic evaluation of the extensor carpi ulnaris in asymptomatic tennis players. PM R 2015;7(3):255–63.

20. Spicer PJ, Romesberg A, Kamineni S, et al. Ultrasound of extensor carpi ulnaris tendon subluxation in a tennis player. Ultrasound Q 2016;32(2):191–3.

21. Allende C, Le Viet D. Extensor carpi ulnaris problems at the wrist–classification, surgical treatment and results. J Hand Surg Br 2005;30(3):265–72.

22. Gruchow HW, Pelletier D. An epidemiologic study of tennis elbow. Incidence, recurrence, and effectiveness of prevention strategies. Am J Sports Med 1979;7(4):234–8.

23. Nirschl RP. Elbow tendinosis/tennis elbow. Clin Sports Med 1992;11(4):851–70.

24. Bunata RE, Brown DS, Capelo R. Anatomic factors related to the cause of tennis elbow. J Bone Joint Surg Am 2007;89(9):1955–63.

25. Nirschl RP, Ashman ES. Elbow tendinopathy: tennis elbow. Clin Sports Med 2003;22(4):813–36.

26. Riek S, Chapman AE, Milner T. A simulation of muscle force and internal kinematics of extensor carpi radialis brevis during backhand tennis stroke: implications for injury. Clin Biomech (Bristol, Avon) 1999; 14(7):477–83.

27. Rossi J, Vigouroux L, Barla C, et al. Potential effects of racket grip size on lateral epicondilalgy risks. Scand J Med Sci Sports 2014;24(6):e462–470.

28. van Kollenburg JA, Brouwer KM, Jupiter JB, et al. Magnetic resonance imaging signal abnormalities in enthesopathy of the extensor carpi radialis longus origin. J Hand Surg Am 2009;34(6):1094–8.

29. Bisset L, Beller E, Jull G, et al. Mobilisation with movement and exercise, corticosteroid injection, or wait and see for tennis elbow: randomised trial. BMJ 2006;333(7575):939.

30. Coombes BK, Bisset L, Brooks P, et al. Effect of corticosteroid injection, physiotherapy, or both on clinical outcomes in patients with unilateral lateral epicondylalgia: a randomized controlled trial. JAMA 2013;309(5):461–9.

31. Krogh TP, Fredberg U, Stengaard-Pedersen K, et al. Treatment of lateral epicondylitis with platelet-rich plasma, glucocorticoid, or saline: a randomized, double-blind, placebo-controlled trial. Am J Sports Med 2013;41(3):625–35.

32. Sayegh ET, Strauch RJ. Does nonsurgical treatment improve longitudinal outcomes of lateral epicondylitis over no treatment? A meta-analysis. Clin Orthop Relat Res 2015;473(3):1093–107.

33. Gautam VK, Verma S, Batra S, et al. Platelet-rich plasma versus corticosteroid injection for recalcitrant lateral epicondylitis: clinical and ultrasonographic evaluation. J Orthop Surg (Hong Kong) 2015;23(1):1–5.

34. Coombes BK, Bisset L, Vicenzino B. Efficacy and safety of corticosteroid injections and other injections for management of tendinopathy: a systematic review of randomised controlled trials. Lancet 2010; 376(9754):1751–67.

35. Olaussen M, Holmedal O, Mdala I, et al. Corticosteroid or placebo injection combined with deep transverse friction massage, Mills manipulation, stretching and eccentric exercise for acute lateral epicondylitis: a randomised, controlled trial. BMC Musculoskelet Disord 2015;16:122.

36. Solheim E, Hegna J, Oyen J. Arthroscopic versus open tennis elbow release: 3- to 6-year results of a case-control series of 305 elbows. Arthroscopy 2013;29(5):854–9.

37. Peart RE, Strickler SS, Schweitzer KM Jr. Lateral epicondylitis: a comparative study of open and arthroscopic lateral release. Am J Orthop (Belle Mead NJ) 2004;33(11):565–7.

38. Dunn JH, Kim JJ, Davis L, et al. Ten- to 14-year follow-up of the Nirschl surgical technique for lateral epicondylitis. Am J Sports Med 2008;36(2):261–6.

39. Baker CL Jr, Baker CL 3rd. Long-term follow-up of arthroscopic treatment of lateral epicondylitis. Am J Sports Med 2008;36(2):254–60.

40. Lattermann C, Romeo AA, Anbari A, et al. Arthroscopic debridement of the extensor carpi radialis brevis for recalcitrant lateral epicondylitis. J Shoulder Elbow Surg 2010;19(5):651–6.

41. Mullett H, Sprague M, Brown G, et al. Arthroscopic treatment of lateral epicondylitis: clinical and cadaveric studies. Clin Orthop Relat Res 2005; 439:123–8.

42. Terra BB, Rodrigues LM, Filho AN, et al. Arthroscopic treatment for chronic lateral epicondylitis. Rev Bras Ortop 2015;50(4):395–402.

43. Oki G, Iba K, Sasaki K, et al. Time to functional recovery after arthroscopic surgery for tennis elbow. J Shoulder Elbow Surg 2014;23(10):1527–31.

44. Baumgard SH, Schwartz DR. Percutaneous release of the epicondylar muscles for humeral epicondylitis. Am J Sports Med 1982;10(4):233–6.

45. Walz DM, Newman JS, Konin GP, et al. Epicondylitis: pathogenesis, imaging, and treatment. Radiographics 2010;30(1):167–84.

46. Vinod AV, Ross G. An effective approach to diagnosis and surgical repair of refractory medial epicondylitis. J Shoulder Elbow Surg 2015;24(8): 1172–7.

47. Stahl S, Kaufman T. The efficacy of an injection of steroids for medial epicondylitis. A prospective study of sixty elbows. J Bone Joint Surg Am 1997; 79(11):1648–52.

48. Gabel GT, Morrey BF. Operative treatment of medial epicondylitis. Influence of concomitant ulnar neuropathy at the elbow. J Bone Joint Surg Am 1995;77(7):1065–9.

49. Vangsness CT Jr, Jobe FW. Surgical treatment of medial epicondylitis. Results in 35 elbows. J Bone Joint Surg Br 1991;73(3):409–11.

50. Grawe BM, Fabricant PD, Chin CS, et al. Clinical outcomes after suture anchor repair of recalcitrant medial epicondylitis. Orthopedics 2016;39(1):e104–7.

51. Abrams GD, Renstrom PA, Safran MR. Epidemiology of musculoskeletal injury in the tennis player. Br J Sports Med 2012;46(7):492–8.

52. Rogowski I, Creveaux T, Sevrez V, et al. How does the scapula move during the tennis serve? Med Sci Sports Exerc 2015;47(7):1444–9.

53. Burkhart SS, Morgan CD, Kibler WB. The disabled throwing shoulder: spectrum of pathology Part III: The SICK scapula, scapular dyskinesis, the kinetic chain, and rehabilitation. Arthroscopy 2003;19(6): 641–61.

54. Ludewig PM, Cook TM. Alterations in shoulder kinematics and associated muscle activity in people with symptoms of shoulder impingement. Phys Ther 2000;80(3):276–91.

55. Laudner KG, Myers JB, Pasquale MR, et al. Scapular dysfunction in throwers with pathologic internal impingement. J Orthop Sports Phys Ther 2006; 36(7):485–94.

56. Mihata T, McGarry MH, Kinoshita M, et al. Excessive glenohumeral horizontal abduction as occurs during the late cocking phase of the throwing motion can be critical for internal impingement. Am J Sports Med 2010;38(2):369–74.

57. Warner JJ, Micheli LJ, Arslanian LE, et al. Scapulothoracic motion in normal shoulders and shoulders with glenohumeral instability and impingement syndrome. A study using Moire topographic analysis. Clin Orthop Relat Res 1992;285:191–9.

58. Kibler WB, Ludewig PM, McClure PW, et al. Clinical implications of scapular dyskinesis in shoulder injury: the 2013 consensus statement from the 'Scapular Summit'. Br J Sports Med 2013;47(14):877–85.

59. Carbone S, Postacchini R, Gumina S. Scapular dyskinesis and SICK syndrome in patients with a chronic type III acromioclavicular dislocation. Results of rehabilitation. Knee Surg Sports Traumatol Arthrosc 2015;23(5):1473–80.

60. Merolla G, De Santis E, Campi F, et al. Supraspinatus and infraspinatus weakness in overhead athletes with scapular dyskinesis: strength assessment before and after restoration of scapular musculature balance. Musculoskelet Surg 2010;94(3):119–25.

61. Kibler WB, Kuhn JE, Wilk K, et al. The disabled throwing shoulder: spectrum of pathology-10-year update. Arthroscopy 2013;29(1):141–161 e126.

62. Wilk KE, Macrina LC, Fleisig GS, et al. Correlation of glenohumeral internal rotation deficit and total rotational motion to shoulder injuries in professional baseball pitchers. Am J Sports Med 2011;39(2): 329–35.

63. Mihata T, Gates J, McGarry MH, et al. Effect of posterior shoulder tightness on internal impingement in a cadaveric model of throwing. Knee Surg Sports Traumatol Arthrosc 2015;23(2):548–54.

64. Mine K, Nakayama T, Milanese S, et al. Effectiveness of stretching on posterior shoulder tightness and glenohumeral internal rotation deficit: a systematic review of randomised controlled trials. J Sport Rehabil 2016;24:1–28.

65. Halbrecht JL, Tirman P, Atkin D. Internal impingement of the shoulder: comparison of findings between the throwing and nonthrowing shoulders of college baseball players. Arthroscopy 1999;15(3):253–8.

66. Myers JB, Laudner KG, Pasquale MR, et al. Glenohumeral range of motion deficits and posterior shoulder tightness in throwers with pathologic internal impingement. Am J Sports Med 2006;34(3):385–91.

67. Burkhart SS, Morgan CD, Kibler WB. The disabled throwing shoulder: spectrum of pathology. Part II: evaluation and treatment of SLAP lesions in throwers. Arthroscopy 2003;19(5):531–9.

68. Snyder SJ, Banas MP, Karzel RP. An analysis of 140 injuries to the superior glenoid labrum. J Shoulder Elbow Surg 1995;4(4):243–8.

69. Grossman MG, Tibone JE, McGarry MH, et al. A cadaveric model of the throwing shoulder: a possible etiology of superior labrum anterior-to-posterior lesions. J Bone Joint Surg Am 2005;87(4):824–31.

70. Kuhn JE, Lindholm SR, Huston LJ, et al. Failure of the biceps superior labral complex: a cadaveric biomechanical investigation comparing the late cocking and early deceleration positions of throwing. Arthroscopy 2003;19(4):373–9.

71. Ben Kibler W, Sciascia AD, Hester P, et al. Clinical utility of traditional and new tests in the diagnosis of biceps tendon injuries and superior labrum anterior and posterior lesions in the shoulder. Am J Sports Med 2009;37(9):1840–7.

72. Sheridan K, Kreulen C, Kim S, et al. Accuracy of magnetic resonance imaging to diagnose superior labrum anterior-posterior tears. Knee Surg Sports Traumatol Arthrosc 2015;23(9):2645–50.

73. Brockmeier SF, Voos JE, Williams RJ 3rd, et al. Outcomes after arthroscopic repair of type-II SLAP lesions. J Bone Joint Surg Am 2009;91(7):1595–603.

74. Neuman BJ, Boisvert CB, Reiter B, et al. Results of arthroscopic repair of type II superior labral anterior posterior lesions in overhead athletes: assessment of return to preinjury playing level and satisfaction. Am J Sports Med 2011;39(9):1883–8.

75. Glasgow SG, Bruce RA, Yacobucci GN, et al. Arthroscopic resection of glenoid labral tears in the athlete: a report of 29 cases. Arthroscopy 1992; 8(1):48–54.

76. Patterson BM, Creighton RA, Spang JT, et al. Surgical trends in the treatment of superior labrum anterior and posterior lesions of the shoulder: analysis of data from the American Board of Orthopaedic Surgery Certification Examination Database. Am J Sports Med 2014;42(8):1904–10.

77. Sayde WM, Cohen SB, Ciccotti MG, et al. Return to play after Type II superior labral anterior-posterior lesion repairs in athletes: a systematic review. Clin Orthop Relat Res 2012;470(6):1595–600.

78. Gorantla K, Gill C, Wright RW. The outcome of type II SLAP repair: a systematic review. Arthroscopy 2010; 26(4):537–45.

79. Kim SH, Ha KI, Kim SH, et al. Results of arthroscopic treatment of superior labral lesions. J Bone Joint Surg Am 2002;84-A(6):981–5.

80. Dillman CJ, Fleisig GS, Andrews JR. Biomechanics of pitching with emphasis upon shoulder kinematics. J Orthop Sports Phys Ther 1993;18(2):402–8.

81. Burkhart SS, Diaz Pagan JL, Wirth MA, et al. Cyclic loading of anchor-based rotator cuff repairs: confirmation of the tension overload phenomenon and comparison of suture anchor fixation with transosseous fixation. Arthroscopy 1997;13(6):720–4.

82. Andrews JR, Broussard TS, Carson WG. Arthroscopy of the shoulder in the management of partial tears of the rotator cuff: a preliminary report. Arthroscopy 1985;1(2):117–22.

83. Payne LZ, Altchek DW, Craig EV, et al. Arthroscopic treatment of partial rotator cuff tears in young athletes. A preliminary report. Am J Sports Med 1997; 25(3):299–305.

84. Tibone JE, Elrod B, Jobe FW, et al. Surgical treatment of tears of the rotator cuff in athletes. J Bone Joint Surg Am 1986;68(6):887–91.

85. Mazoue CG, Andrews JR. Repair of full-thickness rotator cuff tears in professional baseball players. Am J Sports Med 2006;34(2):182–9.

Upper Extremity Injuries in Gymnasts

Megan R. Wolf, MD[a], Daniel Avery, MD[a], Jennifer Moriatis Wolf, MD[b],*

KEYWORDS

- Gymnast • Wrist pain • Carpal instability • Ulnar positive • Ulnar abutment
- Triangular fibrocartilage complex • Scaphoid stress fracture • Grip lock injury

KEY POINTS

- Gymnasts' wrist is a complex entity with multiple potential diagnoses caused by load bearing on the upper extremity.
- Distal radial physeal injury can occur with load in the immature wrist and lead to later ulnar positive variance and ulnar abutment.
- Ulnar abutment and TFCC tears are common causes of ulnar-sided wrist pain in gymnasts.
- Scaphoid stress fractures can occur because of stress with loading at the scaphoid waist.
- Grip lock injuries are unique to gymnastics and are caused when the leather or dowel grip worn on the wrist/hand locks onto a bar and prevents the wrist from rotating.

INTRODUCTION

Gymnastics is a unique sport with varied activity requirements that cause the upper extremity to be used as a weight-bearing extremity. The load demands on the wrist can lead to musculoskeletal issues with chronic use and overuse. In 1989, Mandelbaum and colleagues[1] reported that 87.5% of male gymnasts and 55% of female gymnasts complained of wrist pain with activities requiring compression and impaction of the joint. Of this cohort, 75% of male gymnasts and 33% of female gymnasts noted wrist pain for longer than 3 months. The authors termed these findings "wrist pain syndrome," incorporating ligamentous tears, triangular fibrocartilage complex (TFCC) tears, and secondary chondromalacia of the carpus. Gymnastics as a sport has become more demanding with complex stunts requiring the athletes to begin at a younger age and to train more hours during the week to advance. The abnormal amount of weight bearing on the wrist at a young age has shown changes in the development of the wrist in addition to the more typical overuse complaints in this population of athletes.

DISTAL RADIUS PHYSEAL INJURY
Background

Physeal injuries to the immature distal radius present in a range from mild dorsal wrist pain without radiographic changes to physeal arrest. Because most gymnasts participate in the sport at an early age, the physis is a common site of injury especially with wrist compressive forces reported to be 16 times body weight.[2,3] The immature wrist typically exhibits negative ulnar variance,[4] which naturally distributes a higher load to the distal radius compared with the 80% load seen in neutral variance.[5] Stress injury to the distal radius physis was originally described by Read[6] in three gymnasts with radiographic changes. It is postulated that physeal injury may be the result of compromised blood supply to the metaphyseal and

Disclosure Statement. The authors have nothing to disclose.
[a] Department of Orthopaedic Surgery, University of Connecticut Health Center, 263 Farmington Avenue, MARB4-ORTHO, Farmington, CT 06030-4037, USA; [b] Department of Orthopaedic Surgery and Rehabilitation, University of Chicago Hospitals, 5841 South Maryland Avenue, MC 3079, Chicago, IL 60637, USA
* Corresponding author.
E-mail address: jmwolf@uchicago.edu

hand.theclinics.com

epiphyseal area leading to uncalcified chondrocytes.[7] Chronic compression can lead to full arrest manifested as a shift to ulnar positivity[8,9] or a partial closure appearing similar to a Madelung deformity.[9–11]

Diagnosis

Clinical evaluation should include a thorough history to define the chronicity and the elements that most exacerbate symptoms. Pain, noted as generally dull and aching at the dorsal wrist, is typically experienced with loading in elements, such as floor routines, vaulting, or pommel horse, and relieved with rest. Although pain at rest may be from other causes, it can also be a sign of a more severe injury. On examination, tenderness to palpation at the distal radial physis is noted. Radiographs often show characteristic changes as described by Roy and colleagues[12]: widening of the radial physis, cystic changes of the metaphysis, beaking of the distal aspect of the epiphysis, and haziness within the physis. When radiographs are negative, MRI is recommended to further evaluate the physis and to rule out other causes.

Conservative Modalities

Conservative treatment, as in other overuse-type injuries, centers on avoidance of compressive loading, splinting for immobilization, and often complete rest with no gymnastics participation. There are no known pharmacologic treatments to support an injured physis, and unless pain is experienced at rest, analgesics are not recommended. Reassessment after 6 weeks should be performed to consider the athlete suitable for gradual return. Physical therapy should be prescribed to address the entire upper extremity and contralateral side when improved ability to dissipate forces may prevent recurrence. Return to gymnastic elements should begin gradually, with slowly increasing wrist loading if the athlete remains pain free.

Surgical Treatment

Surgery is reserved for treating the consequences of compressive load on the distal radius physis with injury or arrest, specifically focused on the treatment of resulting positive ulnar variance.[13] Long-term observational studies of gymnasts are scant in literature. Although Claessens and colleagues[14] showed progressive ulnar negativity in gymnasts in 4- to 5-year follow-up, DiFiori and coworkers[15] showed significantly greater ulnar variance compared with normative values at 3-year follow-up. If ulnar-positive variance is noted in association with radial physeal arrest, this should be treated to avoid progressive degeneration with ulnar abutment and articular surface changes and TFCC degeneration (discussed later). Partial closure of the radial physis should be treated only if symptomatic, or if progressive deformity creates unacceptable clinical malalignment. Radial physiolysis and ulnar shortening with or without distal ulna epiphyiodesis is corrective if growth potential remains.[16]

Outcomes

Longitudinal studies for distal radius physeal injuries are minimal. Bak and Boeckstyns[17] described the use of epiphysiodesis of the distal radius and ulna in a 14-year-old gymnast with a 1-year history of wrist pain that interfered with gymnastics, and radiographs showing widening of the radial physis and premature closure of the ulnar aspect. They reported good results with a gymnast who was asymptomatic at 16 months postoperatively and qualified for the national team. Injuries typically present late when premature closure of the physis leads to consequences of ulnar abutment from positive ulnar variance; thus, it is difficult to ascertain how many gymnasts go on to have issues requiring surgical treatment. Treatment of resultant ulnar abutment and/or TFCC tears is described in the following sections.

ULNAR ABUTMENT OF THE WRIST
Background

Excessive transmission of load to the ulnar side of the wrist is called ulnar abutment or ulnar impaction syndrome. With neutral ulnar variance, the distal ulna experiences about 20% of the load of the wrist. With 2 mm of positive ulnar variance, this load can almost double.[5] This is a dynamic change as seen in gymnasts with wrist extension and forearm pronation, such as a handstand, or it is seen at maturity with associated premature radial physeal closure.[8,18] This leads to degeneration of the TFCC and articular surfaces of the distal ulna and lunate.

Diagnosis

Ulna abutment is one of several causes of ulnar-sided wrist pain in the athlete. This entity typically presents with insidious onset of progressive ulnar-sided wrist pain that eventually affects athletic performance. Tenderness to palpation is typically isolated dorsally at the prestyloid recess of the ulna.[19] Loss of wrist and forearm motion may inhibit such elements as the floor exercises, whereas pain with compressive forces affects the vault or pommel horse. Reproduction of pain with the wrist in ulnar deviation as the forearm is taken through a full arc of motion (ulnocarpal stress test[20]) can help confirm the diagnosis. The distal radial ulna joint (DRUJ) should also be assessed because ulnar variance can affect the peak pressure across the DRUJ.[21] Standard radiographic assessment can reveal positive ulnar variance, but if neutral or negative, a pronated, maximum grip radiograph is helpful in confirming dynamic positive ulnar variance.[22] Radiographs may also show cystic or degenerative changes in the proximal ulnar corner of the lunate. In unclear cases or with suspected concomitant pathology, MRI is a useful modality (**Fig. 1**).

Conservative Treatment

Symptomatic ulnar abutment is treated based on the level at which it affects performance. The natural history is one of progressive worsening pain with loading.[23] For mild symptoms, modifying activities, taping, or brace wear may be helpful. As symptoms become more severe, limiting provocative movements in practice can help an athlete still perform in competition. In the chronic setting, intra-articular steroid injections may temporarily alleviate symptoms but should be used with caution in young athletes.

Surgical Treatment

Surgical treatment is aimed at reducing ulnar variance and if present, addressing degeneration or injury of the TFCC. In adolescents who are skeletally immature, arthroscopic debridement of the TFCC combined with modification or avoidance of specific load-bearing gymnastic elements has been described.[1] The standard of surgical

treatment remains ulna shortening osteotomy,[19] reserved for skeletally mature individuals. Plate fixation of the osteotomy requires 4 to 6 weeks of cast immobilization followed by a removable splint, until bone healing is confirmed. Rehabilitation is then required, usually negating same-season return to play. However, this approach corrects positive ulnar variance, prominent ulnar styloid, or associated lunotriquetral instability without violating the TFCC. Secondary procedures are occasionally required for treatment of nonunion or removal of symptomatic hardware.[24]

Outcomes

Specific outcomes for the previously mentioned procedures have not been reported in athletes, much less gymnasts, but results from other populations are overall positive. Tomaino and Weiser[25] reported arthroscopic TFCC debridement combined with ulnar wafer resection in 12 patients noting all were very satisfied or satisfied, complete resolution of pain in 66%, and improved motion and grip strength. Ulnar-shortening osteotomy for ulnar impaction has likewise demonstrated good outcomes. Iwasaki and colleagues[26] reported on 51 patients with 91% having no or minimal pain, significantly improved flexion/extension but not pronation/supination, grip strength similar to the contralateral side, and 57% able to return to their preinjury level of activity.

TRIANGULAR FIBROCARTILAGE COMPLEX TEARS
Background

TFCC is a common cause of ulnar-sided wrist pain in gymnasts. This complex structure supports the ulnar side of the wrist with attachments to the radius, ulnar styloid and fovea, and extensor carpi ulnaris tendon sheath. It is composed of a central disk with deep and superficial peripheral limbs that course on the volar and dorsal aspect, supporting the DRUJ.[27] Injury can occur in isolation or as a result of other processes, such as ulnar abutment or extensor carpi ulnaris subluxation/dislocation. Central articular disk tears usually result from axial load with wrist extended, ulnar deviated, and forearm pronated, which can double the load seen on the ulnar side of the wrist.[28] Peripheral tears are thought to occur with rapid twisting of the wrist.

Diagnosis

Wrist pain caused by TFCC tears can occur acutely (peripheral tears) or have a more insidious onset (central tears). Athletes complain of deep

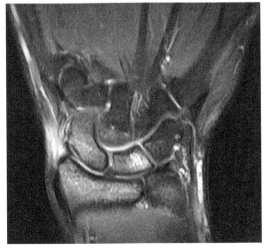

Fig. 1. MRI image showing lunate signal change consistent with ulnar impaction syndrome in a gymnast.

aching pain along the ulnar side of the wrist, pain with forceful gripping, generalized weakness, or a clicking sensation with pronation and supination.[29] Palpable tenderness is located at the ulnar side of the wrist and maximally at the prestyloid recess. Pain may be exacerbated by hyperpronation or supination or with stressing the DRUJ in end range of rotation. Plain radiographic assessment is helpful in evaluating static or dynamic positive ulnar variance. MRI can show cartilage surface changes and tears of the TFCC; however, diagnostic wrist arthroscopy is still the standard for TFCC tears. A recent systematic review by Andersson and colleagues[30] showed the negative predictive value of clinical tests to be 55%, with MRI showing a range between 37% and 90%.

Conservative Treatment

There are various conservative initial treatments of TFCC injuries. Activity modification to avoid exacerbating elements, with or without splinting, may allow continued gymnastics participation. Steroid injections into the ulnocarpal joint are diagnostic and therapeutic, but their use in acute injuries should be judicious because they could impede normal healing. Therapy to work on decreasing inflammation and strengthening of the entire upper extremity, while not specifically addressing the tear, can teach the athlete adaptive use to absorb impact and avoid provocation.

Surgical Treatment

Arthroscopy is the mainstay of diagnosis and treatment.[30] Palmer classified traumatic and degenerative tears into subtypes to which different forms of treatment are delineated.[27,29] The central avascular and peripheral vascular portions dictate different forms of treatment. Tears of the central disk (Palmer I-A) are treated with debridement. A variety of arthroscopic techniques have been shown effective in repairing proximal or distal peripheral tears.[31–35] Palmer I-D, or radial attachment tears, is somewhat controversial because blood supply has been shown to be poor[36,37] giving credence to debridement. However, several other authors have shown successful healing after repair possibly because of abrading the sigmoid notch during repair.[31,38–41] In cases of positive ulnar variance, concomitant ulnar shortening or wafer procedures are considered. Arthroscopic debridement alone requires a short period of immobilization (2 weeks) followed by slow progression back to competition, whereas repair requires 6 to 12 weeks of immobilization before return with protection against forceful pronation/supination.

Outcomes

Outcomes of isolated TFCC treatment are difficult to assess in the literature because of variation and concomitant procedures. Husby and Haugstvedt[42] reported on 35 patients with debridement alone of central or radial tears with 77% assessed as excellent or good by the Mayo Modified Wrist score. Wysocki and colleagues[43] reported on 11 high-level athletes in whom 64% were able to return to sport. However, those who required bearing weight through their wrists were unable to return to competition. However, Mandelbaum and coworkers[1] suggested that arthroscopic treatment was successful in patients with "gymnasts' wrist," which could include TFCC tears.

SCAPHOID STRESS FRACTURES
Background

Repetitive stress on a weight-bearing limb may lead to subthreshold load onto the bone leading to a stress fracture. Stress fractures occur when new or increased activity causes increased bone remodeling, resulting in a relative weakening of the bone as resorption occurs before new bone formation.[44] Furthermore, muscle strength and hypertrophy result before bone remodeling, thus causing an increased force on vulnerable bone.[45]

There are multiple case reports of scaphoid stress fractures in elite level gymnasts, especially in those who have rapidly increased their level of training (**Table 1**).[46–51] Specific load on the scaphoid at the wrist is caused by forced extension, radial deviation, and rotation of the wrist, all motions common in gymnastic activities. Because of the ligamentous attachments proximally and distally on the scaphoid, the scaphoid tends to fail at the waist, which is the point of the greatest bending moment.[52]

Diagnosis

Athletes may present with a history of acute or chronic wrist pain aggravated by extension and focal tenderness over the anatomic snuffbox.[49] Radiographs may be negative at presentation, or may show an area of sclerosis at the scaphoid waist. If clinically suspicious for a stress fracture, MRI typically demonstrates increased signal at the scaphoid waist (**Fig. 2**).

Conservative Modalities

Scaphoid stress fractures may be treated nonoperatively with a thumb spica cast for 8 to 12 weeks, with avoidance of wrist loading during this time. After confirmation of healing using advanced imaging, either computed tomography or MRI,

Table 1
Scaphoid stress fracture case reports

Reference	Patient Age/Sex	Level	Pain Duration	Laterality	Radiographic Presentation	Treatment	Return to Sport
Hanks et al,[47] 1989	18 M	Junior Olympic	2 y	Bilateral	Transverse fracture through waist with sclerotic boarders; bone scan increased uptake	Thumb spica cast 4 mo	8 mo
			1 wk		Bone scan increased uptake	Thumb spica cast 6 wk	Not stated
	18 M	College	2 mo	Unilateral	Normal; bone scan increased uptake	Thumb spica cast 6 wk	Not stated
Manzione and Pizzutillo,[46] 1981	16 M	Nationally ranked	4 wk	Unilateral	Normal; bone scan increased uptake	Thumb spica cast 15 wk	15 wk
Matzkin and Singer,[49] 2000	13 M	State champion	6 mo	Unilateral	Midwaist nondisplaced fracture with sclerosis around waist	Long arm spica cast 8 wk; short arm splint 4 wk	6 mo
Nakamoto et al,[51] 2011	18 M	Not stated	3 mo	Unilateral	Fracture waist and widening radial distal radial epiphysis	Percutaneous screw	16 wk
Yamagiwa et al,[50] 2009	18 M	Nationally ranked	Not stated	Unilateral	Normal; MRI fracture waist	Wrist brace for 2 mo, failed; percutaneous screw	2 mo postoperative
Engel and Feldner-Busztin,[48] 1991	18 M (bilateral)	Not stated	1 y	Bilateral	Bilateral stress fracture waist; bone scan increased uptake	Not stated	Not stated

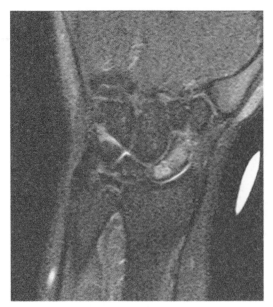

Fig. 2. MRI image demonstrating abnormal signal in the scaphoid consistent with scaphoid stress fracture in a 20-year-old collegiate gymnast. In this case, computed tomography showed no abnormalities.

combined with no tenderness on examination, the gymnast may return to sport gradually.

Surgical Treatment

Operative treatment with screw fixation has been described to treat stress fractures in this population.[50,51] Yamagiwa and colleagues[50] reported on an 18-year-old male nationally ranked gymnast with a scaphoid stress fracture who was treated with percutaneous screw fixation and was able to return to gymnastics 2 months postoperatively. Surgical treatment may provide stabilization of the fracture to prevent displacement and earlier rehabilitation and return to sport (Fig. 3).

Outcomes

Studies of immobilization for scaphoid stress fractures have shown good outcomes, with all athletes returning to gymnastics after radiographic confirmation of healing.[46,47,49] The timing of return ranged from 15 weeks to 8 months after identification of the stress fracture. Scaphoid stress fractures are relatively uncommon except in populations where the upper extremity is loaded as in weight bearing, such as gymnastics. A high suspicion for stress fracture of the scaphoid should be maintained in gymnasts with chronic wrist pain, especially with wrist extension.

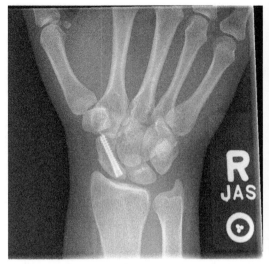

Fig. 3. Headless screw fixation performed after the gymnast failed a trial of nonoperative immobilization.

GRIP LOCK INJURY
Background

In the recent era of gymnastics, athletes have attempted to perform stunts with increasing complexity and power. For events on the high bar in men's gymnastics and uneven bars in women's gymnastics, such activities as the giant swing, which requires increased forces and velocity about the wrist, increased friction on the hand and strength is required. To address this issue, gymnasts have used leather grips, or grips with plastic or wooden dowels to provide protection from friction and increase grip strength (Fig. 4).[53] The use of these grips has led to a gymnastic-specific wrist injury termed a "grip lock injury."

Diagnosis

Grip lock occurs when the leather grip or dowel completely encircles the bar or a portion of the grip becomes caught between the palm and high bar. As the grip catches, the gymnast's hand stops rotating and "locks" onto the bar.[53] The gymnast's body continues rotating around the bar, resulting in sprains, tendon injuries, or fractures. Samuelson and colleagues[53] performed a survey of Illinois colleges and high school gymnastic programs to determine the incidence and mechanism of grip lock injury over a 10-year period. Thirty-eight grip lock injuries were reported among male gymnasts, including 17 high school and 21 collegiate athletes. Of these injuries, 20 were fractures and 3 were sprains. Nineteen of 23 gymnasts reported using dowel grips. The skills in which injury happened were those involving a "cubital grip,"

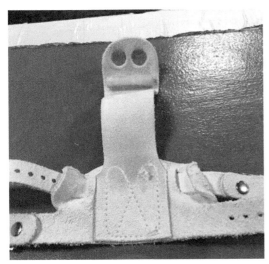

Fig. 4. Leather dowel grip. Gymnasts use leather grips with a plastic or wooden dowel to decrease friction and allow for an increase in grip strength during the high bar or uneven bar events. (*Courtesy of* M. Boyer, MD, MSc, FRCS(C), St Louis, MO.)

or internal rotation of the arm with pronation and flexion of the wrist (**Fig. 5**). Other case reports have described grip lock injuries including open fractures, extensor tendon injury, and extensor tendon strain (**Table 2**).[54–56]

Grip lock injury has been attributed to increased slack in the hand grip equipment.[53] Increased slack may be caused by grips being stretched and worn, too large, or sliding up the wrist. With increased material, the grip is more likely to encircle the bar, thus causing the hand to lock.

Outcomes

Nearly all patients were reported to have returned to gymnastics after a course of nonoperative or operative treatment. One exception was a 24-year-old collegiate gymnast who was found to have attenuation of the extensor digitorum communis tendons to the index finger, middle finger, and ring finger, and adhesions of the extensor indicis proprius, and index finger extensor digitorum communis at the level of the dorsal wrist extensor compartments.[55] This gymnast required two surgeries to optimize extensor tendon function. Residual symptoms are common after these injuries, including extensor tendon lag and loss of motion at the wrist and elbow. Moreover, some athletes have residual pain and limitations in gymnastic participation.[53]

Prevention of grip lock injury is important, to decrease the risk of severe injury in the gymnast. Therefore, grips should be checked before use because it is critical to use a properly fitting grip.

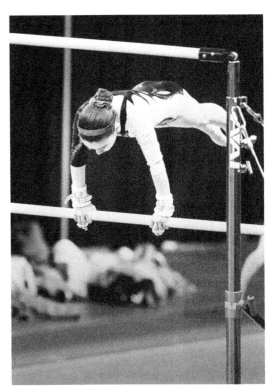

Fig. 5. Uneven bars with leather dowel grip. Gymnast performing a cast maneuver, which requires the gymnast to elevate above the plane parallel to the floor. (*Courtesy of* M. Boyer, MD, MSc, FRCS(C), St Louis, MO.)

Stretched or old grips should be discarded immediately to prevent grip lock injury.

LAXITY RELATED WRIST PAIN
Background

Hypermobility syndrome, first described by Kirk and colleagues[57] in 1967, is defined as joint laxity associated with complaints of the musculoskeletal system. In a study performed in male first division rugby players, the investigators found that the incidence of injury was significantly higher in athletes who were hypermobile compared with athletes with stiffer joints.[58] Gymnasts have been found to have a greater joint laxity compared with other groups.[59] Whether athletes who are hypermobile choose the sport of gymnastics or the laxity is induced with hours of training, joint hypermobility may put them at an increased risk for musculoskeletal complaints, injuries, and overuse injuries.

In a radiographic study, Schernberg[60] concluded that increased soft tissue laxity was associated with a higher incidence of overuse injury versus a control population. Several wrist conditions, such as nondissociative carpal instability, synovial cysts, and chondrocalcinosis, have been linked to

Table 2
Grip lock injury cases

Reference	Patient Age/Sex	Level	Mechanism	Injury	Treatment	Outcome	Return to Sport
Bezek et al,[54] 2009	20 M	Division I	High bar, overgrip position dismount	Ulnar styloid avulsion; EDC strain at musculotendinous junction, PQ strain	Short arm cast 4 wk	35° EIP lag, DRUJ crepitus	5 mo
	18 M	High school senior	High bar, overgrip position dismount	Open both bone forearm fracture; complete rupture IF EDC at musculotendinous junction; stretching EDC IF/MF/RF with enlongation	Operative	MCP extension lac IF/MF/RF, extension contractures digit/wrist; 45° loss wrist flexion	Not stated
Sathyendra and Payatakes,[55] 2013	24 M	College	High bar, overhand grip during giant swing	Nondisplaced ulnar styloid fx; rupture musculotendonous junction EDC; adhesions EIP and IF EDC to compartment floor; intratendinous attenuation extensors to IF/MF/RF	Operative	Extensor lag 60° IF and MF, 35° RF	Did not return
Updegrove et al,[56] 2015	15 M	Not stated	High bar, performing giants	Salter Harris II radius fracture, diaphyseal fracture radius/ulna, avulsion base of third MC	Operative	Full return to function	Not stated

Abbreviation: EDC, extensor digitorum communis; EIP, extensor indicis proprius; IF/MF/RF, index finger, middle finger, and ring finger; MC, metacarpal; MCP, metacarpophalangeal joint; PQ, pronator quadratus.

hypermobility syndrome.[60,61] Garcia-Elias and co-workers studied the kinematic behavior of the scaphoid[62] and perilunate motion[63] in subjects with joint laxity, and noted that global wrist laxity affected scaphoid motion only. Wrist conditions, such as scapholunate injury and midcarpal instability (MCI), may therefore be attributable to laxity in the competitive gymnast.

Wrist Capsulitis

Wrist capsulitis is a disorder of diffuse dorsal wrist pain, tenderness, and swelling. Pain occurs with weight bearing onto the affected extremity, as is common in gymnastics. This may be caused by repetitive impaction or subluxation of the proximal carpal row or dorsal radius and the distal carpal row, which results in inflammation.[28] The ability of the carpal rows to appose may be seen in patients with ligamentous laxity.

Scapholunate Interosseous Ligament Injury

Global laxity and chronic weight bearing on the wrist in extension affects the scaphoid kinematics.[62,63] Scapholunate interosseous ligament (SLIL) injury occurs when the wrist is loaded in extension and ulnar deviation, which results in the capitate driving between the scaphoid and lunate. Snider and colleagues[64] reported three cases of SLIL injury caused by overuse in three gymnasts. These gymnasts were nationally ranked and had no acute wrist injury, but presented for chronic wrist pain and were found to have SLIL disruption. The authors hypothesized that the wrist is placed at risk because of twisting, dismount type of activities that place maximum stress on the radial wrist. All three patients were able to return to gymnastics after arthroscopic debridement and rest.

MIDCARPAL INSTABILITY

MCI is defined as an altered carpal anatomy that leads to hypermobility of the proximal row of the carpus.[61] Lichtman and colleagues[65] described the "ring theory" of wrist kinematics. The authors proposed that the carpus has two distinct rows connected at the scaphotrapezotrapezoidal and the triquetral-hamate (TH) joint. In normal wrist mechanics, radial deviation of the distal carpal row concentrates force at the scaphotrapezotrapezoidal joint, which causes proximal row flexion. In contrast, ulnar wrist deviation concentrates forces at the TH joint, which causes proximal row extension. Disruption of these connections disrupts the balance of these forces and causes dissociative deformity, as is seen in volar intercalated segmental instability and dorsal intercalated segmental instability.

MCI nondissociative is caused by ligamentous laxity as opposed to ligamentous disruption. Palmar MCI is the most common form of MCI, and typically occurs in patients who are ligamentously lax.[61] The volar arcuate, dorsal radiotriquetral, and periscaphoid ligaments are lax, leading to proximal row sag. In ulnar deviation, the normal joint reaction forces are not engaged and the carpus maintains a volar deformity until the TH engages at near maximal ulnar deviation, leading to forceful dorsal translation and a palpable "catch-up clunk."[61] Another type of MCI that may be seen in patients with ligamentous laxity is chronic capitolunate instability. Chronic capitolunate instability is seen after a previous extension injury to the wrist that caused attenuation of the palmar radiocapitate ligament.[61] This injury leads to chronic pain, weakness, and wrist clicking.

Dissociative and nondissociative carpal instabilities may be seen in gymnasts and decrease performance.[28] These changes may be associated with dorsal ganglions, and radioscaphoid, lunotriquetral, or ulnocarpal impactions. Chronic loading of the gymnast's wrist may worsen the underlying laxity, leading to instability, pain, and subsequent inability to compete.

SUMMARY

Wrist pain in the gymnast is a common problem and may have multiple causes. Because of the initiation of training at a young age and repetitive weight bearing on the upper extremity to advance to the elite level, these athletes are prone to wrist injuries. Further research is needed to understand this unique population of athletes and how to prevent and effectively treat these career-ending injuries.

REFERENCES

1. Mandelbaum BR, Bartolozzi AR, Davis CA, et al. Wrist pain syndrome in the gymnast. Pathogenetic, diagnostic, and therapeutic considerations. Am J Sports Med 1989;17(3):305–17.
2. Koh TJ, Grabiner MD, Weiker GG. Technique and ground reaction forces in the back handspring. Am J Sports Med 1992;20(1):61–6.
3. Markolf KL, Shapiro MS, Mandelbaum BR, et al. Wrist loading patterns during pommel horse exercises. J Biomech 1990;23(10):1001–11.
4. Hafner R, Poznanski AK, Donovan JM. Ulnar variance in children–standard measurements for evaluation of ulnar shortening in juvenile rheumatoid arthritis, hereditary multiple exostosis and other

bone or joint disorders in childhood. Skeletal Radiol 1989;18(7):513–6.

5. Palmer AK, Werner FW. Biomechanics of the distal radioulnar joint. Clin Orthop Relat Res 1984;187: 26–35.

6. Read MT. Stress fractures of the distal radius in adolescent gymnasts. Br J Sports Med 1981;15(4): 272–6.

7. Jaramillo D, Laor T, Zaleske DJ. Indirect trauma to the growth plate: results of MR imaging after epiphyseal and metaphyseal injury in rabbits. Radiology 1993;187(1):171–8.

8. DiFiori JP, Caine DJ, Malina RM. Wrist pain, distal radial physeal injury, and ulnar variance in the young gymnast. Am J Sports Med 2006;34(5):840–9.

9. De Smet L, Claessens A, Fabry G. Gymnast wrist. Acta Orthop Belg 1993;59(4):377–80.

10. Brooks TJ. Madelung deformity in a collegiate gymnast: a case report. J Athl Train 2001;36(2):170–3.

11. Vender MI, Watson HK. Acquired Madelung-like deformity in a gymnast. J Hand Surg Am 1988; 13(1):19–21.

12. Roy S, Caine D, Singer KM. Stress changes of the distal radial epiphysis in young gymnasts. A report of twenty-one cases and a review of the literature. Am J Sports Med 1985;13(5):301–8.

13. Little JT, Klionsky NB, Chaturvedi AA, et al. Pediatric distal forearm and wrist injury: an imaging review. Radiographics 2014;34(2):472–90.

14. Claessens A, Lefevre J, Philippaerts R, et al. The ulnar variance phenomenon: a study in young gymnasts. In: Armstrong N, Kirby B, Welsman J, editors. Children and exercise XIX. London: E & FN Spon; 1997. p. 537–41.

15. DiFiori J, Puffer J, Dorey A. Ulnar variance in young gymnasts: a three-year study. Med Sci Sports Exerc 2001;33:S223.

16. Kozin SH, Zlotolow DA. Madelung deformity. J Hand Surg Am 2015;40(10):2090–8.

17. Bak K, Boeckstyns M. Epiphysiodesis for bilateral irregular closure of the distal radial physis in a gymnast. Scand J Med Sci Sports 1997;7(6):363–6.

18. De Smet L, Claessens A, Lefevre J, et al. Gymnast wrist: an epidemiologic survey of ulnar variance and stress changes of the radial physis in elite female gymnasts. Am J Sports Med 1994;22(6):846–50.

19. Jarrett CD, Baratz ME. The management of ulnocarpal abutment and degenerative triangular fibrocartilage complex tears in the competitive athlete. Hand Clin 2012;28(3):329–37.

20. Nakamura R, Horii E, Imaeda T, et al. The ulnocarpal stress test in the diagnosis of ulnar-sided wrist pain. J Hand Surg Br 1997;22(6):719–23.

21. Nishiwaki M, Nakamura T, Nagura T, et al. Ulnar-shortening effect on distal radioulnar joint pressure: a biomechanical study. J Hand Surg Am 2008;33(2): 198–205.

22. Tomaino MM. The importance of the pronated grip x-ray view in evaluating ulnar variance. J Hand Surg Am 2000;25(2):352–7.

23. Bernstein MA, Nagle DJ, Martinez A, et al. A comparison of combined arthroscopic triangular fibrocartilage complex debridement and arthroscopic wafer distal ulna resection versus arthroscopic triangular fibrocartilage complex debridement and ulnar shortening osteotomy for ulnocarpal abutment syndrome. Arthroscopy 2004;20(4):392–401.

24. Sachar K. Ulnar-sided wrist pain: evaluation and treatment of triangular fibrocartilage complex tears, ulnocarpal impaction syndrome, and lunotriquetral ligament tears. J Hand Surg Am 2008; 33(9):1669–79.

25. Tomaino MM, Weiser RW. Combined arthroscopic TFCC debridement and wafer resection of the distal ulna in wrists with triangular fibrocartilage complex tears and positive ulnar variance. J Hand Surg Am 2001;26(6):1047–52.

26. Iwasaki N, Ishikawa J, Kato H, et al. Factors affecting results of ulnar shortening for ulnar impaction syndrome. Clin Orthop Relat Res 2007; 465:215–9.

27. Palmer AK. Triangular fibrocartilage complex lesions: a classification. J Hand Surg Am 1989;14(4): 594–606.

28. Dobyns JH, Gabel GT. Gymnast's wrist. Hand Clin 1990;6(3):493–505.

29. Geissler WB, Burkett JL. Ligamentous sports injuries of the hand and wrist. Sports Med Arthrosc 2014; 22(1):39–44.

30. Andersson JK, Andernord D, Karlsson J, et al. Efficacy of magnetic resonance imaging and clinical tests in diagnostics of wrist ligament injuries: a systematic review. Arthroscopy 2015;31(10): 2014–20.e2.

31. Trumble TE, Gilbert M, Vedder N. Isolated tears of the triangular fibrocartilage: management by early arthroscopic repair. J Hand Surg Am 1997;22(1): 57–65.

32. de Araujo W, Poehling GG, Kuzma GR. New Tuohy needle technique for triangular fibrocartilage complex repair: preliminary studies. Arthroscopy 1996; 12(6):699–703.

33. Corso SJ, Savoie FH, Geissler WB, et al. Arthroscopic repair of peripheral avulsions of the triangular fibrocartilage complex of the wrist: a multicenter study. Arthroscopy 1997;13(1):78–84.

34. Estrella EP, Hung L-K, Ho P-C, et al. Arthroscopic repair of triangular fibrocartilage complex tears. Arthroscopy 2007;23(7):729–37.e1.

35. Geissler W. Arthroscopic management of peripheral ulnar tears of the triangular fibrocartilage complex. In: Slutsky D, editor. Principles and practice of wrist surgery. Philadelphia: Saunders Elsevier; 2010. p. 205–12.

36. Bednar MS, Arnoczky SP, Weiland AJ. The micro-vasculature of the triangular fibrocartilage complex: its clinical significance. J Hand Surg Am 1991;16(6): 1101–5.

37. Chidgey LK. Histologic anatomy of the triangular fibrocartilage. Hand Clin 1991;7(2):249–62.

38. Geissler W. Repair of peripheral radial TFCC tears. In: Geissler W, editor. Wrist arthroscopy. New York: Springer; 2005. p. 42–9.

39. Cooney WP, Linscheid RL, Dobyns JH. Triangular fibrocartilage tears. J Hand Surg Am 1994;19(1): 143–54.

40. Sagerman SD, Short W. Arthroscopic repair of radial-sided triangular fibrocartilage complex tears. Arthroscopy 1996;12(3):339–42.

41. Jantea CL, Baltzer A, Rüther W. Arthroscopic repair of radial-sided lesions of the triangular fibrocartilage complex. Hand Clin 1995;11(1):31–6.

42. Husby T, Haugstvedt JR. Long-term results after arthroscopic resection of lesions of the triangular fibrocartilage complex. Scand J Plast Reconstr Surg Hand Surg 2001;35(1):79–83.

43. Wysocki RW, Richard MJ, Crowe MM, et al. Arthroscopic treatment of peripheral triangular fibrocartilage complex tears with the deep fibers intact. J Hand Surg Am 2012;37(3):509–16.

44. Frost HM. Some ABC's of skeletal pathophysiology. 5. Microdamage physiology. Calcif Tissue Int 1991; 49(4):229–31.

45. Daffner RH, Pavlov H. Stress fractures: current concepts. AJR Am J Roentgenol 1992;159(2):245–52.

46. Manzione M, Pizzutillo PD. Stress fracture of the scaphoid waist. A case report. Am J Sports Med 1981;9(4):268–9.

47. Hanks GA, Kalenak A, Bowman LS, et al. Stress fractures of the carpal scaphoid. A report of four cases. J Bone Joint Surg Am 1989;71(6):938–41.

48. Engel A, Feldner-Busztin H. Bilateral stress fracture of the scaphoid. A case report. Arch Orthop Trauma Surg 1991;110(6):314–5.

49. Matzkin E, Singer DI. Scaphoid stress fracture in a 13-year-old gymnast: a case report. J Hand Surg Am 2000;25(4):710–3.

50. Yamagiwa T, Fujioka H, Okuno H, et al. Surgical treatment of stress fracture of the scaphoid of an adolescent gymnast. J Sports Sci Med 2009;8(4): 702–4.

51. Nakamoto JC, Saito M, Medina G, et al. Scaphoid stress fracture in high-level gymnast: a case report. Case Rep Orthop 2011;2011:492407.

52. Weber ER, Chao EY. An experimental approach to the mechanism of scaphoid waist fractures. J Hand Surg Am 1978;3(2):142–8.

53. Samuelson M, Reider B, Weiss D. Grip lock injuries to the forearm in male gymnasts. Am J Sports Med 1996;24(1):15–8.

54. Bezek EM, VanHeest AE, Hutchinson DT. Grip lock injury in male gymnasts. Sport Heal A Multidiscip Approach 2009;1(6):518–21.

55. Sathyendra V, Payatakes A. Grip lock injury resulting in extensor tendon pseudorupture: case report. J Hand Surg Am 2013;38(12):2335–8.

56. Updegrove GF, Aiyer AA, Fortuna KL. Segmental forearm fracture due to grip-lock injury in male gymnast: a case report. JBJS Case Connect 2015; 5(2):e43.

57. Kirk JA, Ansell BM, Bywaters EG. The hypermobility syndrome. musculoskeletal complaints associated with generalized joint hypermobility. Ann Rheum Dis 1967;26:419–25.

58. Stewart DR, Burden SB. Does generalised ligamentous laxity increase seasonal incidence of injuries in male first division club rugby players? Br J Sports Med 2004;38(4):457–60.

59. Gannon LM, Bird HA. The quantification of joint laxity in dancers and gymnasts. J Sports Sci 1999;17(9): 743–50.

60. Schernberg F. Roentgenographic examination of the wrist: a systematic study of the normal, lax and injured wrist. Part 1: the standard and positional views. J Hand Surg Br 1990;15(2):210–9.

61. Niacaris T, Ming BW, Lichtman DM. Midcarpal instability. Hand Clin 2015;31(3):487–93.

62. Garcia-Elias M, Ribe M, Rodriguez J, et al. Influence of joint laxity on scaphoid kinematics. J Hand Surg Br 1995;20(3):379–82.

63. Freedman D, Garcia-Elias M. The influence of joint laxity on periscaphoid carpal kinematics. J Hand Surg Br 1997;22(4):457–60.

64. Snider MG, Alsaleh KA, Mah JY. Scapholunate interosseus ligament tears in elite gymnasts. Can J Surg 2006;49(4):290–1.

65. Lichtman DM, Schneider JR, Swafford AR, et al. Ulnar midcarpal instability-clinical and laboratory analysis. J Hand Surg Am 1981;6(5):515–23.

Ulnar Neuropathy in Cyclists

Jacob W. Brubacher, MD, Fraser J. Leversedge, MD*

KEYWORDS

• Ulnar nerve • Cubital tunnel • Distal ulnar tunnel • Guyon canal • Cycling • Biking

KEY POINTS

- The form and function of the cyclist exposes the ulnar nerve to both traction and compressive forces at the elbow and wrist, potentially leading to progressive neuropathy.
- Preventing ulnar neuropathy and treating early symptoms include bike fitting, avoiding excessive or prolonged weight bearing through the hands, and the use of padded gloves.
- A comprehensive history and evaluation for ulnar neuropathy is essential owing to the possibility of remote sites of nerve compression including the cervical spine and thoracic outlet.
- The majority of compression neuropathies in cyclists resolve after appropriate rest and conservative treatment; however, should symptoms persist, nerve decompression may be indicated.

INTRODUCTION

Ulnar neuropathy is a common compressive peripheral neuropathy with a reported incidence in the general population of 24.7 cases per 100,000 person-years.[1] Compression most frequently occurs at the cubital tunnel; the incidence of ulnar neuropathy at the elbow is second only to carpal tunnel syndrome as a compressive neuropathy in the upper extremity.[1,2] Previous authors have described both a compressive and a traction-related influence on intraneural pressures with progressive elbow flexion[3–5]; the ulnar nerve is deformed through tension across the flexed elbow and by a structural alteration of the cubital tunnel.[6] Similarly, at the wrist, the ulnar nerve can be influenced adversely by alterations in the dimensions of the distal ulnar tunnel (Guyon canal) such as from a mass (eg, ganglion cyst) or by externally applied pressure.[7,8]

Road cycling has been associated with the development of ulnar neuropathy based on the typical form of the cyclist: a flexed upper body with upper limbs reaching to and braced by the handlebars, thereby directing forces through flexed elbows and contact of the palm and wrist on the handlebars. Ulnar nerve compression in cyclists or 'cyclist's palsy' has been described in the literature.[9–11] A prospective study of long distance cyclists found that 70% of riders experienced motor and/or sensory disturbance during the course of a 4-day, 600 km ride.[10] Similarly, Akuthota and colleagues[12] found significantly prolonged ulnar motor latencies in riders during a 6-day, 420-mile bike tour.

Patients presenting with neurologic symptoms associated with ulnar neuropathy and who reveal a history of recreational or competitive cycling should be evaluated thoroughly. It is important for the clinician to understand the pertinent anatomy and perform a comprehensive clinical examination to consider an accurate diagnosis. Treatment strategies for alleviating symptoms and preventing progressive neuropathy include surgical and nonsurgical interventions, guided by the severity and chronicity of nerve dysfunction.

Department of Orthopaedic Surgery, Duke University, 4709 Creekstone Drive, Suite 200, Durham, NC 27707, USA
* Corresponding author.
E-mail address: fraser.leversedge@duke.edu

Hand Clin 33 (2017) 199–205
http://dx.doi.org/10.1016/j.hcl.2016.08.015
0749-0712/17/© 2016 Elsevier Inc. All rights reserved.

PERTINENT ANATOMY: CUBITAL TUNNEL AND DISTAL ULNAR TUNNEL

Typically, the ulnar nerve originates from the medial cord (C8-T1) of the brachial plexus and courses through the proximal anterior compartment before crossing into the posterior compartment of the brachium through the medial intermuscular septum. The nerve descends the brachium posterior to the intermuscular septum along the medial triceps toward the elbow and the cubital tunnel. Approximately 8 to 10 cm proximal to the medial epicondyle, a thickening of the brachial fascia oriented perpendicular to the longitudinal axis of the arm, the arcade of Struthers, overlies the nerve and is a potential site for ulnar nerve compression, particularly when the nerve is transposed anteriorly. The ulnar nerve traverses the elbow and transitions from the posterior compartment of the arm to the anterior compartment of the forearm via the cubital tunnel (**Fig. 1**). The cubital tunnel is bounded by Osbourne ligament, its roof, by the medial collateral ligament and elbow capsule that form the floor of the tunnel, and by its walls, which consist of the olecranon and medial epicondyle. Anatomic variations include the presence of the anconeus epitrochlearis muscle, present in up to 30% and is superficial to the cubital tunnel, originating at the medial epicondyle and inserting into the medial border of the olecranon. During elbow flexion, the nerve becomes progressively linear and flattened with a significant increase in intraneural pressure.[6,13] The nerve courses distally in the forearm by passing through the ulnar and humeral heads of the flexor carpi ulnaris muscle and descending between the flexor digitorum profundus and the flexor carpi ulnaris muscles. The dorsal sensory branch of the ulnar nerve branches approximately 6 cm proximal to the ulnar head and courses distally and dorsally to supply the dorsal–ulnar wrist and hand, the dorsal and proximal aspects of the ring and small fingers[14] (**Fig. 2**).

The ulnar nerve, dorsal and ulnar to the accompanying ulnar artery at the distal forearm, courses from the forearm into the hand by traversing the distal ulnar tunnel at the wrist. The distal ulnar tunnel, or Guyon canal, is 4 to 5 cm in length and originates at the proximal edge of the volar carpal ligament and continues distally to the fibrous arch of the of the hypothenar muscles.[8] Palpable landmarks relative to the distal ulnar tunnel include the pisiform, found ulnar and proximal, and the hook of hamate radially and distally. The canal entrance is triangular in shape with the apex radially, created by the fibers of the volar carpal ligament inserting into the transverse carpal

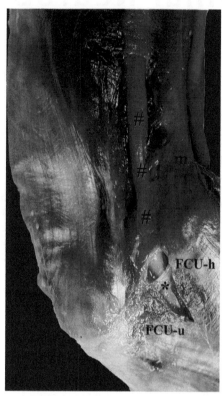

Fig. 1. Medial aspect of the left elbow (top = proximal), demonstrating the course of the ulnar nerve (*hashes*) in the brachium, descending posterior to the medial intermuscular septum (m) and entering the cubital tunnel. The nerve is identified between the humeral (flexor carpi ulnaris [FCU-h]) and ulnar (FCU-u) heads of the FCU origin, and deep to the fibrous aponeurosis that is deep to the muscle (*asterisk*). (*Courtesy of* Martin I. Boyer, MD, Lindley Wall, MD, Fraser Leversedge, MD; with permission.)

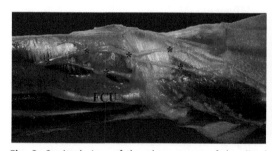

Fig. 2. Sagittal view of the ulnar aspect of the distal right forearm and wrist demonstrating the dorsal sensory branch of the ulnar nerve (DSBUN) (*asterisks*) as it courses dorsally from the ulnar nerve (not shown) and emerges dorsal and radial to the flexor carpi ulnaris (FCU). The DSBUN traverses the ulnocarpal joint at its midsagittal aspect and is superficial to the extensor retinaculum before branching over the dorsal and ulnar wrist. (*Courtesy of* Martin I. Boyer, MD, Lindley Wall, MD, Fraser Leversedge, MD; with permission.)

ligament—the proximal portion of the canal is bounded by the pisiform ulnarly, the volar carpal ligament volarly, and the transverse carpal ligament dorsally[15,16] (**Fig. 3**). More distally, the volar border or roof of the distal ulnar tunnel consists of the palmar aponeurosis, palmaris brevis, and hypothenar adipose tissue. The floor is formed by the flexor digitorum profundus tendons, the pisohamate ligament, the pisometacarpal ligament, and the opponens digiti minimi muscle. The medial wall transitions from the flexor carpi ulnaris tendon and pisiform proximally to the abductor digiti minimi muscle distally. The lateral wall is composed of the extrinsic flexor tendons, the hook of the hamate, and the confluence of the transverse carpal ligament and volar carpal ligament.[8]

The ulnar nerve bifurcates into deep (motor) and superficial (primarily sensory) branch approximately 6 mm distal to the distal pole of the pisiform.[14,17] Typically, the deep motor branch innervates the interossei, third and fourth lumbricals, the adductor pollicis, and the medial (deep) head of the flexor pollicis brevis. The superficial branch of the ulnar nerve innervates the palmaris brevis muscle and provides sensation the palmar side of the small finger and the ulnar-palmar side of the ring finger (**Fig. 4**). Based on this branching pattern of the ulnar nerve within the distal ulnar tunnel, 3 zones of nerve compression have been

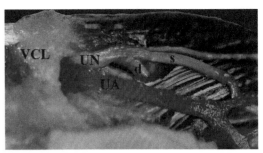

Fig. 4. A palmar view of the relationship of the ulnar artery and nerve as they exit from the volar carpal ligament (VCL) in a right wrist. The ulnar nerve (UN) is dorsal and ulnar to the ulnar artery (UA) and it divides into the superficial (S) and deep (D) branches just distal to the pisiform. The deep motor branch courses dorsally, coursing through the origin of the hypothenar muscles. (*Courtesy of* Martin I. Boyer, MD, Lindley Wall, MD, Fraser Leversedge, MD; with permission.)

described.[18,19] Zone 1 compression of the ulnar nerve occurs proximal to its bifurcation and therefore involves both sensory and motor nerve dysfunction. Zone II involves compression of the deep motor branch only and zone III affects only the superficial branch of the ulnar nerve. Capitani and Beer[20] noted that ulnar nerve compression at the wrist in cyclists can occur in any of these 3 zones, leading to mixed or isolated sensory or motor nerve deficits.

PATIENT EVALUATION

A thorough patient history is imperative with special attention to timing and chronicity of symptoms, inciting and alleviating factors, the quality and duration of symptoms, and use of any protective equipment. A review of the patient's injury history is important because cyclists in particular may have previous injuries that could contribute to nerve compromise such as a clavicle fracture/malunion, cervical spine injury, or upper extremity injury including elbow or hook of the hamate fracture. A high prevalence of thoracic outlet syndrome has been reported in cyclists and this diagnosis should be considered carefully as a differential diagnosis or as a confounding condition associated with ulnar neuropathy.[21] Symptoms in the ulnar nerve distribution are not uncommon with thoracic outlet syndrome owing to the course of the lower trunk that ascends over the first rib before continuing distally into the upper limb, placing the lower trunk at a disadvantage when pathologic changes are present in the triangular outlet created by the anterior and middle scalene muscles and the first rib into which they inert.

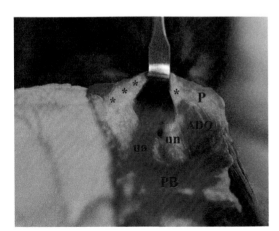

Fig. 3. The distal ulnar tunnel in transverse section viewed from distal to proximal in a right wrist. The palmar boundary or roof of the distal ulnar tunnel, or Guyon's canal, is the volar carpal ligament (*asterisks*), which originates from the pisiform (P) proximally, and the palmaris brevis muscle (PB) is the roof of the distal ulnar tunnel more distally. The ulnar nerve (un) is dorsal and ulnar to the ulnar artery (ua) at this level. ADQ, abductor digiti quinti. (*Courtesy of* Martin I. Boyer, MD, Lindley Wall, MD, Fraser Leversedge, MD; with permission.)

Prolonged compressive neuropathy will cause a predictable biologic cascade of events involving reversible and subsequently irreversible nerve dysfunction.[22] Often, sensory disturbance is noted first, although motor nerve compromise may cause weakness, characteristic ulnar intrinsic atrophy, and possibly a loss of proprioceptive function. Severe and prolonged compression can lead to a loss of protective sensation and an intrinsic motor imbalance primarily affecting the hand with the classic posture of clawing in the ulnar digits presenting as hyperextension of the metacarpophalangeal joints and flexion of the proximal interphalangeal joints.

A comprehensive clinical examination should include the cervical spine and bilateral upper extremities. The examination should begin with inspection for asymmetry between the bilateral extremities with careful attention to presence of atrophy or visible masses, or abnormal posturing of the hand. The cervical spine and the entire limb should be evaluated for potential sites of compression and for confounding conditions that might influence or mimic symptoms of ulnar neuropathy. Comparison to the contralateral limb is essential, particularly because some clinically "silent" findings such as intrinsic atrophy might be appreciated because of asymmetry. Degenerative conditions of the cervical spine may be associated with or aggravated by prolonged extension positioning of the neck common during cycling. Cervical range of motion, examination of cervical roots (motor and sensory), and Spurling and Adson testing should be performed routinely. Range of motion evaluation should include the shoulder, elbow, forearm, wrist, and hand. Sensibility testing can be carried out by subjective light touch, 2-point discrimination, or monofilament testing. Altered sensation over the dorsoulnar aspect of the hand can indicate more proximal compression before departure of the dorsal ulnar sensory branch. Motor evaluation exhibiting weakness in the interossei and thumb adductor whereas strength is preserved in the flexor digitorum profundus to the ring and small can be indicative of ulnar nerve compression at the wrist.

Provocative maneuvers and dynamic assessments may identify sites of nerve compromise. Proximal nerve compression involving the cervical spine, thoracic outlet, or the shoulder region is evaluated through the Spurling and Adson maneuvers, overhead reach, and a Tinel percussion test. At the arm and elbow, the stability of the ulnar nerve at the cubital tunnel should be evaluated through an arc of elbow motion[23] avoiding confusion with a subluxing medial antebrachial cutaneous nerve at the medial epicondyle.[24] The

medial triceps can be a source of ulnar nerve pathology, including a snapping triceps phenomenon that could be exacerbated by bracing of the upper limb on the handlebars during cycling.[25] Attempts to reproduce distal ulnar nerve symptoms through provocation by an ulnar nerve flexion–compression test and a Tinel percussion examination can help to localize nerve pathology. Reproduction of symptoms by direct compression over the distal ulnar tunnel or by Tinel percussion testing at the distal ulnar tunnel may suggest a more distal site of nerve compression. Careful localization of tenderness in the hand and wrist may identify a primary condition that may compromise ulnar nerve function, such as a ganglion cyst at the ulnar wrist, a hook of the hamate fracture or nonunion, or pisotriquetral arthritis.

Radiographs are indicated to support clinical findings and may reveal previous cycling-related injuries such as a clavicle malunion or previous upper extremity fracture. Advanced imaging such as MRI and ultrasound imaging may be helpful adjuncts for identifying areas and causes of focal nerve compression and for studying local anatomy for signs of pathologic changes or anatomic variation that can compromise nerve function. There are many known potential causes of compression in the distal ulnar and these include ganglion cysts, vascular pathology, fractures, accessory muscles or flexor tendon pathology.[26,27] Our clinic uses ultrasound evaluation for nerve pathology, including alterations in nerve structure consistent with compressive neuropathy.[28,29] Electrophysiologic testing should be used in patients who do not respond to conservative measures to address suspected ulnar neuropathy, including temporary cessation of cycling, to assist in confirming the site and severity of nerve compression.

PREVENTION AND NONSURGICAL TREATMENT

The influence of body positioning and the number of potential sources of nerve compression or traction should be recognized when evaluating a cyclist. Slane and colleagues[30] evaluated the influence of glove and hand positions on ulnar nerve pressure. Peak pressures occurred when cyclists did not wear gloves and there was a significant decrease in hypothenar pressure when padded gloves were used.[30] When hands were positioned in the drop handlebar position, hypothenar pressures increased, likely as result of increased forward body weight directed through the wrists.[30] Gloves with thin (3 mm), compliant foam padding gave the greatest pressure reduction; thicker padding did not improve hypothenar pressures.[30]

Alternating the position of the hands was found to be helpful because this maneuver altered the distribution and effects of the pressure.[30] Rauch and colleagues[31] demonstrated the effect of hand and wrist position on altering the amount of nerve contact with hook of the hamate in an MRI study. Wrist hyperextension during cycling places the ulnar nerve in greatest risk of compression.

Often, neurologic symptoms are transient and resolve with rest from the compressive condition associated with cycling; however, cases of persistent symptoms have been reported.[32] Strategies for minimizing nerve compression include avoidance of excessive and prolonged elbow flexion with activity, use of nighttime elbow extension splint to minimize traction forces across the ulnar nerve within the cubital tunnel during elbow flexion, and a neutral wrist splint to reduce adverse tension across the ulnar nerve within the distal ulnar tunnel.[33]

Avoidance of sustained nerve compression is critical for reducing the risk of progressive nerve dysfunction; early recognition can lead to improved outcomes through patient education emphasizing appropriate rest, improved equipment such as padded cycling gloves, altering hand and upper extremity positioning during longer rides, and proper body mechanics through bike fitting including optimal saddle and handle bar positioning.

SURGICAL TREATMENT
Elbow

There is ongoing investigation regarding the surgical management of ulnar neuropathy at the elbow relating primarily to the indications for anterior transposition of the nerve in conjunction with decompression. Numerous studies have attempted to clarify treatment algorithms; however, there is no established methodology for decision making regarding anterior transposition, in part owing to numerous patient factors and surgeon preferences regarding surgical management.[23,34–37] In our practice, a decision to include anterior transposition is influenced by the severity of nerve symptoms, an unstable or subluxing ulnar nerve before or after nerve decompression, the presence of a motor deficit, and the recognition that cyclists have a tendency to position the upper limb such that the influence of traction by weight-bearing through a flexed elbow is increased. If the preoperative physical examination shows nerve instability with elbow flexion, then transposition is likely indicated and has shown improved results in patients under the age of 30 years.[38] The central principal of treatment emphasizes that the nerve must be decompressed at all potential compressive sites, from the arcade of Stuthers in the mid-brachium, to the Osborne ligament and through the heads of the flexor carpi ulnaris. If the nerve is transposed anteriorly, it is critical to inspect the new course of the ulnar nerve through a full arc of elbow motion to ensure that new sites of compression are not created by the transposition itself. This involves resection of the medial intermuscular septum and the fascia between the flexor carpi ulnaris and median-innervated flexor/pronator mass.[33] Our preference is to use an adipose flap described by Rosenwasser that creates a longer flap for maintaining the nerve in its anterior position and that leaves the nerve in a favorable environment, surrounded by subcutaneous fat[39] (**Fig. 5**). Careful dissection should preserve the ulnar nerve's extrinsic vascular supply, traversing superficial sensory nerves (medial brachial cutaneous nerve and medial antebrachial cutaneous nerve) and ulnar nerve branches.

Wrist and Hand

Surgical decompression of the ulnar nerve at the wrist involves exposure of the nerve from the distal forearm fascia through the distal ulnar tunnel.[40] The skin incision crosses the wrist as a Bruner transition to prevent skin contracture. The ulnar nerve is protected by identifying both the superficial and deep branches. All potential sites of compression should be released including the fascia and the tendinous aponeurosis of the hypothenar muscle origin overlying the deep motor branch[33] (**Fig. 6**). Inspection and treatment for

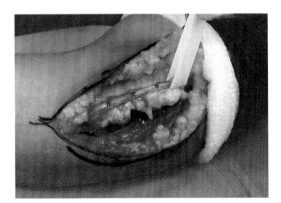

Fig. 5. Intraoperative view of the medial right elbow. The ulnar nerve (*asterisks*) has been decompressed and is positioned in an anteriorly transposed position using a technique that creates an adipose flap using the membranous interval between the superficial and deep layers of the subcutaneous tissue. (*Courtesy of* Martin I. Boyer, MD, Lindley Wall, MD, Fraser Leversedge, MD; with permission.)

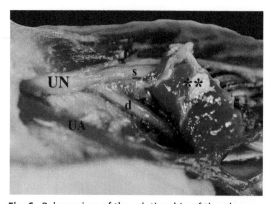

Fig. 6. Palmar view of the relationship of the ulnar artery (UA) and nerve (UN) with its superficial (S) and deep (D) branches as they exit from the volar carpal ligament in a right wrist. Here, the hypothenar origin (*double asterisk*) has been reflected distally to highlight the deep (D) motor branch coursing dorsally. (*Courtesy of* Martin I. Boyer, MD, Lindley Wall, MD, Fraser Leversedge, MD; with permission.)

external sources of compression such as by ganglion cysts, anatomic anomalies, or vascular pathology should be completed.[7,33]

SUMMARY

Ulnar neuropathy is a common and troublesome condition for cyclists, especially those who participate in long distance, multiday rides.[10,12] The form and function of the cyclist predisposes the ulnar nerve to injury, through traction and compressive forces acting on the ulnar nerve through the flexed elbow and by traction and external compression occurring at the distal ulnar tunnel. A careful history and physical examination is essential to confirm the diagnosis and rule out other sites of compression, in particular the cervical spine and thoracic outlet. Prevention and initial treatment of symptoms include careful bike fitting, alternating hand positions, avoidance of excessive weight bearing through hands, and the use of padded gloves. The majority of compression neuropathies in cyclists resolve after appropriate rest and preventive measures have been implemented, however, should symptoms persist, nerve decompression and possible anterior transposition may be indicated.

REFERENCES

1. Mondelli M, Giannini F, Ballerini M, et al. Incidence of ulnar neuropathy at the elbow in the province of Siena (Italy). J Neurol Sci 2005;234(1–2):5–10.
2. Latinovic R, Gulliford MC, Hughes RAC. Incidence of common compressive neuropathies in primary care. J Neurol Neurosurg Psychiatry 2006;77(2): 263–5.
3. Grewal R, Varitimidis SE, Vardakas DG, et al. Ulnar nerve elongation and excursion in the cubital tunnel after decompression and anterior transposition. J Hand Surg Br 2000;25(5):457–60.
4. Wright TW, Glowczewskie F, Wheeler D, et al. Excursion and strain of the median nerve. J Bone Joint Surg Am 1996;78(12):1897–903.
5. Byl C, Puttlitz C, Byl N, et al. Strain in the median and ulnar nerves during upper-extremity positioning. J Hand Surg Am 2002;27(6):1032–40.
6. Gelberman RH, Yamaguchi K, Hollstien SB, et al. Changes in interstitial pressure and cross-sectional area of the cubital tunnel and of the ulnar nerve with flexion of the elbow. An experimental study in human cadavera. J Bone Joint Surg Am 1998; 80(4):492–501.
7. Murata K, Shih J-T, Tsai T-M. Causes of ulnar tunnel syndrome: a retrospective study of 31 subjects. J Hand Surg Am 2003;28(4):647–51.
8. Chen S-H, Tsai T-M. Ulnar tunnel syndrome. J Hand Surg Am 2014;39(3):571–9.
9. Cherington M. Hazards of bicycling: from handlebars to lightning. Semin Neurol 2000;20(2):247–53.
10. Patterson JM, Jaggars MM, Boyer MI. Ulnar and median nerve palsy in long-distance cyclists. A prospective study. Am J Sports Med 2003;31(4):585–9.
11. Eckman PB, Perlstein G, Altrocchi PH. Ulnar neuropathy in bicycle riders. Arch Neurol 1975;32(2): 130–2.
12. Akuthota V, Plastaras C, Lindberg K, et al. The effect of long-distance bicycling on ulnar and median nerves: an electrophysiologic evaluation of cyclist palsy. Am J Sports Med 2005;33(8):1224–30.
13. Yamaguchi K, Sweet FA, Bindra R, et al. The extraneural and intraneural arterial anatomy of the ulnar nerve at the elbow. J Shoulder Elbow Surg 1999; 8(1):17–21.
14. Goto A, Kunihiro O, Murase T, et al. The dorsal cutaneous branch of the ulnar nerve: an anatomical study. Hand Surg 2010;15(3):165–8.
15. Vezeridis PS, Yoshioka H, Han R, et al. Ulnar-sided wrist pain. Part I: anatomy and physical examination. Skeletal Radiol 2010;39(8):733–45.
16. Earp BE, Floyd WE, Louie D, et al. Ulnar nerve entrapment at the wrist. J Am Acad Orthop Surg 2014;22(11):699–706.
17. Ombaba J, Kuo M, Rayan G. Anatomy of the ulnar tunnel and the influence of wrist motion on its morphology. J Hand Surg Am 2010;35(5):760–8.
18. Shea JD, McClain EJ. Ulnar-nerve compression syndromes at and below the wrist. J Bone Joint Surg Am 1969;51(6):1095–103.
19. Gross MS, Gelberman RH. The anatomy of the distal ulnar tunnel. Clin Orthop Relat Res 1985; 196:238–47.

20. Capitani D, Beer S. Handlebar palsy–a compression syndrome of the deep terminal (motor) branch of the ulnar nerve in biking. J Neurol 2002;249(10):1441–5.

21. Smith TM, Sawyer SF, Sizer PS, et al. The double crush syndrome: a common occurrence in cyclists with ulnar nerve neuropathy-a case-control study. Clin J Sport Med 2008;18(1):55–61.

22. Lundborg G, Rydevik B. Effects of stretching the tibial nerve of the rabbit. A preliminary study of the intraneural circulation and the barrier function of the perineurium. J Bone Joint Surg Br 1973;55(2): 390–401.

23. Krogue JD, Aleem AW, Osei DA, et al. Predictors of surgical revision after in situ decompression of the ulnar nerve. J Shoulder Elbow Surg 2015;24(4): 634–9.

24. Cesmebasi A, O'Driscoll SW, Smith J, et al. The snapping medial antebrachial cutaneous nerve. Clin Anat 2015;28(7):872–7.

25. Spinner RJ, Goldner RD. Snapping of the medial head of the triceps and recurrent dislocation of the ulnar nerve. Anatomical and dynamic factors. J Bone Joint Surg Am 1998;80(2):239–47.

26. Moneim MS. Ulnar nerve compression at the wrist. Ulnar tunnel syndrome. Hand Clin 1992; 8(2):337–44.

27. Kuschner SH, Gelberman RH, Jennings C. Ulnar nerve compression at the wrist. J Hand Surg Am 1988;13(4):577–80.

28. Cartwright MS, Walker FO. Neuromuscular ultrasound in common entrapment neuropathies. Muscle Nerve 2013;48(5):696–704.

29. Ellegaard HR, Fuglsang-Frederiksen A, Hess A, et al. High-resolution ultrasound in ulnar neuropathy at the elbow: a prospective study. Muscle Nerve 2015;52(5):759–66.

30. Slane J, Timmerman M, Ploeg H-L, et al. The influence of glove and hand position on pressure over the ulnar nerve during cycling. Clin Biomech (Bristol, Avon) 2011;26(6):642–8.

31. Rauch A, Teixeira PAG, Gillet R, et al. Analysis of the position of the branches of the ulnar nerve in Guyon's canal using high-resolution MRI in positions adopted by cyclists. Surg Radiol Anat 2016;38: 793–9.

32. Brown CK, Stainsby B, Sovak G. Guyon Canal Syndrome: lack of management in a case of unresolved handlebar palsy. J Can Chiropr Assoc 2014;58(4): 413–20.

33. Dy CJ, Mackinnon SE. Ulnar neuropathy: evaluation and management. Curr Rev Musculoskelet Med 2016;9(2):178–84.

34. Gervasio O, Gambardella G, Zaccone C, et al. Simple decompression versus anterior submuscular transposition of the ulnar nerve in severe cubital tunnel syndrome: a prospective randomized study. Neurosurgery 2005;56(1):108–17 [discussion: 117].

35. Nabhan A, Ahlhelm F, Kelm J, et al. Simple decompression or subcutaneous anterior transposition of the ulnar nerve for cubital tunnel syndrome. J Hand Surg Br 2005;30(5):521–4.

36. Chung KC. Treatment of ulnar nerve compression at the elbow. J Hand Surg Am 2008;33(9):1625–7.

37. Mowlavi A, Andrews K, Lille S, et al. The management of cubital tunnel syndrome: a meta-analysis of clinical studies. Plast Reconstr Surg 2000; 106(2):327–34.

38. Henn CM, Patel A, Wall LB, et al. Outcomes following cubital tunnel surgery in young patients: the importance of nerve mobility. J Hand Surg Am 2016;41(4):e1–7.

39. Danoff JR, Lombardi JM, Rosenwasser MP. Use of a pedicled adipose flap as a sling for anterior subcutaneous transposition of the ulnar nerve. J Hand Surg Am 2014;39(3):552–5.

40. Waugh RP, Pellegrini VD. Ulnar tunnel syndrome. Hand Clin 2007;23(3):301–10, v.

Therapy and Rehabilitation for Upper Extremity Injuries in Athletes

Michael S. Gart, MD[a],*, Thomas A. Wiedrich, MD[b]

KEYWORDS

- Rehabilitation • Upper extremity • Athlete • Strength training • Taping • Orthotics
- Alternative therapy

KEY POINTS

- Rehabilitation of the upper extremity athlete differs from other patients because of the high functional demands of competitive sport and potential for reinjury.
- Following injury, several modalities are available to restore range of motion, strength, and sport-specific movements.
- Various orthotic and taping techniques are available to facilitate protected return to play and reduce the risk for reinjury.
- Alternative therapies, including taping, acupuncture, water immersion, and nutritional supplementation, may hasten convalescence after injury.

INTRODUCTION

The central tenet of rehabilitation is to restore the patient to optimal function. In competitive or professional athletes whose function far exceeds that of the general population, the goal of rehabilitation is to restore function sufficient to withstand the demands of their chosen sport.[1] Although injuries to the upper extremity occur in nearly every sport, the specific sport and/or position played can predispose patients to specific injury patterns. Predictable overuse injuries are seen in many overhead athletes from repetitive stress, often at the extremes of range of motion; however, isolated traumatic events occurring during play can result in any number of unpredictable upper extremity injuries. Collaborating with coaches and trainers to better understand the sport-specific or position-specific demands is helpful in individualizing treatment plans to address each patient's needs.

In general, the goals of rehabilitation of the patient-athlete should be the following:

1. Restoration of pain-free range of motion across the injured joint(s)
2. Resistance training to restore strength
3. Higher-intensity, sports-specific exercises
4. Gradual and/or protected return to play

In this article, we discuss general themes in the rehabilitation of athletes, including strength training and orthotics for treating and/or preventing injury, and alternative therapies used in the comprehensive rehabilitation of the upper extremity athlete.

Disclosure Statement: Neither author has any relevant financial relationships to disclose or financial conflicts of interest. This work did not receive funding from any internal or external source.

[a] Division of Plastic and Reconstructive Surgery, Northwestern University Feinberg School of Medicine, 675 North St Clair Street, Suite 19-250, Galter Pavilion, Chicago, IL 60611, USA; [b] Department of Orthopedic Surgery, Chicago Center for Surgery of the Hand, Northwestern University Feinberg School of Medicine, 737 North Michigan Avenue, Suite 700, Chicago, IL 60611, USA

* Corresponding author.

E-mail address: MichaelGartMD@Gmail.com

hand.theclinics.com

PATIENT EVALUATION OVERVIEW

Upper extremity rehabilitation in the competitive athlete presents a unique set of rewards and challenges to the upper extremity surgeon and rehabilitation professionals. The rewards come from working with a patient population that is typically disciplined and invested in their recovery and rehabilitation. The challenges lie in designing a rehabilitation protocol that will adequately prepare the athlete for a return to the demands of his or her sport in a timely fashion. Because many athletes will be returning to the very activities that resulted in their initial injury, careful attention must be paid to reducing the risk for reinjury on their return.

Professional or semiprofessional athletes may not only make their livelihood through competitive sport, but also may define themselves to some degree by their accomplishments on the field. When their abilities are suddenly taken away by injury, patients are at risk for depression or anxiety. Moreover, fear of being told to no longer participate in competitive play may cause more insidious injuries to present late as athletes try to "play through" discomfort. After rehabilitation, fear of reinjury can be significant when a player returns to sport, and can impact their performance and mental well-being. The psychological impacts of injury must not be overlooked in the athlete's rehabilitation program. Psychologists should be involved on an as-needed basis to provide support and offer coping mechanisms to players struggling with depression or anxiety.

REHABILITATION STRATEGIES
Overview

Once inflammation and pain are controlled, the initial focus should be on restoring soft tissue and joint mobility to preinjury levels. Strength training can then proceed and gradually increase in both intensity and duration, culminating in sport-specific movements at high performance. Depending on the specific sport or position, orthotics can be used selectively to facilitate return to play in a protected fashion and can often hasten the convalescence following injury while minimizing the risk of reinjury.

Restoring Range of Motion

When athletes engage in regular or strenuous exercise, delayed-onset muscle soreness (DOMS) and formation of fibrous tissue adhesions can result, leading to a decrease in range of motion.[2,3] Fibrous fascial adhesions can develop in response to injury, inflammation, or inactivity and can diminish soft tissue extensibility, with associated decreases in joint range of motion and loss of normal muscular mechanics.[4–6] In addition to static stretching and range of motion exercises, there are a number of soft tissue mobilization techniques that may be beneficial in restoring full range of motion following an injury.

Instrument-Assisted Soft Tissue Mobilization

Instrument-assisted soft tissue mobilization (IASTM) is a technique derived from massage therapy, whereby pressure is applied to sore or tight muscles to alleviate their symptoms. Despite limited evidence in support of the many benefits attributed to IASTM, its use in active, exercising individuals is on the rise.[6,7]

The Graston Technique is practiced by many therapists and uses specially designed, stainless steel instruments to treat areas of soft tissue fibrosis (**Fig. 1**A). These instruments come in a variety of shapes and sizes to treat all areas of the upper extremity, from shoulder to fingertip (**Fig. 1**B–D). In so-called "self-myofascial release" (SMR), patients can target sore or tight muscle groups by either using their body weight and lying on a foam roller or applying direct pressure with a roller massager (**Fig. 2**). The advantage of SMR is that it can be done on the patient's schedule and does not require a physical therapist.[6,8] SMR is thought to aid recovery by treating DOMS and preventing or eliminating fascial adhesions.[6,9,10] Release of fibrous adhesions is reported to improve circulation, joint range of motion, and muscular performance, thereby reducing the risk for injury.[2]

Strength Training

Once a complete, pain-free range of motion has been achieved, the next step in the rehabilitation process is restoring strength. Numerous strength training techniques have a role in rehabilitation of the upper extremity, depending on the specific injury pattern and goals of therapy. In general, strength training will progress from single-joint exercises at low volume and intensity to sports-specific movements performed at high intensity.

Most standard rehabilitation protocols will use a variety of isometric and isotonic exercises to build strength initially. As rehabilitation progresses, there are several tools available to achieve specific strength goals, including TheraBand Flexbars for strengthening wrist movements (**Fig. 3**) and Bodyblade for stability training (**Fig. 4**). Kinetic chain exercises, which focus on movement patterns that involve the entire upper extremity, are also useful in reproducing more functional, multijoint movements (**Fig. 5**). Although a complete discussion

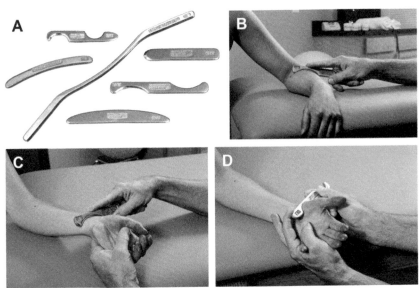

Fig. 1. The Graston Technique. Specialized, stainless steel instruments (*A*) are used for release of fibrous tissue adhesions in the forearm (*B*), wrist (*C*), and hand (*D*). (*Courtesy of* Graston Technique, LLC, Indianapolis, IN; with permission.)

of strength training principles is beyond the scope of this article, we will discuss techniques specific to rehabilitation of athletic populations. For specific rehabilitation protocols, please see related articles elsewhere in this issue.

Periodization

Originally developed in the 1950s, periodization is a rehabilitation strategy that uses regular changes in the training schedule to prevent a plateau in recovery and continue to challenge the patient-athlete. Parameters, such as resistance, repetition, duration, intensity, or movements, can be varied to continually present new challenges to the body and prevent neuromuscular accommodation. These changes can be used to emphasize different skills or development of specific muscle groups depending on the athlete's current demands and where they are in the season of their sport (preseason, postseason, offseason). Several

variations of the periodization model have been described,[11] but the basic principle of constant variation on a set schedule allows continued progression by avoiding muscle accommodation.

Plyometrics

Plyometric movements are characterized by active muscle units being stretched immediately before shortening, usually in an explosive fashion. This stretch-shortening cycle has been reported to increase activation of motor units without the degree of muscle hypertrophy seen with conventional resistance training,[12] and trains muscle-tendon units to generate maximum force in the shortest amount of time.[13,14] When a muscle is stretched, alterations in its contractile properties lead to a higher force production with subsequent contraction than is possible without a "loading" stretch.[14–16] Furthermore, muscle loading elicits a stretch reflex, whereby muscle activation

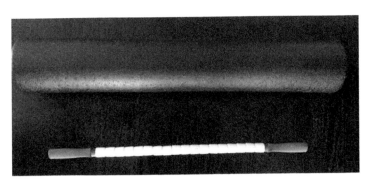

Fig. 2. Foam roller (*above*) and roller massager (*below*).

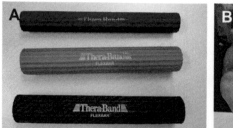
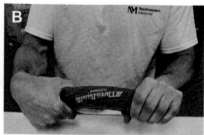
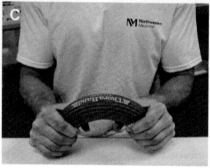

Fig. 3. TheraBand Flexbars (*A*) can be used to strengthen wrist movements, including flexion (*B*) and supination (*C*). (*Courtesy of* The Hygenic Corporation, Akron, OH; with permission.)

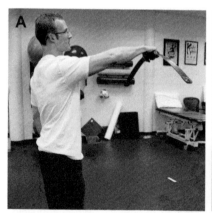
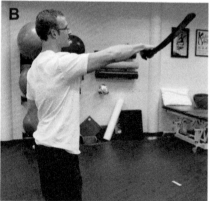

Fig. 4. Bodyblade can be used for stabilization training (*A, B*) in a number of upper extremity positions. (*Courtesy of* Bodyblade, Playa del Rey, CA; with permission.)

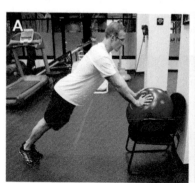
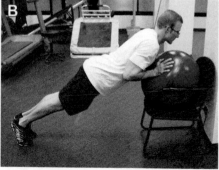

Fig. 5. Stability ball pushups (*A, B*) exercise the upper extremity "kinetic chain" to develop more functional movement patterns.

latencies are shortened in proportion to the magnitude of the loading stress.[17] Last, the stretch of a muscle during the loading phase of a plyometric movement is stored as elastic potential energy by the tendon, which is released during subsequent contraction.[18,19] The combined effect of these changes is a faster and more powerful muscle contraction. Some studies have shown that combining traditional strength training with plyometric movements results in improved power compared with either modality used in isolation.[20]

The goal of plyometric training in rehabilitation of the patient-athlete is to restore sport-specific skills, which often include explosive movements performed at high speed and intensity in multiple planes of movement. Although plyometric exercises can bridge the gap between the lower-intensity, single plane exercises of traditional strength training and competitive sport,[21] they must be used judiciously in rehabilitation after injury. Many plyometric movements expose the joints to substantial forces at high speeds and should be reserved for the terminal phases of rehabilitation, after the athlete has demonstrated sufficient strength and pain-free range of motion.[20] Several rehabilitation protocols include plyometric movements to improve muscle function and facilitate a return to competitive sport,[22–27] and multiple studies have demonstrated a positive effect of plyometric training on several sport-specific tasks, including vertical jump height, running economy, sprint speed, and swimming.[12,28–35] Moreover, there is some evidence to suggest that lower plyometric ability may be predictive of increased injury potential.[36–38] Numerous studies have shown a protective effect of plyometric exercises on knee injuries in female athletes[39–41] and in triathletes.[20,42] Some examples of plyometric movements are shown in **Figs. 6–8**.

It is important to note, however, that most of the published literature on plyometric training and its positive effects on performance, rehabilitation, and injury prevention have focused on the lower extremity; studies on the upper extremity are scarce. Moreover, nearly all of these studies have evaluated healthy, uninjured athletes. At this time, there is no strong evidence available to validate the assumption that plyometric training facilitates a return to sport in the injured athlete, although there are several anecdotal reports of success. Similarly, most of the guidelines on implementing plyometrics in rehabilitation are not evidence based; however, a gradual introduction at lower volume and intensity with sufficient rest periods seems prudent.

ORTHOTICS AND TAPING

During the terminal phases of rehabilitation, when the athlete is preparing for return to play, methods to protect the area of injury from repeated trauma and reinjury are frequently used. Orthotics and taping are typically used to protect an area of healing tissue from impact and/or to limit extremes of motion or forces across a joint. Sporting regulatory bodies (eg, National Collegiate Athletic Association, National Football League, National Basketball Association) may have specifications for the types of orthotics or taping permitted during play, which will factor into the treatment plan. If the treating physician and/or therapist are unfamiliar, communication with team trainers and coaches is helpful in ensuring that a plan for protected return to play is in line with league regulations.

Orthotics

An orthosis is an externally applied device used to modify the structural and/or functional characteristics of a joint or area of injury in an effort to assist healing and facilitate return to performance. In many cases, athletes will require an orthosis for a limited time during rehabilitation or return to play. These include static or dynamic splints and are available as prefabricated splints or custom-made orthotics.

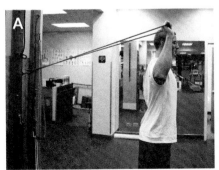
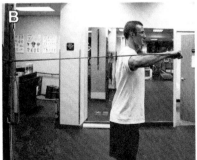

Fig. 6. (*A, B*) Internal shoulder rotation with resistance bands.

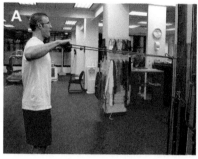
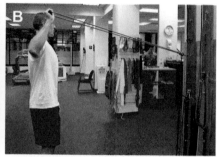

Fig. 7. (*A, B*) External shoulder rotation with resistance bands.

Static, or rigid, splints do not allow movement across a joint and are often used in patients with fractures following acute casting and during return to play until full healing is observed. They are also helpful in immobilizing inflammatory conditions to facilitate soft tissue healing. Prefabricated splints that we commonly use in practice are ring splints to immobilize the proximal interphalangeal (PIP) joint (**Fig. 9**), elbow hinge splints (**Fig. 10**), and wrist splints to prevent hyperextension (**Fig. 11**). If a customized splint is desired, these can be readily fashioned from thermoplastic material. The advantage of a thermoplastic splint is that they are strong yet lightweight, custom-fitted, and easily adjustable.

Dynamic splints allow movement across joints and are useful in rehabilitation of upper extremity injuries, because they permit patients to begin range of motion exercises and strength training while still providing the necessary stabilization. One example is an elbow hinge brace, which allows flexion and extension at the elbow without the risk for varus or valgus stresses (see **Fig. 10**). Dynamic splints can accelerate recovery by avoiding the stiffness and muscle atrophy that is seen with prolonged immobilization. These also can be used during early return to play for additional protection.

Taping

Taping is a popular intervention in rehabilitation for a variety of upper and lower extremity musculoskeletal conditions, and has been shown to reduce pain, improve muscle function, and restore functional movement patterns.[43] In rehabilitation, the use of taping to alleviate pain while performing therapeutic exercises may accelerate recovery and promote adherence to the exercise regimen. Many articles have advocated the use of taping for earlier return to activity and for the prevention of reinjury.[44–47] Broadly speaking, there are 2 categories of taping: nonelastic taping (NET), and kinesiology taping, each of which is discussed in brief detail in the following sections.

Nonelastic taping

NET is highly adhesive with minimal stretch, and is often used to enclose or encapsulate a joint to provide stability and restrict movement (**Fig. 12**). NET is often used in the wrist to limit extremes of flexion and extension, but can be applied across any joint in the upper extremity, from the shoulder to the fingers. It has been demonstrated to be effective at the elbow joint in reducing pain in chronic lateral epicondyalgia.[48] If increased range of protected motion is required, a combination of athletic taping and ELASTIKON tape can be used (**Fig. 13**).

Kinesiology taping

Originally described in the early 1970s, Kinesio taping differs significantly from traditional taping methods in both its application and goals of use.[49] Whereas traditional taping methods enclose or support a joint for added stability and

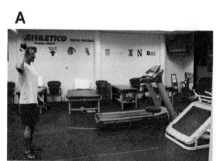
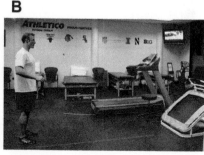

Fig. 8. (*A, B*) Internal rotation Plyoball throws.

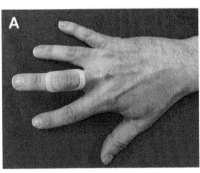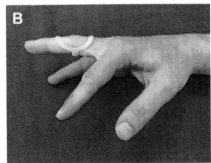

Fig. 9. (*A*, *B*) Prefabricated ring splint to hold proximal interphalangeal joint in extension.

limitation in range of motion, Kinesio taping focuses on the application of tape on and around muscles to support their function. Elastic tape is applied under stretch such that the elastic potential energy of the tape serves to reduce fatigue and increase active range of motion by assisting muscle function. According to the Kinesio Taping Method manual, this traction elevates the epidermis from the underlying mechanoreceptors, reducing nociceptive stimuli.[49] This interplay between the cutaneous afferent signals and motor unit activity is the basis of this method and serves as the foundation for several proposed benefits. In addition to reducing pain, Kinesio taping is thought to increase blood and lymphatic circulation, improve joint realignment, improve proprioception, and possibly reduce the risk of injury.[49,50]

Some studies have demonstrated clinical efficacy in reducing pain[51–55] and range of motion,[45,53,56,57] increasing muscle activity and function,[55,56,58,59] and improving functional performance.[45,60,61] In the upper extremity, most of the available evidence on Kinesio taping has focused on its applications in the shoulder joint, where it appears to reduce pain and improve range of

motion.[62] A randomized, double-blinded trial of college students with rotator cuff tendinopathies found an immediate improvement in pain-free range of shoulder abduction when compared with sham taping, but no other benefits.[55] Kinesio taping also has been reported to increase proprioception and possibly reduce the risk of shoulder injury.[50] However, despite some promising reports

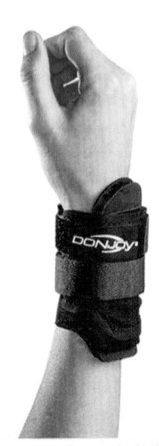

Fig. 11. DonJoy wrist brace used to block hyperextension at the wrist joint. (*Courtesy of* DJO, LLC, Vista, CA; with permission.)

Fig. 10. Hinged elbow brace, which allows elbow flexion and extension while protecting against varus or valgus stresses.

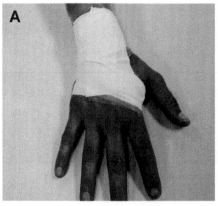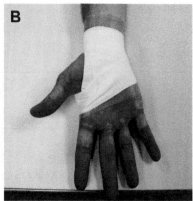

Fig. 12. NET can be applied in a "fan" fashion across the dorsal wrist joint to limit wrist flexion (*A*) or the volar wrist joint to limit wrist extension (*B*).

and its widespread use by therapists and athletes around the world, there is little evidence to support the use of Kinesio taping in clinical practice.[52,55,63]

One recent, well-controlled trial found no change in muscle function with the addition of Kinesio tape.[64] Similarly, a recent review found no benefit when Kinesio taping was compared with sham taping and no intervention or when Kinesio taping was used as an adjunctive method in combination with other therapies.[65] A recent meta-analysis concluded that more methodologically sound research is required before any definitive recommendations for Kinesio taping can be made.[56]

ALTERNATIVE THERAPIES

The use of complementary and alternative medicine (CAM) has steadily been gaining acceptance in Western medicine, and its utilization has steadily increased in recent years.[66–68] Acupuncture and nutritional therapies are frequently used modalities by collegiate and professional athletes.[66–69]

Although previous uses of CAM were supported almost exclusively by anecdotal reports, there is a growing body of more rigorous scientific evidence supporting its use.[68] Here, we discuss in brief detail some of the more common alternative therapy techniques that may benefit athletes during rehabilitation.

Acupuncture

Acupuncture has been practiced in traditional Chinese medicine for more than 2000 years. In this practice, small needles are placed at specific "acupoints" in the body to balance the life energy, or "qi." Many of these acupoints lie along "meridians," channels through which qi flows through the body.[70] The use of acupuncture in Western medicine is practiced in much the same fashion, using the traditional Chinese meridians and acupoints, and is considered to be a safe procedure in experienced hands. In general, individuals are considered to be "responders" or "nonresponders" to acupuncture, and a failure to

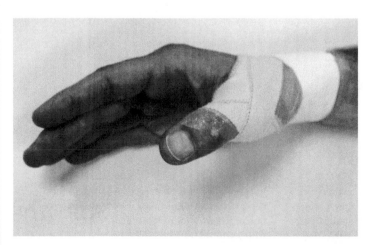

Fig. 13. The first metacarpophalangeal joint can be stabilized with a combination of standard athletic tape if increased range of protected motion is required.

clinically improve within the first 4 sessions may indicate little benefit to further treatment.[70]

Acupuncture has been used for years to enhance performance in recreational and professional athletes.[71–73] In the upper extremity, acupuncture has demonstrated efficacy in treating lateral epicondylalgia,[74–76] rotator cuff tendonitis,[77] and DOMS,[78] and may be useful in the treatment of various myofascial trigger points. Sustained acupuncture therapy has been shown to improve muscle strength in athletes[73]; however, more recent studies have demonstrated increased muscle strength immediately after treatment.[79] The use of acupuncture to improve muscular strength may have implications for its use in rehabilitation, but further study is warranted.

The most common side effects of treatment are localized pain and bruising at the needle insertion sites.[70] With a favorable safety profile and some evidence to support its efficacy in relieving pain and potentially improving muscle strength, acupuncture can be considered an option in rehabilitation of the patient-athlete.

Nutritional Interventions

When an athlete is injured, it is not uncommon for a particular part of the body to require immobilization as part of the initial healing process. Healthy, inactive muscle atrophies at approximately 0.5% per day[80,81]; however, the loss of muscle mass is more pronounced in the first 2 weeks following injury.[82] The loss of muscle strength, which is of more practical significance in most competitive athletes, generally occurs at 3 times the rate of muscle mass (ie, a 10% mass loss corresponds to approximately 30% loss of strength).[83–85] Here, we review some of the nutritional interventions to maintain muscle mass in injured athletes and promote lean muscle gains during the rehabilitation process.

Protein supplementation
Protein supplements are widely consumed by athletes and recreationally active adults to promote lean muscle gain. Although protein supplementation does not appear to improve lean muscle mass in untrained individuals, it may promote muscle hypertrophy, strength gains, and improvements in both aerobic and anaerobic power in trained individuals.[86] A recent review and position statement from the International Society of Sports Nutrition (ISSN) found that protein intakes of 1.4 to 2.0 g/kg per day were not only safe, but improved physical adaptation to exercise.[87]

In addition to the total amount of protein consumed, the timing of consumption is important in maximizing the effect on muscle synthesis and prevention of disuse atrophy. It has been experimentally determined that maximal protein synthesis occurs with the ingestion of 20 to 40 g of protein immediately after exercise,[88–93] followed by repeat ingestion of 20 g every 3 hours for the 12-hour window following exercise.[89,92] Practically speaking, this translates to frequent, protein-rich meals consumed throughout the day in the acute injury period and during the strength training portions of rehabilitation to mitigate disuse atrophy and promote muscle mass and strength gains.

Creatine
The performance-enhancing effects of creatine supplementation have been studied extensively in resistance strength training.[94,95] Inside skeletal myocytes, creatine is converted into phosphocreatine, where it serves as an energy buffer and phosphate source to replenish ATP.[94] Supplementation with creatine has been shown to increase strength, lean muscle mass, skeletal muscle function, and exercise performance.[94,96] Chronic supplementation with creatine at recommended dosages of 4 to 5 g per day have consistently shown not to have any adverse effect on health in patients without preexisting renal disease.[97–100] For the athlete looking to maximize strength gains in the rehabilitation period, creatine can be considered a safe and effective addition to the nutritional protocol.

Beta-alanine
Beta-alanine (BA) is a nonproteogenic amino acid that is both endogenously produced and acquired through dietary intake of poultry and meats.[101] It is the rate-limiting substrate in the synthesis of carnosine, an intracellular protein found in skeletal muscle that serves to sequester free protons and regulate intramuscular pH, mitigating the effects of exercise-induced lactic acidosis and improving muscular performance.[102] It is also thought to act as a free-radical scavenger and reduce oxidative stresses on exercising muscle.[103] Over the past decade, it has become one of the most popular sports nutrition ingredients on the market. In a recent review and position statement from the ISSN, BA was found to be safe in recommended doses (4–6 g/d in divided doses of 2 g or less) and improve exercise performance, with more profound effects during shorter, high-intensity exercises.[101] Although more research is needed to determine what, if any, the role for BA in rehabilitation may be, the promising performance results coupled with minimal side effects (paresthesias) make BA supplementation something to consider in a strength training protocol, particularly as

higher-intensity, sports-specific movements are introduced.

Beta-hydroxy-methylbutyrate

Beta-hydroxy-methylbutyrate (HMB) is a metabolite of the branched-chain amino acid leucine, which has long been known to increase strength and lean body mass.[104–106] Recent research has suggested that these effects may be mediated through the HMB metabolite,[107] and subsequent studies of HMB have shown efficacy in enhancing muscular recovery,[108,109] lean body mass,[108,110] strength,[107] power,[107,111] and aerobic performance.[112,113] In a recent review and position statement from the ISSN, HMB was found to reduce skeletal muscle damage associated with training and enhance recovery; promote skeletal muscle hypertrophy, strength, and power gains at a dose of 38 mg/kg of body mass; and inhibit protein breakdown while promoting protein synthesis.[113] Based on the available evidence, chronic consumption of HMB is safe in all age groups and may be considered during rehabilitation to inhibit muscle breakdown, promote muscle growth, and speed recovery following exercise.

Omega-3 fatty acids

Recent data suggest that fish oil–derived omega-3 fatty acids supplemented at 4 g per day (1.86 g eicosapentaenoic acid per day and 1.50 g docosahexaenoic acid per day) may augment an athlete's anabolic response to amino acids and increase muscle protein synthesis by 60%.[114,115] Moreover, chronic supplementation with fish oils can result in greater training-induced strength gains.[116] Both of these effects are thought to act independently of the proposed anti-inflammatory actions of omega-3 fatty acids. In the postinjury, inflammatory state, fish oil supplementation may serve a dual purpose for the rehabilitating athlete by reducing inflammation and promoting lean mass and strength gains.

Postexercise Water Immersion

The intense training associated with many competitive sports can result in exercise-induced muscle damage and DOMS. Athletic trainers routinely use postexercise water immersion using cold water baths, warm water ("whirlpool") baths, or "contrast-water therapy" (alternating hot and cold) to mitigate the effects of strenuous exercise on subsequent athletic performance. One comparative study demonstrated superiority of cold water immersion for postexercise recovery compared with contrast-water therapy or no intervention.[117] Another recent study found no difference in functional recovery of swimmers using cool or warm water immersion.[118] Although the literature comparing the efficacy of these different modalities is scant, a recent Cochrane review found some evidence that cold water immersion reduces DOMS compared with passive interventions involving rest alone or no intervention.[119]

SUMMARY

Rehabilitation of the patient-athlete presents unique challenges, but can be a very rewarding endeavor. Each athlete has unique demands of his or her sport that require a specific rehabilitation program to prepare the athlete for return to sport and minimize the risk of reinjury. In this article, we have outlined some of the more commonly used methods in rehabilitation of the athlete with upper extremity injury to provide a framework for providers working with athletic populations.

ACKNOWLEDGMENTS

The authors thank Nicole Kauppila, Lauren Levitt, and Sean McNeil of Athletico Physical Therapy in Chicago, Illinois, for their assistance in obtaining photographs for this article.

REFERENCES

1. Prokop LL. Upper-extremity rehabilitation: conditioning and orthotics for the athlete and performing artist. Hand Clin 1990;6(3):517–24.
2. Cheung K, Hume P, Maxwell L. Delayed onset muscle soreness: treatment strategies and performance factors. Sports Med 2003;33(2):145–64.
3. Halperin I, Aboodarda SJ, Button DC, et al. Roller massager improves range of motion of plantar flexor muscles without subsequent decreases in force parameters. Int J Sports Phys Ther 2014; 9(1):92–102.
4. Cheatham SW, Kolber MJ, Cain M, et al. The effects of self-myofascial release using a foam roll or roller massager on joint range of motion, muscle recovery, and performance: a systematic review. Int J Sports Phys Ther 2015;10(6):827–38.
5. Curran PF, Fiore RD, Crisco JJ. A comparison of the pressure exerted on soft tissue by 2 myofascial rollers. J Sport Rehabil 2008;17(4):432–42.
6. Schroeder AN, Best TM. Is self myofascial release an effective preexercise and recovery strategy? A literature review. Curr Sports Med Rep 2015; 14(3):200–8.
7. Crane JD, Ogborn DI, Cupido C, et al. Massage therapy attenuates inflammatory signaling after exercise-induced muscle damage. Sci Transl Med 2012;4(119):119ra113.
8. MacDonald GZ, Penney MD, Mullaley ME, et al. An acute bout of self-myofascial release increases

range of motion without a subsequent decrease in muscle activation or force. J Strength Cond Res 2013;27(3):812–21.

9. Behara B, Jacobson BH. The acute effects of deep tissue foam rolling and dynamic stretching on muscular strength, power, and flexibility in division I linemen. J Orthop Trauma 2015. [Epub ahead of print].

10. Healey KC, Hatfield DL, Blanpied P, et al. The effects of myofascial release with foam rolling on performance. J Strength Cond Res 2014;28(1):61–8.

11. Issurin VB. Benefits and limitations of block periodized training approaches to athletes' preparation: a review. Sports Med 2016;46(3):329–38.

12. Saunders PU, Telford RD, Pyne DB, et al. Short-term plyometric training improves running economy in highly trained middle and long distance runners. J Strength Cond Res 2006;20(4):947–54.

13. Bobbert MF, Gerritsen KG, Litjens MC, et al. Why is countermovement jump height greater than squat jump height? Med Sci Sports Exerc 1996;28(11):1402–12.

14. Rassier DE, Herzog W. Force enhancement and relaxation rates after stretch of activated muscle fibres. Proc Biol Sci 2005;272(1562):475–80.

15. Bosco C, Komi PV, Ito A. Prestretch potentiation of human skeletal muscle during ballistic movement. Acta Physiol Scand 1981;111(2):135–40.

16. Rassier DE, Herzog W. Relationship between force and stiffness in muscle fibers after stretch. J Appl Physiol (1985) 2005;99(5):1769–75.

17. Chmielewski TL, Myer GD, Kauffman D, et al. Plyometric exercise in the rehabilitation of athletes: physiological responses and clinical application. J Orthop Sports Phys Ther 2006;36(5):308–19.

18. Roberts TJ. The integrated function of muscles and tendons during locomotion. Comp Biochem Physiol A Mol Integr Physiol 2002;133(4):1087–99.

19. Roberts TJ, Marsh RL, Weyand PG, et al. Muscular force in running turkeys: the economy of minimizing work. Science 1997;275(5303):1113–5.

20. Hill J, Leiszler M. Review and role of plyometrics and core rehabilitation in competitive sport. Curr Sports Med Rep 2011;10(6):345–51.

21. Cordasco FA, Wolfe IN, Wootten ME, et al. An electromyographic analysis of the shoulder during a medicine ball rehabilitation program. Am J Sports Med 1996;24(3):386–92.

22. Cascio BM, Culp L, Cosgarea AJ. Return to play after anterior cruciate ligament reconstruction. Clin Sports Med 2004;23(3):395–408, ix.

23. Myer GD, Paterno MV, Ford KR, et al. Neuromuscular training techniques to target deficits before return to sport after anterior cruciate ligament reconstruction. J Strength Cond Res 2008;22(3):987–1014.

24. Myer GD, Paterno MV, Hewett TE. Back in the game: a four-phase return-to-sport program for athletes with problem ACLS. Rehab Manag 2004;17(8):30–3.

25. Wilk KE, Arrigo C. Current concepts in the rehabilitation of the athletic shoulder. J Orthop Sports Phys Ther 1993;18(1):365–78.

26. Wilk KE, Meister K, Andrews JR. Current concepts in the rehabilitation of the overhead throwing athlete. Am J Sports Med 2002;30(1):136–51.

27. Wilk KE, Voight ML, Keirns MA, et al. Stretch-shortening drills for the upper extremities: theory and clinical application. J Orthop Sports Phys Ther 1993;17(5):225–39.

28. Chelly MS, Ghenem MA, Abid K, et al. Effects of in-season short-term plyometric training program on leg power, jump- and sprint performance of soccer players. J Strength Cond Res 2010;24(10):2670–6.

29. DiStefano LJ, Padua DA, Blackburn JT, et al. Integrated injury prevention program improves balance and vertical jump height in children. J Strength Cond Res 2010;24(2):332–42.

30. Kotzamanidis C. Effect of plyometric training on running performance and vertical jumping in prepubertal boys. J Strength Cond Res 2006;20(2):441–5.

31. Markovic G, Jukic I, Milanovic D, et al. Effects of sprint and plyometric training on muscle function and athletic performance. J Strength Cond Res 2007;21(2):543–9.

32. Ozbar N, Ates S, Agopyan A. The effect of 8-week plyometric training on leg power, jump and sprint performance in female soccer players. J Strength Cond Res 2014;28(10):2888–94.

33. Potdevin FJ, Alberty ME, Chevutschi A, et al. Effects of a 6-week plyometric training program on performances in pubescent swimmers. J Strength Cond Res 2011;25(1):80–6.

34. Ramirez-Campillo R, Alvarez C, Henriquez-Olguin C, et al. Effects of plyometric training on endurance and explosive strength performance in competitive middle- and long-distance runners. J Strength Cond Res 2014;28(1):97–104.

35. Spurrs RW, Murphy AJ, Watsford ML. The effect of plyometric training on distance running performance. Eur J Appl Physiol 2003;89(1):1–7.

36. Kiesel K, Plisky PJ, Voight ML. Can serious injury in professional football be predicted by a preseason functional movement screen? N Am J Sports Phys Ther 2007;2(3):147–58.

37. O'Connor FG, Deuster PA, Davis J, et al. Functional movement screening: predicting injuries in officer candidates. Med Sci Sports Exerc 2011;43(12):2224–30.

38. Okada T, Huxel KC, Nesser TW. Relationship between core stability, functional movement, and

performance. J Strength Cond Res 2011;25(1):
252–61.

39. Hewett TE, Ford KR, Myer GD. Anterior cruciate ligament injuries in female athletes: part 2, a meta-
analysis of neuromuscular interventions aimed at
injury prevention. Am J Sports Med 2006;34(3):
490–8.

40. Hewett TE, Lindenfeld TN, Riccobene JV, et al. The
effect of neuromuscular training on the incidence of
knee injury in female athletes. A prospective study.
Am J Sports Med 1999;27(6):699–706.

41. Hewett TE, Stroupe AL, Nance TA, et al. Plyometric
training in female athletes. Decreased impact
forces and increased hamstring torques. Am J
Sports Med 1996;24(6):765–73.

42. Bonacci J, Green D, Saunders PU, et al. Plyometric
training as an intervention to correct altered neuro-
motor control during running after cycling in triathletes: a preliminary randomised controlled trial.
Phys Ther Sport 2011;12(1):15–21.

43. McConnell J. A novel approach to pain relief pre-
therapeutic exercise. J Sci Med Sport 2000;3(3):
325–34.

44. Beynnon BD, Renstrom PA. The effect of bracing
and taping in sports. Ann Chir Gynaecol 1991;
80(2):230–8.

45. Jaraczewska E, Long C. Kinesio taping in stroke:
improving functional use of the upper extremity in
hemiplegia. Top Stroke Rehabil 2006;13(3):31–42.

46. Rovere GD, Curl WW, Browning DG. Bracing and
taping in an office sports medicine practice. Clin
Sports Med 1989;8(3):497–515.

47. Webber A. Acute soft-tissue injuries in the young
athlete. Clin Sports Med 1988;7(3):611–24.

48. Vicenzino B, Brooksbank J, Minto J, et al. Initial effects of elbow taping on pain-free grip strength and
pressure pain threshold. J Orthop Sports Phys Ther
2003;33(7):400–7.

49. Kase K, Wallis J, Kase T, et al. Clinical therapeutic
applications of the kinesio taping method. 3rd edition. Tokyo: Kinesio USA, LLC; 2013.

50. Burfeind SM, Chimera N. Randomized control trial
investigating the effects of kinesiology tape on
shoulder proprioception. J Sport Rehabil 2015;
24(4):405–12.

51. Garcia-Muro F, Rodriguez-Fernandez AL, Herrero-
de-Lucas A. Treatment of myofascial pain in the
shoulder with Kinesio taping. A case report. Man
Ther 2010;15(3):292–5.

52. Gonzalez-Iglesias J, Fernandez-de-Las-Penas C,
Cleland JA, et al. Short-term effects of cervical kinesio taping on pain and cervical range of motion
in patients with acute whiplash injury: a randomized clinical trial. J Orthop Sports Phys Ther
2009;39(7):515–21.

53. Kalichman L, Vered E, Volchek L. Relieving symptoms of meralgia paresthetica using Kinesio taping:

a pilot study. Arch Phys Med Rehabil 2010;91(7):
1137–9.

54. Saavedra-Hernandez M, Castro-Sanchez AM,
Arroyo-Morales M, et al. Short-term effects of kinesio taping versus cervical thrust manipulation in patients with mechanical neck pain: a randomized
clinical trial. J Orthop Sports Phys Ther 2012;
42(8):724–30.

55. Thelen MD, Dauber JA, Stoneman PD. The clinical
efficacy of kinesio tape for shoulder pain: a randomized, double-blinded, clinical trial. J Orthop
Sports Phys Ther 2008;38(7):389–95.

56. Williams S, Whatman C, Hume PA, et al. Kinesio
taping in treatment and prevention of sports injuries: a meta-analysis of the evidence for its effectiveness. Sports Med 2012;42(2):153–64.

57. Yoshida A, Kahanov L. The effect of kinesio taping
on lower trunk range of motions. Res Sports Med
2007;15(2):103–12.

58. Briem K, Eythorsdottir H, Magnusdottir RG, et al.
Effects of kinesio tape compared with nonelastic
sports tape and the untaped ankle during a sudden inversion perturbation in male athletes.
J Orthop Sports Phys Ther 2011;41(5):328–35.

59. Fratocchi G, Di Mattia F, Rossi R, et al. Influence of
kinesio taping applied over biceps brachii on isoki-
netic elbow peak torque. A placebo controlled
study in a population of young healthy subjects.
J Sci Med Sport 2013;16(3):245–9.

60. Chang HY, Chou KY, Lin JJ, et al. Immediate effect
of forearm Kinesio taping on maximal grip strength
and force sense in healthy collegiate athletes. Phys
Ther Sport 2010;11(4):122–7.

61. Yasukawa A, Patel P, Sisung C. Pilot study: investigating the effects of kinesio taping in an acute pediatric rehabilitation setting. Am J Occup Ther
2006;60(1):104–10.

62. Taylor RL, O'Brien L, Brown T. A scoping review of
the use of elastic therapeutic tape for neck or upper extremity conditions. J Hand Ther 2014;27(3):
235–45 [quiz: 246].

63. Callaghan MJ, Selfe J. Patellar taping for patellofe-
moral pain syndrome in adults. Cochrane Database Syst Rev 2012;(4):CD006717.

64. Poon KY, Li SM, Roper MG, et al. Kinesiology tape
does not facilitate muscle performance: a decep-
tive controlled trial. Man Ther 2015;20(1):130–3.

65. Parreira Pdo C, Costa Lda C, Hespanhol LC Jr,
et al. Current evidence does not support the use
of kinesio taping in clinical practice: a systematic
review. J Physiother 2014;60(1):31–9.

66. Barnes PM, Bloom B, Nahin RL. Complementary
and alternative medicine use among adults and
children: United States, 2007. Natl Health Stat
Report 2008;12:1–23.

67. Barnes PM, Powell-Griner E, McFann K, et al. Complementary and alternative medicine use among

adults: United States, 2002. Adv Data 2004;343: 1–19.

68. Macznik AK, Schneiders AG, Sullivan SJ, et al. What "CAM" we learn about the level of evidence from 60 years of research into manipulative and body-based therapies in sports and exercise medicine? Complement Ther Med 2014;22(2):349–53.

69. Nichols AW, Harrigan R. Complementary and alternative medicine usage by intercollegiate athletes. Clin J Sport Med 2006;16(3):232–7.

70. Wadsworth LT. Acupuncture in sports medicine. Curr Sports Med Rep 2006;5(1):1–3.

71. Akimoto T, Nakahori C, Aizawa K, et al. Acupuncture and responses of immunologic and endocrine markers during competition. Med Sci Sports Exerc 2003;35(8):1296–302.

72. Dhillon S. The acute effect of acupuncture on 20-km cycling performance. Clin J Sport Med 2008; 18(1):76–80.

73. Huang LP, Zhou S, Lu Z, et al. Bilateral effect of unilateral electroacupuncture on muscle strength. J Altern Complement Med 2007;13(5):539–46.

74. Fink M, Wolkenstein E, Karst M, et al. Acupuncture in chronic epicondylitis: a randomized controlled trial. Rheumatology (Oxford) 2002;41(2):205–9.

75. Haker E, Lundeberg T. Acupuncture treatment in epicondylalgia: a comparative study of two acupuncture techniques. Clin J Pain 1990;6(3):221–6.

76. Molsberger A, Hille E. The analgesic effect of acupuncture in chronic tennis elbow pain. Br J Rheumatol 1994;33(12):1162–5.

77. Kleinhenz J, Streitberger K, Windeler J, et al. Randomised clinical trial comparing the effects of acupuncture and a newly designed placebo needle in rotator cuff tendinitis. Pain 1999;83(2): 235–41.

78. Hubscher M, Vogt L, Bernhorster M, et al. Effects of acupuncture on symptoms and muscle function in delayed-onset muscle soreness. J Altern Complement Med 2008;14(8):1011–6.

79. Hubscher M, Vogt L, Ziebart T, et al. Immediate effects of acupuncture on strength performance: a randomized, controlled crossover trial. Eur J Appl Physiol 2010;110(2):353–8.

80. Phillips SM, Glover EI, Rennie MJ. Alterations of protein turnover underlying disuse atrophy in human skeletal muscle. J Appl Physiol (1985) 2009; 107(3):645–54.

81. Wall BT, van Loon LJ. Nutritional strategies to attenuate muscle disuse atrophy. Nutr Rev 2013;71(4): 195–208.

82. Wall BT, Morton JP, van Loon LJ. Strategies to maintain skeletal muscle mass in the injured athlete: nutritional considerations and exercise mimetics. Eur J Sport Sci 2015;15(1):53–62.

83. Farthing JP, Krentz JR, Magnus CR. Strength training the free limb attenuates strength loss during unilateral immobilization. J Appl Physiol (1985) 2009;106(3):830–6.

84. Wall BT, Dirks ML, van Loon LJ. Skeletal muscle atrophy during short-term disuse: implications for age-related sarcopenia. Ageing Res Rev 2013; 12(4):898–906.

85. Wall BT, Snijders T, Senden JM, et al. Disuse impairs the muscle protein synthetic response to protein ingestion in healthy men. J Clin Endocrinol Metab 2013;98(12):4872–81.

86. Pasiakos SM, McLellan TM, Lieberman HR. The effects of protein supplements on muscle mass, strength, and aerobic and anaerobic power in healthy adults: a systematic review. Sports Med 2015;45(1):111–31.

87. Campbell B, Kreider RB, Ziegenfuss T, et al. International Society of Sports Nutrition position stand: protein and exercise. J Int Soc Sports Nutr 2007;4:8.

88. Cuthbertson D, Smith K, Babraj J, et al. Anabolic signaling deficits underlie amino acid resistance of wasting, aging muscle. FASEB J 2005;19(3): 422–4.

89. Moore DR, Robinson MJ, Fry JL, et al. Ingested protein dose response of muscle and albumin protein synthesis after resistance exercise in young men. Am J Clin Nutr 2009;89(1):161–8.

90. Pennings B, Boirie Y, Senden JM, et al. Whey protein stimulates postprandial muscle protein accretion more effectively than do casein and casein hydrolysate in older men. Am J Clin Nutr 2011; 93(5):997–1005.

91. Pennings B, Groen B, de Lange A, et al. Amino acid absorption and subsequent muscle protein accretion following graded intakes of whey protein in elderly men. Am J Physiol Endocrinol Metab 2012;302(8):E992–9.

92. Witard OC, Jackman SR, Breen L, et al. Myofibrillar muscle protein synthesis rates subsequent to a meal in response to increasing doses of whey protein at rest and after resistance exercise. Am J Clin Nutr 2014;99(1):86–95.

93. Yang Y, Breen L, Burd NA, et al. Resistance exercise enhances myofibrillar protein synthesis with graded intakes of whey protein in older men. Br J Nutr 2012;108(10):1780–8.

94. Bemben MG, Lamont HS. Creatine supplementation and exercise performance: recent findings. Sports Med 2005;35(2):107–25.

95. Perez-Schindler J, Hamilton DL, Moore DR, et al. Nutritional strategies to support concurrent training. Eur J Sport Sci 2015;15(1):41–52.

96. Tarnopolsky MA. Caffeine and creatine use in sport. Ann Nutr Metab 2010;57(Suppl 2):1–8.

97. Kim HJ, Kim CK, Carpentier A, et al. Studies on the safety of creatine supplementation. Amino Acids 2011;40(5):1409–18.

98. Lugaresi R, Leme M, de Salles Painelli V, et al. Does long-term creatine supplementation impair kidney function in resistance-trained individuals consuming a high-protein diet? J Int Soc Sports Nutr 2013;10(1):26.

99. Persky AM, Rawson ES. Safety of creatine supplementation. Subcell Biochem 2007;46:275–89.

100. Shao A, Hathcock JN. Risk assessment for creatine monohydrate. Regul Toxicol Pharmacol 2006;45(3): 242–51.

101. Trexler ET, Smith-Ryan AE, Stout JR, et al. International Society of Sports Nutrition position stand: beta-alanine. J Int Soc Sports Nutr 2015;12:30.

102. Suzuki Y, Nakao T, Maemura H, et al. Carnosine and anserine ingestion enhances contribution of nonbicarbonate buffering. Med Sci Sports Exerc 2006;38(2):334–8.

103. Klebanov GI, Teselkin Yu O, Babenkova IV, et al. Effect of carnosine and its components on free-radical reactions. Membr Cell Biol 1998;12(1): 89–99.

104. Anthony JC, Anthony TG, Layman DK. Leucine supplementation enhances skeletal muscle recovery in rats following exercise. J Nutr 1999;129(6): 1102–6.

105. Anthony JC, Yoshizawa F, Anthony TG, et al. Leucine stimulates translation initiation in skeletal muscle of postabsorptive rats via a rapamycin-sensitive pathway. J Nutr 2000;130(10):2413–9.

106. Norton LE, Layman DK. Leucine regulates translation initiation of protein synthesis in skeletal muscle after exercise. J Nutr 2006;136(2):533s–7s.

107. Nissen S, Sharp R, Ray M, et al. Effect of leucine metabolite beta-hydroxy-beta-methylbutyrate on muscle metabolism during resistance-exercise training. J Appl Physiol (1985) 1996;81(5):2095–104.

108. Jowko E, Ostaszewski P, Jank M, et al. Creatine and beta-hydroxy-beta-methylbutyrate (HMB) additively increase lean body mass and muscle strength during a weight-training program. Nutrition 2001;17(7–8):558–66.

109. Knitter AE, Panton L, Rathmacher JA, et al. Effects of beta-hydroxy-beta-methylbutyrate on muscle damage after a prolonged run. J Appl Physiol (1985) 2000;89(4):1340–4.

110. Gallagher PM, Carrithers JA, Godard MP, et al. Beta-hydroxy-beta-methylbutyrate ingestion, Part I: effects on strength and fat free mass. Med Sci Sports Exerc 2000;32(12):2109–15.

111. Kraemer WJ, Hatfield DL, Volek JS, et al. Effects of amino acids supplement on physiological adaptations to resistance training. Med Sci Sports Exerc 2009;41(5):1111–21.

112. Vukovich MD, Dreifort GD. Effect of beta-hydroxy beta-methylbutyrate on the onset of blood lactate accumulation and V(O)(2) peak in endurance-trained cyclists. J Strength Cond Res 2001;15(4): 491–7.

113. Wilson JM, Fitschen PJ, Campbell B, et al. International Society of Sports Nutrition position stand: beta-hydroxy-beta-methylbutyrate (HMB). J Int Soc Sports Nutr 2013;10(1):6.

114. Smith GI, Atherton P, Reeds DN, et al. Dietary omega-3 fatty acid supplementation increases the rate of muscle protein synthesis in older adults: a randomized controlled trial. Am J Clin Nutr 2011; 93(2):402–12.

115. Smith GI, Atherton P, Reeds DN, et al. Omega-3 polyunsaturated fatty acids augment the muscle protein anabolic response to hyperinsulinaemia-hyperaminoacidaemia in healthy young and middle-aged men and women. Clin Sci (Lond) 2011;121(6):267–78.

116. Rodacki CL, Rodacki AL, Pereira G, et al. Fish-oil supplementation enhances the effects of strength training in elderly women. Am J Clin Nutr 2012; 95(2):428–36.

117. Ingram J, Dawson B, Goodman C, et al. Effect of water immersion methods on post-exercise recovery from simulated team sport exercise. J Sci Med Sport 2009;12(3):417–21.

118. Soultanakis HN, Nafpaktiitou D, Mandaloufa SM. Impact of cool and warm water immersion on 50-m sprint performance and lactate recovery in swimmers. J Sports Med Phys Fitness 2015;55(4): 267–72.

119. Bleakley C, McDonough S, Gardner E, et al. Cold-water immersion (cryotherapy) for preventing and treating muscle soreness after exercise. Cochrane Database Syst Rev 2012;(2):CD008262.

Index

Hand Clin 33 (2017) 221–228
http://dx.doi.org/10.1016/S0749-0712(16)30124-X
0749-0712/17

Printed and bound by CPI Group (UK) Ltd, Croydon, CR0 4YY

21/10/2024

01777182-0001